Guide to Healthy Restaurant Eating

Third Edition

Hope S. Warshaw, MMSc, RD, CDE, BC-ADM

American Diabetes Association.
Cure • Care • Commitment®

tor, *Book Publishing,* John Fedor; *Managing Editor,* Abe Ogden; *Editor,* Rebecca ning; *Production Manager,* Melissa Sprott; *Composition,* Circle Graphics, Inc.; er *Design,* Koncept, Inc.; *Printer,* Transcontinental Printing.

Printed in Canada
3 5 7 9 10 8 6 4 2

The suggestions and information contained in this publication are generally consistent with the *Clinical Practice Recommendations* and other policies of the American Diabetes Association, but they do not represent the policy or position of the Association or any of its boards or committees. Reasonable steps have been taken to ensure the accuracy of the information presented. However, the American Diabetes Association cannot ensure the safety or efficacy of any product or service described in this publication. Individuals are advised to consult a physician or other appropriate health care professional before undertaking any diet or exercise program or taking any medication referred to in this publication. Professionals must use and apply their own professional judgment, experience, and training and should not rely solely on the information contained in this publication before prescribing any diet, exercise, or medication. The American Diabetes Association—its officers, directors, employees, volunteers, and members—assumes no responsibility or liability for personal or other injury, loss, or damage that may result from the suggestions or information in this publication.

♾ The paper in this publication meets the requirements of the ANSI Standard Z39.48-1992 (permanence of paper).

ADA titles may be purchased for business or promotional use or for special sales. To purchase this book in large quantities, or for custom editions of this book with your logo, contact Lee Romano Sequeira, Special Sales & Promotions, at the address below, or at LRomano@diabetes.org or 703-299-2046.

American Diabetes Association
1701 North Beauregard Street
Alexandria, Virginia 22311

Library of Congress Cataloging-in-Publication Data

Warshaw, Hope S., 1954-
Guide to healthy restaurant eating / Hope S. Warshaw.—3rd ed.
p. cm.
Includes bibliographical references and index.
ISBN 1-58040-246-1 (pbk.)
1. Diabetes—Diet therapy. 2. Food exchange lists. 3. Restaurants. I. American Diabetes Association. II. Title.

RC662.W3155 2006
616.4'620654—dc22

2005016440

To people with diabetes who, on a daily basis,
strive to control blood glucose to stay healthy
and prevent diabetes complications.
May the knowledge and information
you gain from this book help you
stay healthy and complication free.

— HSW

Contents

Alphabetical Index of Restaurants

Preface to the Third Edition

Three years have elapsed since the second edition of the *Guide to Healthy Restaurant Eating* was published. Have restaurant offerings and the amount of nutrition information available changed since then? Yes and no.

More nutrition information is available than ever before from what I refer to as "walk up and order" national chain restaurants. These are the restaurants in which you walk up to the counter or drive up to the window and place your food order. This abundance of information is evidenced by the increased thickness of this book's spine. The *Guide to Healthy Restaurant Eating* now includes nutrition information for nearly 5,000 menu items. That's commendable disclosure!

On the downside, however, little additional information is available from those "sit down and order" national chain restaurants. They boast about providing the nutrition information for a few of their healthier, low-carbohydrate or low-fat items, but they remain hush-hush and filled with excuses when it comes to full nutrition disclosure for the bulk of their menu offerings. That's not commendable!

There continues to be virtually no information available from independent chains, single unit restaurants, or most ethnic restaurants beyond a few of the national fast-food Mexican, Chinese, and Italian chains. This is understandable, because it is expensive to obtain and provide nutrition information.

What hasn't changed much—even though there's a lot of talk about the epidemics of obesity and type 2 diabetes—is the huge portions served in restaurants. Plenty of portions are enough for two or more, and you're consistently prompted to overeat with meal deals, two-for-one specials, mounds of French fries, and all-you-can-eat buffet restaurants.

This means you'll continue to need all the portion control pointers included in the pages ahead. Portion control is one of your best defensive strategies to limit overeating.

You'll also welcome the many tips to "guesstimate" restaurant portions in the "Put Your Best Guess Forward" section (page 31) and throughout this book. With so many more people tightly managing their blood glucose levels and adjusting their medications (usually insulin) based on the grams of carbohydrate they eat, good "guesstimating" skills are essential.

In our fast-paced, convenience-focused world, Americans continue to choose restaurant meals, eaten in or out of the restaurant, to get the job of eating done. Current trends indicate that we will likely be eating more restaurant meals and spending more of our food dollars on restaurant foods in the future as well.

I hope you find the third edition of the *Guide to Healthy Restaurant Eating* helpful in your quest to eat nutritious foods, control your blood glucose, and stay healthy for many years to come. I encourage you to continue to ask for nutrition information from restaurants that still do not provide it. If enough of us keep asking, eventually they'll give us the facts. I also urge you to support federal and state legislative efforts to require national chain restaurants to tell us the nutrition content of the foods they serve. These initiatives have the potential to help all of us make healthier food choices.

In health,
Hope S. Warshaw, MMSc, RD, CDE, BC-ADM

Acknowledgments

This book would have been impossible to create without the cooperation and assistance from many people at the corporate headquarters of many restaurant chains and the willingness of many other chains to provide their nutrition information on their Web sites. On behalf of the people with diabetes who will use and benefit from the information in the pages ahead, I am indebted to these restaurant chains. They set an example of public responsibility for the rest of the chain restaurant industry.

No book is completed by just the author alone. In this case, many manuscript pages and a large nutrient database became a book with many people's help. I am grateful to Paula Payne, RD, who assisted with the development of the nutrient database and other aspects of the book. Thanks also to all those at ADA who supported this effort: Rebecca Lanning, Editor; Abe Ogden, Managing Editor; John Fedor, Director, Book Publishing; and Len Boswell, Vice President, Publications.

A last thanks goes to my professional colleagues who consistently lend their ears and ideas. They continue to be a source of inspiration and encouragement.

Today's Diabetes Eating Goals

During the 1990s diabetes eating goals underwent a minor revolution. In fact, the phrase "a diabetic diet" is now a misnomer. No such diet exists. No longer must you ax sugary foods and sweets from your list of acceptable foods. Now you can savor the taste of a few slices of pizza at your local pizza parlor or cruise to the drive-thru for a hamburger and french fries when time is not on your side. The bottom line is that current diabetes eating goals encourage you to eat healthfully and to do what it takes to keep your blood glucose levels in the normal range as much as possible. Your diabetes plan should work around your needs and lifestyle and not vice versa. Your health care providers have many more tools today to help you formulate a diabetes plan that works for you. The end goal, of course, is to prevent or slow down long-term diabetes complications, such as eye, heart, and kidney problems. These occur, to a great degree, because of high blood glucose levels day after day.

Diabetes Eating Goals in a Nutshell

In 1994 the American Diabetes Association (ADA) put forth six nutrition goals. These were again reinforced in the 2002 nutrition goals:

1. Hold blood glucose (blood sugar) as near to normal as possible. Balance what you eat with insulin

or diabetes pills (if you need diabetes medicine to control your blood glucose) and physical activity.

2. Keep or get your blood lipid (blood fat) levels as close to levels recommended by ADA as possible. Blood lipids include cholesterol, low-density lipoproteins (LDL, or "bad" cholesterol), high-density lipoproteins (HDL, or "good" cholesterol), and triglycerides (the form in which your body stores fat in fat cells for ready energy).
3. Eat enough calories to stay at or get to a healthy weight for you. If you are a child or teenager or if you are pregnant or breastfeeding, eat the right number of calories to grow and develop normally.
4. Prevent or treat problems caused by high or low blood glucose. For instance, eat on time to prevent low blood glucose (hypoglycemia).
5. Prevent, slow down, or treat long-term diabetes problems. For example, eat less saturated fat to prevent heart problems, or eat a moderate amount of protein to slow kidney problems if you have them.
6. Improve your overall health by choosing foods and eating the way all Americans are encouraged to eat. This means eating what you know is healthy for your whole family.

Those are the nutrition goals. But what foods should you eat to reach these goals? Here are general pointers to focus on:

- Eat more (six or more servings) grains, beans, and starchy vegetables each day. Make three of the servings whole grains.
- Eat more fruits and vegetables. Strive for 2 1/2 cups of vegetables and 2 cups of fruit a day.

- Include at least three servings of fat-free or low-fat dairy foods each day—milk, yogurt, and cheese—within your calorie allotment. They provide calcium and other important nutrients.
- Eat a moderate amount of meat and other protein foods. Two 3-oz servings each day are enough for most people. Not only does eating less meat help you eat less protein, it also makes it easier for you to eat less total fat, saturated fat, and cholesterol.
- Go light on fats and oils. Limit oils high in saturated fat and trans fat, such as coconut and palm oils. Limit partially hydrogenated fats, which contain trans fats. Trans fats find their way into restaurant food mainly in fried and prepared foods. Limiting fried foods is a good way to limit trans fats when you eat in restaurants.
- Limit foods high in cholesterol (such as whole-milk dairy foods, egg yolks, and organ meats).
- Enjoy small amounts of sugary foods and sweets once in a while. If you have some pounds to shed or your blood glucose or blood fats are not in a good range, eat sweets more sparingly. If you're on the slim side, you can splurge on sweets a bit more often if you want to.
- Drink no more than one alcoholic drink a day if you are a woman and two drinks a day if you are a man. One drink is defined as 1 1/2 oz of hard liquor (a shot), 12 oz of beer, or 5 oz of wine.

Everybody Sings the Same Song

Take note: ADA recommendations for healthy eating echo the way all Americans are encouraged to eat—even Americans at risk for heart disease or some cancers.

Whether it's the American Heart Association, the American Cancer Society, or the U.S. government, every organization is singing the same nutrition song.

This means that as a person with diabetes, you don't need to stick out like a sore thumb because you strive to eat healthfully. That's not to make healthy eating sound simple or not to acknowledge that at times you feel like a fish swimming upstream because so many Americans chow down on downright unhealthy foods and large portions of them. Remember, it's not easy to eat healthfully. And that is particularly true with restaurant foods.

How Much Should You Eat?

Base what you eat each day on what you like to eat, as long as you eat these foods in reasonable amounts. The quantities of food you eat and when you eat need to match your lifestyle and schedule. Another critical element is to determine what foods and times for meals and snacks work best to help you keep your blood glucose, blood lipids, and blood pressure in control. Lastly, what's best for your diabetes is what allows you to feel good day to day and what helps prevent or slow down the development of diabetes problems.

No set number of calories is right for everyone with diabetes. The number of calories you need depends on many factors. A few of them are your height, your age, your current weight and whether you want to lose weight or are at a healthy weight, whether you have a hard or easy time losing weight, your daily activity level, the type of physical activity you do, and more. Always have a meal plan and method of meal planning that fit you and your lifestyle. To develop a meal plan and/or healthy eating goals that you are comfortable with and one that factors in your individual needs, work with a registered dietitian (RD) with diabetes expertise, such as a certified diabetes educator (CDE). A dietitian can help you learn how to work almost any food into a healthy eating plan or to solve your meal planning dilemmas. For instance, maybe you travel several days a week and eat all your meals in restaurants. (To find diabetes education programs near you, see "Help Is Nearby," on page 6.) Several books on the topic of food, nutrition, and meal planning published by the ADA give more in-depth information about how much and what you should eat.

Myriad Approaches to Meal Planning

Once you know what and how much you should eat, you and your dietitian can zero in on a meal planning approach that fits your needs. If you want a simple approach, for example, then the diabetes food pyramid may be best for you. Or if you are willing to check your blood glucose several times a day and do some math, then you might opt for carbohydrate counting.

You may be familiar with the diabetes exchange system as the way some people with diabetes learn to plan meals. The ADA and the American Dietetic Association's *Exchange Lists for Meal Planning* date back to 1950. The exchange system has been revised a number of times. The last revision was in 2003. Today, the exchange system is no longer the only way to do diabetes meal planning. You can use the diabetes food pyramid, carbohydrate gram counting, fat gram counting, or the point system, to name a few options. The right meal planning approach for you is the one that you can learn and put to work. One approach might be right for you when you first develop diabetes, and then down the road another approach may work best as you change the way you manage your diabetes.

Any Meal Planning Approach Works in Restaurants

No matter which meal planning approach you use, you can take advantage of the information in this book. If you opt for the exchange system or the diabetes food pyramid, use the food servings or exchanges noted in the charts. If you do carbohydrate counting, then the grams of carbohydrate and grams of dietary fiber are where you want to focus. Zero in on the calories and fat if fat gram counting is part of your meal planning method.

Help Is Nearby

Whether you have just found out you have diabetes or you have been doing the diabetes balancing act for years, you can always learn more. Get to know a diabetes educator. A diabetes educator can help you tailor your diabetes management plan and offer tips for dealing with diabetes. The following resources are a good start to link you up with quality diabetes care:

- To find a Recognized Diabetes Education Program (a teaching program approved by the American Diabetes Association) near you, call 1-800-DIABETES (1-800-342-2383), look at ADA's Internet home page http://www.diabetes.org, or go straight to http://www.diabetes.org/education/eduprogram.asp.

- To find diabetes educators (who may be dietitians, nurses, pharmacists, counselors, or other health professionals) near you, call the American Association of Diabetes Educators (AADE) toll-free at 1-800-TEAMUP4 (1-800-832-6874) or go to AADE's Internet site at www.aadenet.org and go to "Find an Educator."

Here's more good news: It may now be easier for you to take advantage of the services of a diabetes educator or diabetes education program (known in Medicare parlance as Diabetes Self-Management Training) as well as a dietitian. Medicare now covers diabetes education and nutrition counseling (known as Medical Nutrition Therapy) for diabetes in many new settings for those with Medicare Part B. Also, in nearly all states across the country, private insurers and managed care organizations that are regulated by the state must cover diabetes education and nutrition counseling. If you have questions about whether or not your diabetes education will be covered, contact your nearby diabetes education program or dietitian, health care company, your state insurance commissioner's office, the local Medicare office, or the American Diabetes Association.

Restaurant Pitfalls and Strategies for Self-Defense

To eat out healthfully is no small task. You need willpower and perseverance. It's tough enough to eat healthfully in your own house. But even more challenges confront you when you have to pick and choose from a menu and are not able to sneak a peek in the kitchen. You can't march into the kitchen and hold the cook's hand when he or she ladles more butter or shakes more salt onto your once healthy vegetables.

Healthy restaurant eating is, no doubt, a challenge. That's because there are lots of pitfalls—from sky-high portions to the use of large quantities of fat and salt. The good news is that you can choose to eat healthfully in 99 percent of restaurants. *Choose* is the critical word here. It's important to learn the pitfalls of restaurant eating and tuck the strategies to eat more healthfully in restaurants into your brain.

Pitfalls of Restaurant Eating

- **You think of restaurant ventures as special occasions.** Yes, once upon a time, people only ate in restaurants to celebrate a birthday, Mother's Day, or an anniversary. Not today. The average American eats four or more meals away from home each week. And personally you may top that number. When you eat that many meals away from home each week, your waistline quickly spreads if you treat each meal as a special occasion or even finish the portion served in most restaurants. Today, restaurant meals for most people are just part of our fast-paced life. They're hardly special occasions.

- **You're not the cook.** The cook is in the kitchen and you can't peek. Your methods of control are to ask questions about the food on the menu, to make special requests to get an item delivered the way you want it, and to practice portion control both when you order and when you eat.
- **Fats are here, there, and everywhere.** Remember, fat makes food taste good and stay moist. Restaurants, therefore, love it. Fat is in high-fat ingredients, such as butter, sour cream, or cream; in high-fat foods, such as cheese, bacon, or potato chips; and in high-fat cooking methods, such as deep-fat frying, breading and frying, and sautéing. And it's at the table in fried Chinese noodles, tortilla chips, or butter. You need to master the craft of being a fat sleuth. You'll get plenty of tips ahead.
- **Sodium can skyrocket.** Along with fat, salt makes food taste good. It is also used in many pre-prepared restaurant foods to keep them safe. So, many restaurants pour it aplenty. If you're watching your sodium intake, you'll need to shy away from certain items and make some special requests.
- **Portions are oversized.** Restaurants simply serve too much food. Unfortunately, they and many Americans believe more is better. The portions are often enough for two. You need to develop and use strategies that help you not overeat.
- **Meat (protein) is front and center.** A primary focus of the American diner is summed up in the catch-

phrase "Where's the beef?" Whether it is fish, chicken, or beef, the protein often takes center stage in restaurant meals. And most plates contain too much of it. A steak is often 8 oz or more cooked. A chicken breast is often a whole chicken breast. A goal to eat healthier is to put the meat on the side of your plate and fill the rest of your plate with healthier sides—vegetables and whole-grain starches.

Americans Eat Out: How Much and How Often?

An average American today spends almost half of every food dollar on food eaten away from home. In 1950, according to the National Restaurant Association, the average American spent only a quarter of his or her food dollar eating away from home. The average American today eats four or more meals out of the house each week. Lunch is the meal eaten out most often, with dinner a close second. Breakfast is eaten out least often. And men eat out more than women. Fast-food restaurants—from hamburger joints to pizza and sub shops—represent about a quarter of all restaurants. As for ethnic food, Americans' favorites are Mexican, Chinese, and Italian.

Let's face it, restaurant meals—eaten in or out—are just part of dealing with our fast-paced world. You might ask, "Is that a problem if I have diabetes?" The answer is no, as long as you learn to eat healthy restaurant meals most of the time. And remember, whether you eat in the restaurant or take food out to the soccer field, your office, or the kitchen table, you face the same decisions. In fact, you have to make similar choices in today's supermarkets, because they have begun to look a bit like restaurants, with ready-to-eat parts of meals, complete meals, sandwiches, premade salads, and salad bars. Of course, one advantage in the supermarket is that frequently the nutrition facts stare you in the face. Not so in restaurants. At best, you have to hunt them down.

Ten Strategies to Eat Out Healthfully

1. **Develop a can-do attitude.** Too many of us think in negative equations: Eating out equals pigging out; a restaurant meal is a special occasion; eating out means blowing your "diet." These attitudes defeat your efforts to eat healthfully. It's time to develop a can-do attitude about restaurant meals. Build confidence to believe that you can enjoy a healthy meal when you eat out. Slowly begin to change how you order and the types of restaurants in which you choose to eat.
2. **Decide when to eat out—or not.** Take a look at how often you eat out. If your count verges on the excessive, then ask yourself why you eat out so frequently and how you can reduce your restaurant meals. Also, if you eat out more frequently, you need to keep splurges to a minimum. If you eat out only once a month, you might take a few more liberties—perhaps with an alcoholic drink or a dessert.
3. **Zero in on the site.** Seek out restaurants that offer at least a smattering of healthier options. Remember, there is an advantage to eating in chain restaurants. You know the menu all too well. This can help you plan ahead, no matter which one of the chain's locations you pop into.
4. **Set your game plan.** On your way to the restaurant—whether it's a quick fast-food lunch

or a leisurely weekend dinner—envision a healthy and enjoyable outcome. Plan your strategy, or at least what you might have if you aren't familiar with the restaurant, before you cross the threshold. Don't become a victim of hasty choices or be swayed by the sights and smells.

5. **Become a fat sleuth.** Learn to focus on fats. Fat is the densest form of calories, and it often gets lost in the sauce, so to speak—or on the salad, on the bread, or in the chips. Watch out for high-fat ingredients—butter, cream, sour cream. Be alert for high-fat foods—cheese, avocado, sausage. Steer clear of high-fat preparation methods—frying of any kind. Look out for high-fat dishes—Mexican chimichangas, broccoli with cheese sauce, or stuffed potato skins, for starters.
6. **Let your food plan be your guide.** Choose foods with your healthy eating plan in mind. Try to fulfill each food group with menu items or substitute foods to make your meal complete. For instance, replace a serving of milk or a fruit serving, which are often hard to get in restaurants, with another starch serving so that you will keep your carbohydrate intake consistent—an important diabetes goal.
7. **Practice portion control from the start.** The best way not to eat too much is to order less. Order with your stomach in mind, not your eyes. You need to outsmart the menu to get the right amount of food for you.
8. **Be creative with the menu.** You outsmart the menu by being creative. You also control portions by being creative. Remember, no sign at the entrance says, "All who enter must order an entree." Your options are to take advantage of appetizers,

soups, and salads; to split menu items, including the entree, with your dining partner; to order one or two fewer dishes than the number of people at the table and eat family or Asian style; or to mix and match two entrees to achieve nutritional balance. For example, in a steak house, one person orders the steak, baked potato, and salad bar and the other orders just the potato and salad bar, then they split the steak. In an Italian restaurant, one person orders pasta with a tomato-based sauce and the other orders a chicken or veal dish with a vegetable.

9. **Get foods made to order.** Don't be afraid to ask for what you want, even in a fast-food restaurant. Restaurants today need your business and want you back. Make sure your requests are practical—leave an item such as potato chips off the plate; substitute mustard for mayonnaise on a sandwich; make a sandwich on whole-wheat bread rather than on a croissant; or serve the salad dressing on the side. Restaurants can abide these requests. However, don't expect to have your special requests greeted with a smile at noon in a fast-food restaurant or when you try to remake a menu item. Be reasonable and pleasant.
10. **Know when enough is enough.** Many of us grew up being members of the clean-plate club. Now you need to reserve a membership in the "leave-a-few-bites-on-your-plate club." To keep from overeating, don't order too much, order creatively, and push your plate away when you meet your calorie needs. Remember, take-home containers are at-the-ready in most restaurants.

Restaurant Dilemmas and Diabetes

Many people who eat restaurant meals have concerns about their health and need to ask questions. So, as a person with diabetes, your questions and special requests are nothing out of the ordinary. However, as someone with diabetes, you deal with dilemmas beyond just the food, due to your schedule for medications and your blood glucose control. This section provides you with guidance to face these additional challenges.

Delayed Meals

A big challenge, if you take a diabetes medication that can cause your blood glucose to get too low (see Table 1, p. 16), may be how to manage delayed meals. For example, if you are used to eating lunch between noon and 12:30 pm, how can you safely delay your meal until 1:00 or 1:30 pm when your friends or business associates want to meet? Or what should you do if you want to dine at 7:30 pm on a Saturday night, when your usual dinner time during the week is 6:00 pm?

A big and positive change in the management of diabetes today is that there are new oral blood glucose–lowering medications and new types of insulin that better mesh with the realities of life in the 21st century. Several of these medications help your health care providers, diabetes educators, and you work out a medication schedule that best controls your blood glucose

TABLE 1 Diabetes Medications and Hypoglycemia

Diabetes medications that can cause hypoglycemia	Diabetes medications that do not cause hypoglycemia
Sulfonylureas: Amaryl, Glucotrol, Glucotrol XL, glyburide, glipizide, DiaBeta, Glynase, Micronase Combination pill: Glucovance (combination of metformin and glyburide; the glyburide portion can cause hypoglycemia), Metaglip (combination of metformin and glipizide; the glipizide portion can cause hypoglycemia) Meglitinides: repaglinide (Prandin) d-phenylalanine: nateglinide (Starlix) Insulin: all	Metformin: Glucophage, Glucophage XR, Riomet Alpha-glucosidase inhibitors: Precose and Glyset Glitazones: Avandia and Actos Combination pill: Avandamet (combination of Avandia and metformin)

while allowing you the flexibility you need to live your life in the manner that best suits your needs. What's important in developing a medication plan is that you communicate your lifestyle and schedule to your health care providers and diabetes educators. If they don't know your habits, then they are less able to help you develop a medication plan that suits you.

The biggest concern in delaying meals is if you have taken a diabetes medication that can cause your blood glucose to go too low if you don't eat on time. Prior to the availability of new blood glucose–lowering oral medications and newer insulins, this was more of a concern than it is today. But it is certainly still a concern for you if your blood glucose can get too low. On page 16 is a list of the diabetes medications that can cause blood glucose to go too low (cause hypoglycemia) and those that cannot. If you take one or more of the medications that can cause low blood glucose then you need to pay special attention to your meal times.

Do keep in mind, though, that several of the newer diabetes medications that can cause hypoglycemia are rapid-acting, such as the insulins lispro (Humalog), aspart (Novolog), and the newest glulisine (Apidra) and the oral pills Prandin and Starlix. Their job is to quickly lower your blood glucose after you eat. If you take one of these medications along with other medications that are not likely to cause low blood glucose, then you should take these rapid-acting medications a few minutes before you start to eat rather than at your usual meal time. (See the section on rapid-acting insulins, below.)

If you take a pre-mixed combination of insulin, such as 70/30 or 75/25, or just take insulin twice a day, such as a mixture of NPH or Lente and regular, it becomes more important for you to eat on time to prevent low blood glucose. A disadvantage of these insulin regimens is that they do not allow much flexibility in meal times. If you regularly need more flexibility in your schedule, then talk to your health care providers and diabetes educators about your needs. Today there are much more flexible insulin regimens including the use of an insulin pump or the use of the insulin glargine (Lantus) with one of the rapid-acting insulins (Humalog, Novolog, or Apidra). All of these insulins are available in pens.

Practical Tips to Using Rapid-Acting Insulin with Restaurant Meals

More and more people who take insulin are on a flexible insulin regimen. Usually, they take Lantus once or twice a day and rapid-acting insulin just before they eat. More people are also using insulin pumps. These so-called flexible insulin regimens can make insulin dosing for restaurant meals easier.

Recent observations suggest that rapid-acting insulin doesn't get absorbed and lower blood glucose as quickly as practitioners first believed when it came on the market in 1996. Today most experts agree that the maximum blood glucose–lowering effect of rapid-acting insulin occurs closer to two hours after an injection rather than 45–90 minutes. If this is true for you, the optimal time to take rapid-acting insulin is about 10 to 15 minutes before you eat, rather than with the first bite or 15 minutes after you start to eat.

Another big key to blood glucose control is to give yourself enough insulin to cover the rise of blood glucose from the food you eat. Like many people, you may find yourself in a reactive mode when it comes to dosing insulin. This means that you take it in response to high blood glucose rather than taking enough insulin just before a meal to cover the rise of blood glucose in the hours after you eat. That's usually between two and four hours, depending on what and how much you eat. Experts agree that it's much harder to bring high blood glucose back down into the normal range than to control the rise of blood glucose with sufficient insulin taken before the meal.

Although taking rapid-acting insulin 10 to 15 minutes before a meal and carefully calculating your dose according to the carbohydrate you will eat are ideal for blood glucose control, you may not always be able to do so, for one reason or another, when you eat restaurant meals. These practical tips can help you keep your blood glucose in better control when you eat restaurant meals:

High blood glucose before a meal: Take some rapid-acting insulin a half hour before your meal to give the insulin time to lower your blood glucose. It might take longer than this to come down, but at least it will be on the downswing.

Low blood glucose before a meal: If your blood glucose is low before a meal (below about 80 mg/dl), wait to take your insulin. Give the carbohydrate about 15 minutes to raise your blood glucose before you take the insulin to cover your food.

Uncertain carbohydrate intake: If you don't know how much carbohydrate you will eat at a meal, consider splitting your rapid-acting insulin dose. Take enough insulin 15 minutes before the meal to cover a minimum amount of carbohydrate that you know you will eat, say 30 to 45 grams. Then, as the meal goes on and you know how much more carbohydrate you will eat, take more insulin to cover that amount. This method is easiest if you are on an insulin pump or if you use an insulin pen and don't mind an extra injection.

Drawn-out meals: Pump users who plan to have a long, drawn-out restaurant meal and/or a meal that is higher in fat may want to consider using one of the optional bolus delivery tools on their insulin pump. Most insulin pumps allow you to deliver a bolus over time rather than all at once or to deliver some insulin immediately and some over the next few hours.

Learn from your experiences: Because of the large variation in responses to blood glucose from food and insulin among individuals, you can learn how to fine-tune your control by recording your experiences for future reference. Keep notes of your responses to various foods and activities in a notebook, computer file, or your logbook. Chart this information: foods you eat and the amounts, the amount of insulin you take to cover the food, your blood glucose levels before and after you eat (2 hours, 4 hours, 6 hours), and any lessons you learn to apply the next time around. Although perfect control is near to impossible, your personal database can help you adjust to many different situations you encounter in everyday life.

Steps to Take If Low Blood Sugar Is Possible

If you will delay a meal and you take a longer acting pill or insulin that can cause your blood glucose to get too low, take precautions to prevent this. Follow these steps.

Check your blood glucose at the usual time of your meal.

- If it is high (>150 mg/dl*), you can wait a short time before you eat without concern. But do check again if you feel your blood glucose is getting too low before your meal.
- If your blood glucose level is around your pre-meal goal (90–130 mg/dl) and you feel it will fall too low

*The numbers used for blood glucose values in this book are based on plasma glucose goals, not whole blood. Today, most blood glucose meters read results as plasma, not whole blood.

before you get to eat, eat some carbohydrate (start with 15 grams) to make sure your blood glucose doesn't go too low before your meal.

- If you delay your meal more than one hour and your blood glucose is around your pre-meal goal, you may need to eat more than 15 grams of carbohydrate to keep it from going too low before your meal.

It is always a smart idea to keep quick and easy carbohydrate foods in places such as your desk, briefcase, purse, locker, or glove compartment. Also, it is good to carry glucose tablets. They help you treat an impending low blood glucose before it gets too low. After all, you never know what will happen in restaurants, especially a sit-down restaurant. The restaurant might not have your reservation, they might not be able to seat you quickly, your meal-mate might be late, the kitchen might be slow, or there may be a mix up with your order. And the list goes on. As the saying goes, "It's better to be safe than sorry."

Suggested foods that are easy to carry and contain carbohydrate are dried fruit, cans of juice, pretzels, milk, yogurt, gum drops, gummy bears, or snack crackers. Check the nutrition facts label on the food to determine the amount equivalent to 15 grams of carbohydrate.

If your blood glucose is lower than 80 mg/dl and/or you feel the symptoms of low blood glucose, then you should use 15 grams of some source of carbohydrate to treat your hypoglycemia. Try to eat your meal soon after.

These suggestions offer you general rules of thumb. Check with your health care providers or diabetes educator to learn what are the best alternatives for you based on your diabetes medication plan. But if your diabetes medication plan is not fitting with your lifestyle, recognize that there are alternatives.

Alcohol

Clearly there are numerous reasons not to drink alcohol. Alcohol is high in calories (unhealthy calories). It can cause low blood glucose if you take an oral diabetes medication or insulin that can cause low blood glucose. It can lead to health problems with overuse, can slow your responses, and can be dangerous if you drink and drive. However, if your blood glucose and blood lipids are in good control and you drink sensibly, there is no reason you cannot enjoy some alcohol. And a common time to drink alcohol is when you eat in a restaurant. Here's how to drink smartly with diabetes.

Tips to Sip By

- Don't drink when your blood glucose is below 80 mg/dl or you have symptoms of hypoglycemia.
- Remember that alcohol can cause low blood glucose soon after you drink it (if your medicine is working hardest and/or you need to eat). It can continue to cause low blood glucose 8–12 hours after you drink it, especially if you drink in excess, take too much medicine, or don't eat enough.
- Don't drink on an empty stomach. Either munch on a carbohydrate source (popcorn or pretzels) as you drink or wait to drink until you get your meal.
- Alcohol can also make blood glucose too high. This is true for anyone with diabetes, no matter how they control it. High blood glucose can be caused by the calories from carbohydrate in the alcoholic beverage, such as wine or beer, or in a mixer, such as orange juice.

- Avoid mixers that add lots of carbohydrates and calories—tonic water, regular soda, syrups, juices, and liqueurs.
- Check your blood glucose to help you decide whether you should drink and when you need to eat something.
- Wear or carry identification that states you have diabetes.
- Sip a drink to make it last.
- At a meal have a noncaloric, nonalcoholic beverage by your side to quench your thirst.
- If you do not take a diabetes medicine that can cause low blood glucose and you have some pounds to shed, you can substitute an alcoholic drink for fats in your meal plan.
- If you do not have to lose weight, then just have an occasional drink and don't worry about the extra calories.
- Do not drive for several hours after you drink alcohol. Never drink and drive.

Sugars and Sweets

It is common to want a sweet dessert to end a restaurant meal. As you know by now, you can fit sweets into your diabetes food plan as long as you substitute them for other foods or compensate for their extra carbohydrates, fat, and calories with your diabetes medicines to keep your blood glucose close to normal. To set healthy goals with sweets, you also need to consider your weight and blood fats. Work with a dietitian to figure out how to fit sweets into your meal plan. In the meantime, here are a few pointers.

Hints for Sweet Tooths

- Prioritize your personal diabetes goals. Which is most important for you: blood glucose control, weight loss, or lower blood fats? Your priorities dictate how you strike a balance with sugars and sweets.
- Choose a few favorite desserts. Decide how often to eat them and how to fit them into your meal plan.
- Perhaps it is best for you to limit desserts just to when you eat in restaurants. That way you keep sweets out of your home.
- Split a dessert in a restaurant or take half home if possible. Portions are generally too big.
- Take advantage of smaller portions available in restaurants or ice cream spots—kiddie, small, or regular are the words to look for.
- Use the nutrition information you find in this book and information you find in restaurants to learn about the calorie, carbohydrate, fat, saturated fat, and cholesterol content of desserts.
- When you eat a sweet, check your blood glucose about two hours later to see how it has been affected. You might find, for instance, that because of the fat content, the same quantity of ice cream raises your blood glucose more slowly than does frozen yogurt, which contains less fat and more carbohydrate.
- Keep an eye on your hemoglobin A1C (your longer-range blood glucose measure) and your blood fat (lipid) levels to see whether eating more sweets leads to a worsening in these numbers.

These are basic guidelines and suggestions to deal with diabetes restaurant dilemmas. Each person with diabetes is different. So talk with your health care provider and diabetes educator to get information pertinent to the way you manage your diabetes.

Restaurants Help or Hinder Your Healthy Eating Efforts

The pendulum swings back and forth on how helpful restaurants are nutritionally. During the 1980s and early 1990s, when the voices of people concerned about what they ate and about their health were loud, restaurants developed healthier options. Lower-calorie and lower-fat menu items were introduced. Restaurateurs willingly made lower-fat milk and reduced-calorie salad dressings available. Some restaurants even marked their menus with little hearts or other notations to indicate which menu items met specific health criteria.

The pendulum in restaurants then swung back in the late 1990s and early 2000s. McDonald's dropped the McLean hamburger and meal-sized salads. Belly-busting portions became commonplace again. Taco Bell's Border Lights line bombed because it was introduced toward the end of this round of the health craze. We were back in the era of giant burgers, supersized meals, and more all-you-can-eat buffets.

In the last few years, due to another round of interest in low-carb diets and, more important, childhood and adult obesity, some restaurant chains have begun taking action about nutrition. For example, McDonald's has stopped offering supersizing, Ruby Tuesday has developed healthier options and provides some nutrition information, and Subway has taken on healthier eating in a big way.

Unfortunately, a majority of Americans still cast all health and nutrition cares to the wind when they set foot in a restaurant. And you can see where that is leading us. Today over 65 percent of American adults are overweight and type 2 diabetes is growing exponentially.

The "no cares" nutrition attitude makes it harder for those who are health conscious. But don't feel pessimistic. Lower-fat milk, reduced-calorie salad dressings, and lower-fat frozen desserts are still widely available, and there's a greater ease in making special requests. With skills and a bit of fortitude, you can eat healthfully at most restaurants. Granted, you still have to pick and choose among the menu offerings.

Remember, too, that your voice still matters. You can make a difference.

Chains That Give the Nutrition Lowdown

Since the first edition of this book was published in 1997, the amount of information available via the Internet has exploded. And nutrition information for restaurant foods is no exception. It is now relatively easy to access nutrition information for the fast-food hamburger chains—from the large McDonald's and Burger King to the smaller Carl's Jr. and Sonic. Among the categories of restaurants and chains that make nutrition information available on their Web sites are those selling pizza, chicken, Mexican food, desserts and ice cream, subs and sandwiches, and donuts and bagels.

The types of restaurants that, for the most part, either do not have or do not provide nutrition information are chain sit-down restaurants. Several of these restaurants are all too happy to give you nutrition information about their few healthier items. But somehow they don't have the information or are unwilling to disclose the nutrition information for the complete menu.

Why don't some restaurants provide nutrition information? There are a few reasons. First, it's expensive to obtain nutritional analyses on all menu items. Second, restaurants that do not provide information tend to change their menus frequently. As soon as they printed nutrition information, it would need to be revised. Third, they want you to stay blindfolded to the nutrition lowdown on their foods. An important point here is that you—a person with diabetes concerned about your health—need to keep asking for nutrition information at restaurants that don't give it.

How to Get the Latest Nutrition Lowdown

If you do not find a particular restaurant chain in this book or there is a new menu item introduced for a restaurant that is included, here are a few hints on how to get the nutrition information.

- If you have access to the Internet, use it. We have provided Internet addresses for all the restaurants that have them. We have also indicated the ones that have nutrition information on their Web sites.
- If you don't have Internet access, ask for nutrition information at the store location you frequent. You might get lucky and have a nutrition pamphlet put right into your hands. Sometimes they have run out or just don't keep them in stock. Make sure you check the date on the nutrition pamphlet to be sure it is current.

- If the restaurant does not have the information, ask where you can call or write for it. You might need to call or write the corporate headquarters and have them send you a pamphlet.
- If you have a question about the nutrition content or ingredients used in a few items, contact the company either through the Internet or by phone.

A Bit of Help from Your Government

The nutrition facts panel on most canned and packaged foods in the supermarket hardly seems new. But they have only been in their current format for just over a decade. The Nutrition Labeling and Education Act (NLEA), which is the federal legislation that changed the nutrition label and increased the number of foods with information, requires restaurants to comply with several aspects of this law. Restaurants must provide nutrition information to customers when nutrition and health claims are made on signs and placards. If any restaurant makes a health claim about a food, that it is "low-fat," for instance, the nutrition information has to comply with the meaning of the term according to the NLEA. This helps you know that when you see the word "healthy" to describe a can of beans or a fast-food sandwich, it has the same meaning. Restaurants from small one-unit sandwich shops to McDonald's have to abide by these regulations. Table 2 (see page 29) gives terms you might see on restaurant menu items and their definitions.

The law permits restaurants to make

- specific claims about a menu item's nutritional content.

TABLE 2 Meaning of Nutrition Claims* on Restaurant Menus, Signs, and Placards

Nutrition Claim	Meaning
Cholesterol-Free	Less than 2 mg of cholesterol per serving and 2 g or less of saturated fat per serving
Low-Cholesterol	20 mg or less of cholesterol per serving and 2 g or less of saturated fat per serving
Fat-Free	Less than 0.5 g of fat per serving
Low-Fat	3 g or less of fat per serving
Light or Lite	Cannot be used by restaurants as a nutrient content claim, but can be used to describe a menu item, such as "lighter fare" or "light size"
Sodium-Free	Less than 5 mg of sodium per serving
Low-Sodium	140 mg or less of sodium per serving
Sugar-Free	Less than 0.5 g of sugar per serving
Low-Sugar	May not be used as a nutrient claim
Healthy	The food item is low in fat, low in saturated fat, has limited amounts of cholesterol and sodium, and provides significant amounts of one or more key nutrients—vitamins A and C, iron, calcium, protein, or fiber.
Heart Healthy (These claims will indicate that a diet low in saturated fat and cholesterol may reduce the risk of heart disease.)	The item is low in fat, saturated fat, and cholesterol, and provides without fortification (added nutrients) significant amounts of one or more key nutrients—vitamins A and C, iron, calcium, protein, or fiber. OR The item is low in fat, saturated fat, and cholesterol, and provides without fortification (added nutrients) significant amounts of one or more key nutrients—vitamins A and C, iron, calcium, protein—and is a significant source of soluble fiber.

*The definitions of these claims are the same as those used for food labels in the supermarket.

- one of the approved health claims about the relationship between a nutrient or food and a disease or health condition. The criteria to make the health claim must be met.

If the restaurant makes a nutrition or health claim, it must provide you with the nutrition information to back it up. The claim can be substantiated by a nutrition database, nutrition information in the cookbook from which the recipe was made, or another source that provides nutrition information. Further, restaurants do not have to give you the information in the nutrition label format you are familiar with from the supermarket. They can provide it in any format they choose.

Now there is a move afoot to require chain restaurants with more than a certain number of outlets to provide nutrition information. Legislation has been introduced in several states and at the federal level in both the House and the Senate. The Center for Science in the Public Interest has done a good job of promoting the need for this information. More information about this topic is available at www.cspinet.org.

Put Your Best Guess Forward

When you've got the nutrition facts in hand, it makes knowing the nutrients you eat a snap. And the listings in this book help a great deal when you choose to eat in one of the more than 60 restaurants whose information is provided in the pages ahead.

The reality is, however, that nutrition facts are simply not available from some of the restaurants in which you may choose to eat. They might be sit-down chain restaurants unwilling to provide information or smaller local chains that weren't large enough to include in this book. Or they might be independent single-location restaurants who are unlikely to have any nutrition information. Assessing the nutrient content of what you eat in these restaurants is more of a challenge. The following tips should help you learn to put your best guess forward.

Tips to Put Your Best Guess Forward

- Have measuring equipment at home and use it. Have a set of measuring spoons and measuring cups, as well as an inexpensive food scale. Weigh and measure foods at home sometimes. Do this regularly as you familiarize yourself with the portions you should eat. Then on occasion, say once a month, weigh and measure foods, especially the starches, fruits, and meats. Weighing and measuring foods at home regularly helps you keep portions in control and helps you more precisely estimate them in restaurants. Estimating with the precise portion size helps you estimate the nutrient content most correctly.

- Use these "handy" hand guides to estimate portions:
  - Tip of the thumb (to first knuckle)—1 teaspoon
  - Whole thumb—1 tablespoon
  - Palm of your hand—3 ounces (this is the portion size of cooked meat that most people need at a meal). Other 3-ounce portion guides: the size of a deck of regular size playing cards or the size of a household bar of soap.
  - Tight fist—1/2 cup
  - Loose fist or open handful—1 cup

    Note: These guidelines hold true for most women's hands, but some men's hands are much larger. Check the size of your hands out for yourself with real weighing and measuring equipment.
- Use the scales in the produce aisle of the supermarket to educate yourself about the servings of food you may be served in a restaurant, such as baked white or sweet potatoes, an ear of corn, or a banana. Weigh individual pieces of these foods. Check out how many ounces a usual potato or an ear of corn is that you may be served in a restaurant. Note that you are weighing these foods raw, but their weight doesn't change that much when cooked.
- If there are no data for a particular restaurant you frequent, use the information available from other similar restaurants in the pages of this book. If you want to get a feel for the nutrient content of a food like french fries, baked potato, stuffing, pizza, or bagels, look at the serving size and nutrition information for those foods in restaurants that are in-

cluded. You might want to take a few examples and then do an average. For example: if you regularly eat at a local pizza shop rather than a national chain and they have no nutrition information, take the nutrition information from this book for two slices of medium-sized regular crust cheese pizza from three restaurants. Then do an average. You will come pretty close to the nutrition content of the two slices of cheese pizza you eat.

- You can also use the nutrition information from the nutrition facts of foods in the supermarket to estimate what you might eat in a restaurant. You might find some similar foods in the frozen or packaged convenience foods area. Again, take a couple of examples and then average.
- If you regularly eat particular ethnic foods for which you find no nutrition information, you might want to get a few cookbooks out of the library (or use your own) that contain recipes for the foods you enjoy. Then use a nutrient database or book with nutrition information (see pages 34–35) to determine the estimated nutrient content for each ingredient. Do this for a couple of similar recipes. Then get an average to help you estimate the nutrient content of what you are eating in the restaurant. This might work well for ethnic foods such as Indian, Mexican, or Chinese.

Most people regularly eat just 50 to 100 foods, including restaurant foods. People tend to frequent the same restaurants and order similar items. For this reason, it makes sense to spend some time estimating the nutrient content of your favorite restaurant items for which nutrition information is not available. Once you have this figured out, put it in a notebook or develop a computer file that you print out and keep with you.

Keep in mind that most restaurants serve portions that are larger than most average-sized people need to eat. So, even if you choose healthy foods that combine to make a healthy meal, you will likely also need to limit the amount you eat. Portion control is clearly not an easy task. Learn some techniques by reading the "Strategies for Self-Defense" on pages 12–14.

A word to the wise: avoid all-you-can-eat restaurants and other settings that simply promote overeating, such as hotel breakfast buffets or salad or food bars. This is best if you don't have much willpower or it bothers you to think that the restaurant is making money on you because you will not walk out feeling like a stuffed turkey. However, if you feel these settings work well because they help you control portions, use them to your advantage.

If you frequently eat particular items in large chain restaurants for which nutrition information is not available in this book, contact the restaurants. Several restaurants noted that while they were unwilling to provide the nutrition information for all their items for this book, if a customer contacted them, they would provide information for several items.

Resources for Nutrition Information of Foods

BOOKS:

The Diabetes Carbohydrate and Fat Gram Guide, by Lea Ann Holzmeister, RD, CDE. American Diabetes Association, 2nd edition, 2000, 480 pages. This book provides the carbohydrate count, as well as other nutrition information, for thousands of foods including fruits; vegetables and other produce; meats, poultry and seafood; desserts; many foods you know by their brand name; frozen entrees; and more.

The Doctor's Pocket Calorie, Fat, and Carb Counter, by Allan Borushek. Allan Borushek and Associates, 2005, 308 pages. This book lists calorie, fat, and carbohydrate information for thousands of basic and brand-name foods. (See www.calorieking.com to order the book or to download food and restaurant databases.)

Calories and Carbohydrates, by Barbara Kraus. Signet, 15th edition, 2003, 496 pages. Carbohydrate and calorie counts for more than 8,500 items are included in this food dictionary. It covers brand-name and basic foods of every variety.

The Corinne T. Netzer Carbohydrate Counter, by Corinne T. Netzer. Dell, 7th edition, 2001, 496 pages. This book features carbohydrate counts for thousands of foods, including fresh and frozen produce, dairy products, breads, grains, pastas, sweets, fast foods, and more.

INTERNET:

www.nal.usda.gov. From this Web site, the United State National Agricultural Library, you can download a nutrient database of 6,000 basic foods for free. Go to Publications and Databases, and then click on Databases. Select USDA Nutrient Databases for Standard Reference, and then click Information to download. This database is also available online at www.nal.usda.gov/fnic/foodcomp/

www.calorieking.com

www.nutritiondata.com

www.dietfacts.com

How This Book Works for You

You might open this book and be thrilled to see many of the restaurants you frequent. Then again, you might wonder why a certain restaurant that you've never laid eyes on is included, or why your favorite hamburger or pizza stop is nowhere to be found.

Each July, a restaurant trade association magazine, *Restaurants and Institutions,* publishes a list of the top 400 restaurant chains. The more than 60 chain restaurants in this book were selected based on the number of locations they operate and whether the business was growing or in the red.

If one of your favorite restaurants is not included, it is for one of the following reasons:

- The restaurant might not have been willing or able to provide sufficient menu and/or nutrition information to warrant their inclusion. This is especially true for sit-down restaurants.
- The restaurant chain may not be large enough across the country, although it appears to you that in your area there are many locations.

Where to Find the Restaurant

Clearly, you know to look in "Burgers and More" to find McDonald's or Wendy's, or in "Pizza, Pasta, and All Else Italian" to find Domino's or Pizza Hut. But because Boston Market's menu today includes more than just chicken, you might not guess that it is in the section "Sit-Down Family Fare." Let's just say we used the "best fit" approach. Nine times out of ten you'll guess correctly. But if you don't find a restaurant in the chapter where you think it should be, then check the alphabetical listing of restaurants on page ix in the beginning of the book.

Close but Not Exact

You should be aware that the nutrition information from restaurants is close but not exact. Many restaurants state that their nutrition information is based on the specified ingredients and preparation. However, the same restaurant has locations all over the country, and different regions purchase their ingredients and foods from different food wholesalers. For example, a Wendy's in California might purchase lettuce, tomatoes, and hamburger buns from one food supplier, whereas a Wendy's in Connecticut will buy foods from another company. The same is true internationally. The nutrition analysis of these items is close, but not identical. However, it is close enough to help you to make food decisions and manage your blood glucose.

Restaurant foods are also prepared by different people. Even in the same restaurant, on different days you might get more or less cheese on your pizza, more pickles or ketchup on your hamburger, or a slightly smaller or larger steak even though you order the 6-oz filet. Wherever humans are involved, portions aren't exact. Consider these differences if one day you notice that your blood glucose goes up more or less than you expect from a restaurant meal you've eaten again and again.

Beverages and Condiments

There are two categories of items that are not listed separately in the information provided for each restaurant. The first is beverages. Regularly sweetened drinks, such as carbonated beverages (soda, or pop), lemonade, noncarbonated fruit drinks, and the like, are not listed individually because from a nutrition standpoint, they are loaded with sugar and provide almost no nutritional value. Most restaurants also serve a similar variety of noncaloric beverages as well as milk and orange juice. To avoid repeating information on the same products, we've put the nutrition information for the most commonly served regular and diet beverages in Table 3 on page 40.

The second category of items not listed for individual restaurants is common condiments, such as ketchup, mustard, mayonnaise, and honey. Don't despair; we've put the nutrition information for these condiments in Table 4 on page 42.

The Nutrition Numbers Ahead

All the nutrition information you need to know to fit foods into your eating plan is in the pages ahead, unless the information was not available from the restaurant. Whether you use the diabetes exchange system or the diabetes food pyramid, do carbohydrate counting or fat gram counting for meal planning,

TABLE 3 Nutrition Information for Beverages

Beverage	Amount	Cal.	Fat (g)	Sat. Fat (g)	Chol. (mg)	Sod. (mg)	Carb. (g)	Pro. (g)	Servings/Exchanges
Beer (regular)	12 oz	140	0	0	0	11	13	1	1 carb, 2 fat*
Beer (light)	12 oz	99	0	0	0	18	5	1	2 fat*
Coffee, black (regular and decaffeinated)	8 oz	5	0	0	0	4	1	0	free
Coke (regular)	12 oz	144	0	0	0	6	43	0	3 carb
Coke (diet)	12 oz	1	0	0	0	6	0	0	free
Iced Tea (unsweetened)	12 oz	4	0	0	0	6	1	0	free
Liquor (any type)	1 1/2 oz	96	0	0	0	0	0	0	2 fat*
Lemonade (regular)	12 oz	160	0	0	0	0	42	0	3 carb
Milk (whole)	8 oz	150	8	5	33	120	12	8	1 whole milk
✓Milk (reduced-fat/2%)	8 oz	120	5	3	18	122	12	8	1 low-fat milk

Milk (low-fat/1%)	8 oz	102	2	2	12	107	12	8	1 fat-free milk, 1/2 fat
✓Milk (fat-free)	8 oz	83	0	0	4	126	12	8	1 fat-free milk
Milk, chocolate (low-fat)	8 oz	157	3	2	8	152	26	8	1 fat-free milk, 1 carb
✓Apple juice	8 oz	117	0	0	0	7	29	0	2 fruit
✓Orange juice	8 oz	110	0	0	0	2	25	2	2 fruit
Pepsi (regular)	12 oz	144	0	0	0	6	43	0	3 carb
Pepsi (diet)	12 oz	1	0	0	0	6	0	0	free
Sprite (regular)	12 oz	148	0	0	0	3	37	0	2 1/2 carb
Sprite (diet)	12 oz	1	0	0	0	6	0	0	free
Tea (hot, nothing added)	8 oz	2	0	0	0	7	1	0	free
Wine, white	6 oz	120	0	0	0	9	1	0	2 fat*
Wine, red	6 oz	120	0	0	0	114	3	1	2 fat*

*Talk to your diabetes educator or health care provider about whether you can work alcoholic beverages into your meal plan and how to do so.

✓Healthiest Bets

TABLE 4 Nutrition Information for Condiments

Condiment	Amount	Cal.	Fat (g)	Sat. Fat (g)	Chol. (mg)	Sod. (mg)	Carb. (g)	Pro. (g)	Servings/Exchanges
Bacon, thinly sliced	1 slice	36	3	1	5	101	0	2	1 fat
Butter	1 t	30	4	2	10	39	0	0	1 fat
Cheese, American	1-oz slice	106	9	6	27	405	1	6	1 high-fat meat
Cheese, Swiss	1-oz slice	107	8	5	26	74	1	8	1 high-fat meat
Cheese, mozzarella, whole-milk	1/4 cup shredded/1 oz	80	6	4	22	106	1	6	1 medium-fat meat
Cream Cheese (regular)	1 T	50	5	3	15	45	1	1	1 fat
Cream Cheese (light)	1 T	30	3	2	5	80	1	2	1/2 fat
Half & Half	1/2 oz/1 T	20	2	1	6	6	1	0	free
Honey	1 t	22	0	0	0	0	6	0	1/2 carb
Honey Mustard	1 t	15	1	n/a	n/a	75	2	0	free

Ketchup	1 T	16	0	0	0	137	4	0	free
Margarine (regular stick)	1 t	34	4	1	0	44	0	0	1 fat
Margarine (regular tub)	1 t	34	4	1	0	51	0	0	1 fat
Margarine (light)	1 t	17	2	0	0	17	0	0	free
Mayonnaise (regular)	1 T	100	11	2	8	78	0	0	2 fat
Mayonnaise (light)	1 T	40	4	0	5	15	1	0	1 fat
Mustard	1 t	5	0	0	0	65	0	0	free
Non-Dairy Creamer	1/2 oz/1 T	16	1	0	0	5	2	0	free
Olive Oil	1 t	40	5	2	0	0	0	0	1 fat
Pancake Syrup (regular)	1 T	50	0	0	0	13	13	0	1 carb
Pancake Syrup (light)	1 T	25	0	0	0	56	7	0	1/2 carb
Pancake Syrup (low-calorie)	1 T	23	0	0	0	57	6	0	1/2 carb

(*Continued*)

TABLE 4 Nutrition Information for Condiments (*Continued*)

Condiment	Amount	Cal.	Fat (g)	Sat. Fat (g)	Chol. (mg)	Sod. (mg)	Carb. (g)	Pro. (g)	Servings/Exchanges
Relish, pickle-type	1 T	19	0	0	0	164	5	0	free
Salsa, tomato-based	1 T	3	0	0	0	112	1	0	free
Sour Cream (regular)	1 T	26	3	2	5	6	1	0	1/2 fat
Sour Cream (light)	1 T	18	1	0	5	10	1	1	free
Soy Sauce	1 t	3	0	0	0	343	1	0	free
Vinegar (all types)	1 t	2	0	0	0	0	1	0	free

n/a, not available

the numbers are here. This is the nutrition information you'll find, in this order:

- Calories
- Fat (in grams) and
  - Percentage of calories from fat. Look at this in relation to grams of fat. Keep in mind that the percentage of calories from fat might be high, but the grams of fat might be low, or vice versa.
  - Saturated fat (in grams). Saturated fat is the type of fat that raises blood cholesterol levels. Try to keep your saturated fat intake to 10 percent or less of your total calories.
- Cholesterol (in milligrams)
- Sodium (in milligrams)
- Carbohydrate (in grams)
  - Dietary fiber (in grams). Dietary fiber is a component of carbohydrate. Generally, Americans don't eat enough dietary fiber. Try to eat 20–35 grams of dietary fiber each day.
- Protein (in grams)
- Food servings/exchanges. Servings and exchanges are virtually the same. They have been calculated using the *2003 Exchange Lists for Meal Planning,* published by the ADA and the American Dietetic Association, and the book *Diabetes Meal Planning Made Easy,* 2nd edition, published by ADA in 2000.

A "best-fit" approach was used to calculate servings or exchanges. There is no one right way to fit restaurant foods into your meal plan. Figuring out what food group the grams of carbohydrate come from is the biggest challenge to figuring servings or exchanges. This is how it was approached: When it appears that the grams of carbohydrate come from a starch—be it potato, bread, or starchy vegetable—the servings or exchanges are called starches. If the carbohydrate comes from vegetable, fruit, or milk, the servings or exchanges are designated as such.

A food group in the *2003 Exchange Lists for Meal Planning* is the "other carbohydrate" group. This group contains foods such as sweets, frozen desserts, spaghetti sauce, jam, and maple syrup, to name a few. The calories and carbohydrates in many of these foods come from simple sugars. Therefore, in calculating the servings or exchanges for this book, we've called foods that fit into the "other carbohydrate" group "carb." Exchanges for fast-food shakes and frozen and regular desserts, for example, are calculated as carbs.

When it comes to meat dishes, the servings or exchanges were calculated based on the group that the meat itself fits into regardless of how it's prepared. For example, fish fillet sandwiches and chicken fingers are considered to fall into the lean meat group even though they have a lot of fat by the time they are served. On the other hand, sausage in any form is classified as a high-fat meat because that's the food group sausage fits into.

It is worth noting that some restaurants that provide nutrition information also provide exchanges. These were not used in this book. We calculated exchanges/servings based on ADA methodology. We have often found inconsistencies between the restaurant's exchange calculations and the ones obtained using ADA guidelines.

Putting It All Together

Perhaps one of the hardest parts of meal planning is figuring out how to put together healthy, well-balanced meals. This is a particular challenge in restaurants. To show you how to design healthier restaurant meals, we've put together two sample meals for most of the restaurants. We applied the following criteria to put together the meals. (Please note that the criteria might be less strict than what you would consider for a healthy meal at home. That's because restaurant meals tend to be higher in calories and fat, and in some instances in some restaurants it was virtually impossible to meet these criteria, especially for fat and sodium. Also, keep in mind that you can make special requests to have higher fat or sodium ingredients left out, so that the items that you eat are healthier.) No meals were designed for several of the restaurants, including all those in the "Sweets and Frozen Treats" chapter, because of their limited menus.

The Light 'n Lean Choice

- 400–700 calories (based on about 1,200–1,600 calories per day)
- 30–40 percent of calories from fat
- 100–200 milligrams of cholesterol (total per day should be 300 milligrams or less)
- 1,000–1,800 milligrams of sodium (total per day should be no more than 2,300 milligrams)

The Healthy 'n Hearty Choice

- 600–1,000 calories (based on about 1,800–2,400 calories per day)
- 30–40 percent of calories from fat
- 100–200 milligrams of cholesterol (total per day should be 300 milligrams or less)
- 1,000–1,800 milligrams of sodium (total per day should be no more than 2,300 milligrams)

Healthiest Bets

With nutrition information in hand, we've also made it easy for you to zero in on healthier restaurant offerings. We've marked these "Healthiest Bets" with a ✓. Remember, foods that are not marked as Healthiest Bets are not necessarily foods you should never eat. Healthiest Bets just steer you toward healthier choices.

When you're putting together healthy meals, don't look at only the Healthiest Bets. You can feel free to mix and match healthier and less healthy foods to make up overall healthy meals. Also keep in mind that if you split or share some less healthy bets, such as shakes, desserts, or fried items, they then fit into Healthiest Bets. That's why you'll see some Healthiest Bets and some less healthy items mixed and matched in the sample meals for each restaurant. What's most important is that you eat a healthy balance over the course of the day and from week to week. So if you want a juicy hamburger and french fries for lunch one day a month, go ahead and enjoy.

The Healthiest Bets were chosen on the basis of the following criteria:

- Breakfast entrees: Less than 400 calories per serving, with less than 15 grams of fat (3 fat exchanges [about 30 percent fat]) and 1,000 milligrams of sodium.
- Lunch or dinner entrees, including entree salads: Less than 600–750 calories, with less than 20 grams of fat (4 fat exchanges [about 30 percent fat]) and 1,000 milligrams of sodium.
- Pizza, sandwiches (including breakfast sandwiches), hamburgers, etc.: Less than 500 calories per reasonable serving (for example, 2 slices of pizza), 20 grams

of fat (4 fat exchanges [about 30% fat]), and 1,000 milligrams of sodium.

- Side items: For items such as fruit, vegetables (raw and cooked), grains, legumes, starches, and meats, no more than 5 grams of fat (1 fat exchange). For fried items, such as french fries, hash browns, chicken pieces, fried chicken, onion rings, and potato chips, less than 10 grams of fat (2 fat exchanges); less than 500 milligrams of sodium per serving.
- Soups: Less than 10 grams of fat (2 fat exchanges) and 1,000 milligrams of sodium per serving.
- Salad dressings, cream cheeses, spreads, and condiments: Less than 50 calories, 5 grams of fat (1 fat exchange), and 250 milligrams of sodium per tablespoon.
- Breads (such as rolls, biscuits, bagels, bread, croissants, scones, donuts, muffins, pretzels, and scones): Less than 400 calories, 10 grams of fat (2 fat exchanges), and 800 milligrams of sodium per serving.
- Desserts: Less than 300 calories, 10 grams of fat (2 fat exchanges), and 30 grams of carbohydrate per serving.
- Beverages (such as milk, juice, milk shakes, and special coffees): Less than 300 calories, 30 grams of carbohydrate, and 5 grams of fat (1 fat exchange). Less than 400 milligrams of sodium. (Coffee and diet beverages, though minimal in calories, were not checked as Healthiest Bets.)

Bon Appetit!

Breakfast Eats, Drinks, Snacks, and More

RESTAURANTS

Auntie Anne's Hand-Rolled Soft Pretzels
Cinnabon World Famous Cinnamon Rolls
Dunkin' Donuts
Einstein Bros Bagels
Jamba Juice
Krispy Kreme Doughnuts
Starbucks
Tim Hortons

Note: Restaurants in this chapter devote their menus to bagels, donuts, coffees, hot and cold drinks, shakes, pretzels, and more. They are the usual American breakfast spots. Look in "Burgers, Fries, and More" for fast-food breakfasts. Look in "Sit-Down Family Fare" for restaurants that serve breakfast and brunch as well as lunch and dinner. Look in "Soups, Sandwiches, and Subs" for Au Bon Pain and Panera Bread, which also serve breakfast items.

The healthy meal choices for the restaurants in this section have slightly fewer calories and other nutrients than the criteria noted on page 47. That's because meals you eat in these restaurants are most likely breakfasts, light meals, or snacks.

NUTRITION PROS

- Bagels have become a popular breakfast item. Before you apply a spread, they are low in fat. That's

Healthy Tips

- ★ Stick with coffee without a lot of added cream, whole milk, or sugar. They add fat and empty calories. Use a sugar substitute. Today you often have three choices—Splenda, Equal, and Sweet 'N Low.
- ★ Try half of a soft-baked pretzel as an accompaniment to a salad or as a snack.
- ★ Opt for one of the light bagel spreads, but keep in mind that they are hardly calorie or fat free. Spread them thinly.
- ★ Cake donuts have slightly less fat than yeast donuts.
- ★ Do eat breakfast. Skipping breakfast just keeps your engine in low gear and may help you rationalize overeating at meals during the rest of the day. Plus, if you take diabetes medications that can cause low blood glucose, skipping breakfast is not a smart move.
- ★ In breakfast sandwiches, choose ham or cheese and pass on bacon or sausage.
- ★ Read the fine print when you see the words "low-fat," "fat-free," or "sugar-free." They don't mean there are no calories or no carbohydrate. In fact, some of these foods can contain more carbohydrate and/or more calories than the regular food.
- ★ If jam or jelly is an option, take it. Jams and jellies have no fat. Spread them thinly all the same.

good. However, they have gotten bigger and bigger. Today's bagels can be equal to about four slices of bread. You might consider a half or two-thirds at a sitting if you need to control your carbohydrate intake. Also apply spreads thinly and wisely.

- Light cream cheese spreads are available in most bagel shops.
- Soft-baked pretzels unadulterated with lots of fat or sugar are a healthy snack or side item. But half might be plenty, so share it.
- Whole wheat pretzels and bagels are a source of dietary fiber.
- No longer is it donuts-only at Dunkin' Donuts and other donut shops. They serve bagels, low-fat muffins, and various coffees too.
- Muffin mania has died down, but you'll still find them at many breakfast spots. Often low-fat muffins are available. Even a regular muffin is a better choice than some donuts or loaded bagels. But do watch the size. They can be huge.
- English muffins and yeast rolls are healthy choices as long as you use only a light amount of butter or margarine.
- One of the quickest and healthiest breakfast foods—dry or cooked cereal with fat-free (skim) milk—is rarely served. When it's an option, grab it.

NUTRITION CONS

- Bagels can quickly become high fat and high calorie if they are topped with a quarter inch of high-fat cream cheese or spread.
- Bagels in most bagels shops average at least 3–4 oz and 250–340 calories. They're often equal to at least three or four slices of bread, not two.

- Pretzels sound healthy, but their calories and fat rise when they are rolled in lots of glaze or butter, or dipped in cheese sauce, cream cheese, or caramel.
- Croissants are high fat by nature—that's how they become flaky. You add insult to injury when you stuff a croissant with items such as bacon, sausage, cheese, tuna salad, or chicken salad.
- Donuts are high in fat (but surprisingly, not as bad as you might think). Save them for a once-in-a-while splurge.
- Biscuits are loaded with fat. When sausage, bacon, egg, and/or cheese is sandwiched between them, they give you your fat for one day in one fell swoop.
- The fancy coffees and teas—both hot and iced, from mochas to frappuccinos to chais—are not just coffee and tea. The sugar and fat, if whole milk, half and half, or whipped cream are used, are blended through and through.

Get It Your Way

- ★ Order bagel spreads on the side so that you can control how much is spread.
- ★ Order butter or margarine on the side.
- ★ Opt for fat-free milk in specialty coffees.
- ★ Order a sandwich on a bagel or roll, not on a high-fat croissant.

Auntie Anne's Hand-Rolled Soft Pretzels

❖ Auntie Anne's Hand-Rolled Soft Pretzels provides nutrition information for all its menu items on its Web site at www.auntieannes.com.

Light 'n Lean Choice

Jalapeno Pretzel, without butter

Calories	270	Sodium (mg)	780
Fat (g)	1	Carbohydrate (g)	58
% calories from fat	3	Fiber (g)	2
Saturated fat (g)	0	Protein (g)	8
Cholesterol (mg)	0		

Exchanges: 4 starch

Healthy 'n Hearty Choice

Sour Cream & Onion Pretzel, without butter

Calories	310	Sodium (mg)	920
Fat (g)	1	Carbohydrate (g)	66
% calories from fat	3	Fiber (g)	2
Saturated fat (g)	0	Protein (g)	9
Cholesterol (mg)	0		

Exchanges: 4 1/2 starch

(*Continued*)

Auntie Anne's Hand-Rolled Soft Pretzels

	Amount	Cal.	Fat (g)	% Cal. Fat	Sat. Fat (g)	Chol. (mg)	Sod. (mg)	Carb. (g)	Fiber (g)	Pro. (g)	Servings/Exchanges
DIPPING SAUCES											
Caramel Dip	3 T	135	3	20	1.5	5	110	27	0	1	1 1/2 carb, 1/2 fat
Cheese Sauce	2 1/2 T	100	8	72	4	10	510	4	0	3	2 fat
Chocolate Flavored Dip	2 1/2 T	130	4	28	1.5	2	65	24	1	1	1 1/2 carb, 1 fat
Hot Salsa Cheese	2 1/2 T	100	8	72	4	10	550	4	0	2	2 fat
Light Cream Cheese	2 1/2 T	70	6	77	4	25	140	1	0	3	1 1/2 fat
✓Marinara Sauce	2 1/2 T	10	0	0	0	0	180	4	0	0	free
Strawberry Cream Cheese	2 1/2 T	110	10	82	6	35	105	4	0	2	2 1/2 fat
Sweet Mustard	2 1/2 T	60	2	30	1	40	120	8	0	0	1/2 carb
DUTCH ICE											
Auntie Anne's Lemonade	22 oz	180	0	0	0	0	0	43	0	0	3 carb

Blue Raspberry Dutch Ice	20 oz	230	0	0	0	0	30	55	0	0	3 1/2 carb
Blue Raspberry Dutch Ice	14 oz	165	0	0	0	0	20	38	0	0	2 1/2 carb
Grape Dutch Ice	20 oz	260	0	0	0	0	30	62	0	0	4 carb
Grape Dutch Ice	14 oz	180	0	0	0	0	20	43	0	0	3 carb
Kiwi-Banana Dutch Ice	20 oz	270	0	0	0	0	40	63	0	0	4 carb
Kiwi-Banana Dutch Ice	14 oz	190	0	0	0	0	30	44	0	0	3 carb
Lemonade Dutch Ice	14 oz	315	0	0	0	0	0	77	0	0	5 carb
Lemonade Dutch Ice	20 oz	450	0	0	0	0	0	110	0	0	7 carb
Mocha Dutch Ice	14 oz	400	10	23	9	0	100	74	0	0	5 carb
Mocha Dutch Ice	20 oz	570	15	24	12.5	0	150	105	0	0	7 carb
Orange Crème Dutch Ice	20 oz	400	0	0	0	0	50	92	0	0	6 carb
Orange Crème Dutch Ice	14 oz	280	0	0	0	0	35	64	0	0	4 carb
Pina Colada Dutch Ice	20 oz	535	0	0	0	0	50	125	0	0	8 carb

✓ = Healthiest Bets

(Continued)

DUTCH ICE (*Continued*)	Amount	Cal.	Fat (g)	% Cal. Fat	Sat. Fat (g)	Chol. (mg)	Sod. (mg)	Carb. (g)	Fiber (g)	Pro. (g)	Servings/Exchanges
Pina Colada Dutch Ice	14 oz	220	0	0	0	0	15	53	0	0	3 1/2 carb
Strawberry Dutch Ice	14 oz	220	0	0	0	0	40	50	0	0	3 1/2 carb
Strawberry Dutch Ice	20 oz	315	0	0	0	0	60	72	0	0	4 1/2 carb
Wild Cherry Dutch Ice	20 oz	300	0	0	0	0	35	69	0	0	4 1/2 carb
Wild Cherry Dutch Ice	14 oz	210	0	0	0	0	25	48	0	0	3 carb
DUTCH SHAKES											
Chocolate Dutch Shake	14 oz	580	27	42	18	105	380	75	0	10	5 carb, 4 fat
Chocolate Dutch Shake	20 oz	860	41	43	26	155	576	113	0	14	7 1/2 carb, 8 fat
Coffee Dutch Shake	20 oz	890	41	41	26	155	456	115	0	14	7 1/2 carb, 8 fat
Coffee Dutch Shake	14 oz	590	27	41	18	105	304	77	0	10	5 carb, 4 fat
Strawberry Dutch Shake	14 oz	610	27	40	18	105	304	78	0	10	5 carb, 4 1/2 fat
Strawberry Dutch Shake	20 oz	910	41	41	26	155	456	118	0	14	7 1/2 carb, 8 fat

Vanilla Dutch Shake	20 oz	770	41	48	26	155	460	87	0	15	5 1/2 carb, 8 fat
Vanilla Dutch Shake	14 oz	510	27	48	17	105	300	58	0	10	4 carb, 4 1/2 fat
DUTCH SMOOTHIES											
Blue Raspberry Dutch Smoothie	14 oz	230	8	31	5	30	100	34	0	3	2 carb, 3 fat
Blue Raspberry Dutch Smoothie	20 oz	400	14	32	9	55	180	61	0	5	4 carb, 2 fat
Grape Dutch Smoothie	20 oz	400	14	32	9	55	180	65	0	5	4 carb, 1 1/2 fat
Grape Dutch Smoothie	14 oz	230	8	31	5	30	100	36	0	3	2 carb, 3 fat
Kiwi-Banana Dutch Smoothie	14 oz	240	8	30	5	30	100	38	0	3	2 1/2 carb, 1 1/2 fat
Kiwi-Banana Dutch Smoothie	20 oz	430	14	29	9	55	180	68	0	5	4 1/2 carb, 3 fat
Lemonade Dutch Smoothie	20 oz	540	14	23	9	55	150	95	0	5	6 1/2 carb, 3 fat

✔ = Healthiest Bets

(Continued)

DUTCH SMOOTHIES (*Continued*)	Amount	Cal.	Fat (g)	% Cal. Fat	Sat. Fat (g)	Chol. (mg)	Sod. (mg)	Carb. (g)	Fiber (g)	Pro. (g)	Servings/Exchanges
Lemonade Dutch Smoothie	14 oz	300	8	24	5	30	80	53	0	3	3 1/2 carb, 1 1/2 fat
Mocha Dutch Smoothie	14 oz	330	13	35	9	30	130	50	0	3	3 carb, 2 1/2 fat
Mocha Dutch Smoothie	20 oz	590	23	35	16	55	240	90	0	5	6 carb, 4 1/2 fat
Orange Crème Dutch Smoothie	20 oz	500	14	25	9	55	180	83	0	5	5 1/2 carb, 2 1/2 fat
Orange Crème Dutch Smoothie	14 oz	280	8	26	5	30	100	46	0	3	3 carb, 2 fat
Pina Colada Dutch Smoothie	14 oz	260	8	28	5	30	90	44	0	3	3 carb, 3 fat
Pina Colada Dutch Smoothie	20 oz	470	14	27	9	55	170	79	0	5	5 carb, 3 fat
Strawberry Dutch Smoothie	20 oz	450	14	28	9	55	180	72	0	5	4 1/2 carb, 3 fat

Strawberry Dutch Smoothie	14 oz	250	8	29	5	30	100	40	0	3	3 carb, 1 1/2 fat
Wild Cherry Dutch Smoothie	20 oz	450	14	28	9	55	170	74	0	5	5 carb, 1 1/2 fat
Wild Cherry Dutch Smoothie	14 oz	250	8	29	5	30	90	41	0	3	3 carb, 3 fat
PRETZELS WITH BUTTER											
✓Almond	1	400	8	18	5	20	400	72	2	9	3 starch, 1 1/2 carb, 1 1/2 fat
Cinnamon Sugar	1	450	9	18	5	25	430	83	3	8	3 starch, 2 1/2 carb, 2 fat
Garlic	1	350	5	13	2.5	10	850	68	2	9	3 starch, 1 carb, 1 fat
Glazin Raisin	1	510	4	7	2	10	480	107	4	11	4 starch, 2 1/2 carb, 1 fat
Jalapeno	1	310	5	15	2.5	10	940	59	2	8	3 starch, 1/2 carb, 1 fat
Maple Crumb	1	550	6	10	2	10	550	112	3	10	3 starch, 4 carb, 1 fat

✓ = Healthiest Bets

(Continued)

PRETZELS WITH BUTTER (*Continued*)	Amount	Cal.	Fat (g)	% Cal. Fat	Sat. Fat (g)	Chol. (mg)	Sod. (mg)	Carb. (g)	Fiber (g)	Pro. (g)	Servings/Exchanges
Original	1	370	4	10	2	10	930	72	3	10	3 starch, 1 1/2 carb, 1 fat
Parmesan Herb	1	440	13	27	7	30	660	72	9	10	3 starch, 1 1/2 carb, 2 fat
Pretzel Dog	1	290	16	50	7	40	600	25	1	10	1 1/2 starch, 2 fat
Sesame	1	410	12	26	4	15	860	64	7	12	4 starch, 2 1/2 fat
✓Smart Bites	1	10	1	90	0	0	30	2	1	1	2 starch, 1 fat
Smart Bites	15	150	8	48	0	0	450	30	15	15	2 starch, 1 fat
Sour Cream and Onion	1	340	5	13	3	10	930	66	2	9	4 starch, 1 carb, 1 fat
Stix	4	247	3	11	4	7	620	48	2	7	3 starch, 1/2 fat
Whole Wheat	1	370	5	12	1.5	10	1120	72	7	11	4 starch, 1/2 carb, 1 fat
PRETZELS WITHOUT BUTTER											
✓Almond	1	350	2	5	0.5	0	390	72	2	9	4 starch, 1/2 carb
✓Cinnamon Sugar	1	350	2	5	0	0	410	74	2	9	3 starch, 2 carb

Garlic	1	320	1	3	0	0	830	66	2	9	3 starch, 1 1/2 carb
Glazin Raisin	1	470	1	2	0	0	460	104	3	11	4 starch, 3 carb
Jalapeno	1	270	1	3	0	0	780	58	2	8	3 starch, 1 carb
Maple Crumb	1	520	3	5	0	0	550	112	3	10	3 starch, 4 1/2 carb, 1/2 fat
Original	1	340	1	3	0	0	900	72	3	10	3 starch, 1 1/2 carb
Parmesan Herb	1	390	5	12	2.5	10	780	74	4	11	3 starch, 2 carb, 1 fat
Sesame	1	350	6	15	1	0	840	63	3	11	4 starch, 1 fat
Sour Cream and Onion	1	310	1	3	0	0	920	66	2	9	3 starch, 1 1/2 carb
✓Stix	4	227	1	4	0	0	600	48	2	7	2 starch, 1 carb
Whole Wheat	1	350	2	5	0	0	1100	72	7	11	4 starch, 1/2 carb

✓ = Healthiest Bets

Cinnabon World Famous Cinnamon Rolls

❖ Cinnabon World Famous Cinnamon Rolls has a Web site—www.cinnabon.com. It does not, however, provide nutrition information on the Web site. Some information was made available by phone.

Light 'n Lean Choice

Apple Minibon

Calories	385	Sodium (mg)	261
Fat (g)	5	Carbohydrate (g)	53
% calories from fat	12	Fiber (g)	1
Saturated fat (g)	1	Protein (g)	6
Cholesterol (mg)	n/a		

Exchanges: 3 1/2 starch, 1 fat

Healthy 'n Hearty Choice

Caramel Pecan Minibon

Calories	339	Sodium (mg)	337
Fat (g)	13	Carbohydrate (g)	49
% calories from fat	35	Fiber (g)	2
Saturated fat (g)	3	Protein (g)	6
Cholesterol (mg)	n/a		

Exchanges: 3 starch, 2 1/2 fat

Cinnabon World Famous Cinnamon Rolls

	Amount	Cal.	Fat (g)	% Cal. Fat	Sat. Fat (g)	Chol. (mg)	Sod. (mg)	Carb. (g)	Fiber (g)	Pro. (g)	Servings/Exchanges
BONS & ROLLS											
✓Apple Minibon	1	385	5	12	1	n/a	261	53	1	5	2 starch, 1 1/2 carb, 1 fat
Caramel Pecan Minibon	1	339	13	35	3	n/a	337	49	2	6	1 starch, 2 carb, 2 1/2 fat
Chocolate Minibon	1	345	13	34	3	n/a	300	52	2	6	1 1/2 starch, 2 carb, 2 1/2 fat
CinnaPacks	1 pack	1100	56	46	10	n/a	6000	141	8	16	4 starch, 5 1/2 carb, 10 fat
Cinnastix	1	379	21	50	6	n/a	413	41	1	6	1 starch, 2 carb, 4 fat
Classic Cinnamon Roll	1	813	32	35	8	n/a	801	117	4	15	2 starch, 6 carb, 6 fat

✓ = Healthiest Bets; n/a = not available

Dunkin' Donuts

❖ Dunkin' Donuts provides nutrition information for all its menu items on its Web site at www.dunkindonuts.com.

Light 'n Lean Choice

1 English Muffin with Egg/Cheese
4 oz Orange Juice

Calories	335	Sodium (mg)	1,011
Fat (g)	9	Carbohydrate (g)	47
% calories from fat	24	Fiber (g)	1
Saturated fat (g)	4.5	Protein (g)	16
Cholesterol (mg)	140		

Exchanges: 2 starch, 1 fruit, 2 lean meat

Healthy 'n Hearty Choice

2 Glazed Yeast Donuts
8 oz low-fat milk

Calories	462	Sodium (mg)	607
Fat (g)	18	Carbohydrate (g)	62
% calories from fat	35	Fiber (g)	2
Saturated fat (g)	5	Protein (g)	14
Cholesterol (mg)	12		

Exchanges: 3 carb, 3 fat, 1 milk

Dunkin' Donuts

	Amount	Cal.	Fat (g)	% Cal. Fat	Sat. Fat (g)	Chol. (mg)	Sod. (mg)	Carb. (g)	Fiber (g)	Pro. (g)	Servings/Exchanges
BAGELS											
✓Blueberry	1	330	3	8	0.5	0	600	66	2	10	4 starch
✓Cinnamon Raisin	1	330	3	8	0.5	0	430	65	3	10	4 starch
✓Everything	1	370	6	15	0.5	0	650	67	3	14	4 1/2 starch
✓Harvest	1	350	6	15	1	0	500	61	7	13	4 1/2 starch
✓Multigrain	1	380	6	14	1	0	650	68	5	14	4 1/2 starch
✓Onion	1	320	4	11	0.5	0	610	61	3	12	4 starch
✓Plain	1	320	3	8	0.5	0	650	62	2	12	4 starch
✓Poppyseed	1	370	7	17	0.5	0	650	65	3	14	4 1/2 starch, 1 fat
Reduced Carb	1	380	12	28	4.5	20	780	45	14	25	3 starch, 1 lean meat, 1 1/2 fat

✓ = Healthiest Bets

(*Continued*)

BAGELS (*Continued*)	Amount	Cal.	Fat (g)	% Cal. Fat	Sat. Fat (g)	Chol. (mg)	Sod. (mg)	Carb. (g)	Fiber (g)	Pro. (g)	Servings/Exchanges
Salsa	1	310	3	9	0.5	0	790	60	2	13	4 starch
Salt	1	320	3	8	0.5	0	4520	62	2	12	4 starch
✓Sesame	1	380	8	19	0.5	0	650	64	3	14	5 starch
✓Sourdough	1	370	3	7	0.5	0	760	71	2	15	4 1/2 starch
✓Wheat	1	330	4	11	1	0	610	62	4	12	4 starch
BREAKFAST SANDWICHES											
Bacon Egg Cheese Bagel	1	510	14	25	6	150	1300	69	2	26	4 1/2 starch, 1 medium-fat meat, 1 high-fat meat
Bacon Egg Cheese Croissant	1	440	27	55	10	155	830	32	1	18	2 starch, 1 medium-fat meat, 1 high-fat meat, 2 fat
Bacon Egg Cheese English Muffin	1	330	12	33	6	155	1210	34	1	19	2 starch, 1 medium-fat meat, 1 high-fat meat
Bacon Ham Egg Cheddar	1	570	18	28	8	175	1490	69	2	35	4 1/2 starch, 2 high-fat meat

Egg Cheese Bagel	1	470	10	19	4.5	140	1190	71	2	23	4 starch, 1 medium-fat meat, 1 high-fat meat
Egg Cheese Biscuit	1	370	20	49	7	140	1190	32	1	15	2 starch, 2 high-fat meat, 1/2 fat
Egg Cheese Croissant	1	390	23	53	8	145	630	32	1	14	2 starch, 2 high-fat meat, 1 1/2 fat
Egg Cheese English Muffin	1	280	9	29	4.5	140	1010	34	1	15	2 starch, 1 medium-fat meat, 1 fat
Ham Egg Cheese Bagel	1	510	11	19	5	160	1460	71	2	30	4 1/2 starch, 2 medium-fat meat
Ham Egg Cheese Croissant	1	430	24	50	9	165	900	32	1	21	2 starch, 2 high-fat meat, 1 1/2 fat
Ham Egg Cheese English Muffin	1	310	10	29	5	160	1270	34	1	21	2 starch, 2 medium-fat meat
Sausage Egg Cheese Bagel	1	680	29	38	11	185	1700	72	2	33	4 1/2 starch, 3 high-fat meat, 1 fat

✓ = Healthiest Bets

(Continued)

BREAKFAST SANDWICHES (*Continued*)	Amount	Cal.	Fat (g)	% Cal. Fat	Sat. Fat (g)	Chol. (mg)	Sod. (mg)	Carb. (g)	Fiber (g)	Pro. (g)	Servings/Exchanges
Sausage Egg Cheese Biscuit	1	570	39	62	13	185	1700	32	1	24	2 starch, 3 high-fat meat, 3 fat
Sausage Egg Cheese Croissant	1	600	41	62	14	190	1140	32	1	24	2 starch, 3 high-fat meat, 3 fat
Sausage Egg Cheese English Muffin	1	480	27	51	10	185	1520	35	1	24	2 starch, 3 high-fat meat, 1/2 fat
CAKE DOUGHNUTS											
✓Apple Crumb	1	290	15	47	13	15	320	41	1	3	3 carb
Chocolate Coconut	1	300	19	57	6	0	370	31	1	4	2 carb, 3 fat
Chocolate Frosted	1	290	16	50	3.5	0	370	33	1	3	2 carb, 3 fat
Cinnamon	1	330	20	55	5	25	340	34	1	4	2 carb, 4 fat
Double Chocolate	1	310	17	49	3.5	0	370	37	2	3	2 carb, 3 fat

✓Frosted Lemon	1	240	14	53	3.5	0	150	28	0	2	2 carb, 2 fat
Glazed	1	350	19	49	5	25	340	41	1	4	3 carb, 3 fat
✓Glazed Ginger Bread	1	260	11	38	2.5	20	320	35	1	3	2 carb, 2 fat
✓Glazed Lemon	1	240	14	53	3.5	0	150	28	0	2	2 carb, 2 1/2 fat
Old Fashion	1	300	19	57	5	25	330	28	1	4	2 carb, 3 fat
Powdered	1	330	19	52	5	25	330	36	1	4	3 carb, 2 1/2 fat
Whole Wheat Glazed	1	310	19	55	4	0	380	32	2	4	2 carb, 3 1/2 fat
COOKIES											
✓Chocolate Chunk	2	220	11	45	7	35	105	28	1	3	2 carb, 2 fat
✓Chocolate Chunk w/ Walnuts	2	230	12	47	6	35	110	27	1	3	2 carb, 2 fat
✓Oatmeal Raisin Pecan	2	220	10	41	5	30	110	29	1	3	2 carb, 2 fat
✓White Chocolate Chunk	2	230	12	47	7	35	120	28	1	3	2 carb, 2 fat

✓ = Healthiest Bets

(*Continued*)

	Amount	Cal.	Fat (g)	% Cal. Fat	Sat. Fat (g)	Chol. (mg)	Sod. (mg)	Carb. (g)	Fiber (g)	Pro. (g)	Servings/Exchanges
COOLATTA											
Coffee w/ 2% milk	16 oz	190	2	9	1.5	10	80	41	0	4	2 1/2 carb
Coffee w/ cream	16 oz	350	22	57	14	75	65	40	0	3	2 1/2 carb, 4 fat
Coffee w/ milk	16 oz	210	4	17	2.5	15	80	42	0	4	3 carb
Coffee w/ skim milk	16 oz	170	0	0	0	0	80	41	0	4	2 carb
Lemonade	16 oz	240	0	0	0	0	35	59	0	0	4 carb
Orange Mango	16 oz	270	0	0	0	0	25	66	2	1	4 carb
Strawberry Fruit	16 oz	290	0	0	0	0	30	72	1	0	4 1/2 carb
Vanilla Bean	16 oz	440	17	35	15	0	95	70	1	1	4 carb, 3 fat
CREAM CHEESE											
Chive	4 T	170	17	90	11	45	230	4	2	4	3 fat
Garden Vegetable	4 T	170	15	79	11	45	340	4	0	2	3 1/2 fat

Lite	4 T	110	9	74	7	30	230	6	0	4	1 1/2 fat
Plain	4 T	190	17	81	13	55	190	4	0	4	3 1/2 fat
Salmon	4 T	170	17	90	11	45	180	2	0	4	3 1/2 fat
Shedd's Buttermatch Blend	1 T	80	9	100	2	0	100	0	0	0	2 fat
Strawberry	4 T	190	17	81	9	45	150	9	0	4	3 1/2 fat
DANISH											
✓Apple	1	250	10	36	2.5	5	220	36	0	4	2 carb, 2 fat
✓Cheese	1	270	14	47	4.5	15	210	32	0	4	2 carb, 2 1/2 fat
✓Strawberry Cheese	1	250	12	43	3.5	10	200	33	0	4	2 carb, 2 fat
FANCIES											
Apple Fritter	1	300	14	42	3	0	360	41	1	4	2 1/2 carb, 2 1/2 fat
Bow Tie Donut	1	300	17	51	3.5	0	340	34	1	4	2 carb, 3 fat
Chocolate Frosted Roll	1	290	15	47	3	0	340	36	1	4	2 carb, 3 fat

✓ = Healthiest Bets

(Continued)

FANCIES (*Continued*)	Amount	Cal.	Fat (g)	% Cal. Fat	Sat. Fat (g)	Chol. (mg)	Sod. (mg)	Carb. (g)	Fiber (g)	Pro. (g)	Servings/Exchanges
Coffee Roll	1	270	14	47	3	0	340	33	1	4	2 carb, 2 1/2 fat
Éclair	1	270	11	37	2.5	0	290	39	1	3	2 1/2 carb, 2 fat
Glazed Fritter	1	260	14	48	3	0	330	31	1	4	2 carb, 2 1/2 fat
Maple Frosted Coffee Roll	1	290	14	43	3	0	340	36	1	4	2 carb, 3 fat
HOT ESPRESSO DRINKS											
Cappuccino	10 oz	80	5	56	2.5	20	70	7	0	4	1 milk
Cappuccino w/ Soy Milk	10 oz	70	3	39	0	0	80	6	1	4	1 milk
Cappuccino w/ Soy Milk & Sugar	10 oz	120	3	23	0	0	80	20	1	4	1/2 carb, 1 milk
Cappuccino w/ Sugar	10 oz	130	5	35	2.5	15	65	21	0	4	1/2 carb, 1 milk, 1 fat
Caramel Swirl Latte	10 oz	230	6	23	3.5	25	140	36	0	8	2 carb, 1 milk
Caramel Swirl Latte w/ Soy Milk	10 oz	210	4	17	0	0	160	34	1	8	1 1/2 carb, 1 milk

✔Espresso	2 oz	0	0	0	0	0	5	1	0	0	free
✔Espresso w/ Sugar	2 oz	30	0	0	0	0	5	7	0	0	1/2 carb
Latte	10 oz	120	6	45	3.5	25	95	10	0	6	1 milk, 1/2 fat
✔Latte w/ Soy Milk	10 oz	90	4	40	0	0	110	8	1	6	1 milk
✔Latte w/ Soy Milk & Sugar	10 oz	150	4	24	0	0	110	22	1	6	1/2 carb, 1 milk
Latte w/ Sugar	10 oz	160	6	34	3.5	25	95	22	0	6	1 carb, 1 milk
Mocha Swirl Latte	10 oz	230	7	27	4	25	110	37	1	6	2 carb, 1 milk
Mocha Swirl Latte w/ Soy Milk	10 oz	210	5	21	1	0	130	35	2	7	1 1/2 carb, 1 milk
ICED ESPRESSO DRINKS											
Iced Caramel Swirl Latte	16 oz	240	7	26	4	25	150	37	0	8	2 carb, 1 milk
Iced Caramel Swirl Latte w/ Soy Milk	16 oz	210	4	17	0	0	160	34	1	8	1 1/2 carb, 1 milk

✔ = Healthiest Bets

(Continued)

ICED ESPRESSO DRINKS (*Continued*)	Amount	Cal.	Fat (g)	% Cal. Fat	Sat. Fat (g)	Chol. (mg)	Sod. (mg)	Carb. (g)	Fiber (g)	Pro. (g)	Servings/Exchanges
✓Iced Latte	16 oz	120	7	53	4	25	105	11	0	6	1/2 carb, 1 milk
✓Iced Latte w/ Soy Milk	16 oz	90	4	40	0	0	115	8	1	6	1 milk
✓Iced Latte w/ Soy Milk & Sugar	16 oz	140	4	26	0	0	115	20	1	6	1/2 carb, 1 milk
✓Iced Latte w/ Sugar	16 oz	170	7	37	4	25	110	23	0	6	1 carb, 1 milk
Iced Mocha Swirl Latte	16 oz	240	8	30	4.5	25	125	38	1	7	1 1/2 carb, 1 milk, 1 fat
Iced Mocha Swirl Latte w/ Soy Milk	16 oz	210	5	21	1	0	130	35	2	7	1 carb, 1 milk, 1 fat
MUFFIN											
Banana Walnut	1	540	25	42	3.5	65	520	69	3	10	4 1/2 carb, 4 fat
Blueberry	1	470	17	33	3	60	500	73	2	8	5 carb, 2 fat
Chocolate Chip	1	630	26	37	8	70	560	89	2	10	5 1/2 carb, 4 fat
Coffee Cake	1	580	19	29	3	65	520	78	1	9	5 carb, 4 fat

Corn	1	510	18	32	3.5	75	860	77	1	8	5 carb, 2 1/2 fat
Cranberry Orange	1	440	17	35	3	65	480	66	3	8	4 carb, 3 fat
Honey Bran Raisin	1	480	15	28	2.5	60	480	79	5	8	5 carb, 2 fat
Reduced Fat Blueberry	1	440	12	25	3	55	650	75	2	8	5 carb, 1 1/2 fat
MUNCHKINS											
✓Cinnamon Cake	4	270	15	50	3.5	25	210	31	1	3	2 carb, 2 1/2 fat
✓Glazed	5	200	9	41	2	0	220	27	1	3	2 carb, 1 1/2 fat
✓Glazed Cake	3	280	13	42	3	20	190	38	1	3	2 1/2 carb, 2 fat
✓Glazed Chocolate Cake	3	200	10	45	2	0	250	26	1	3	1 1/2 carb, 2 fat
✓Jelly Filled	5	210	9	39	2	0	240	30	1	3	2 carb, 1 1/2 fat
✓Lemon Filled	4	170	8	42	1.5	0	190	23	0	2	1 1/2 carb, 1 fat
Plain Cake	4	270	16	53	4	25	240	27	1	3	1 1/2 carb, 3 fat
✓Powdered Cake	4	270	14	47	3.5	25	210	31	1	3	2 carb, 2 1/2 fat
✓Sugar Raised	7	220	12	49	2.5	0	290	26	1	4	1 1/2 carb, 2 1/2 fat

✓ = Healthiest Bets

(*Continued*)

	Amount	Cal.	Fat (g)	% Cal. Fat	Sat. Fat (g)	Chol. (mg)	Sod. (mg)	Carb. (g)	Fiber (g)	Pro. (g)	Servings/Exchanges
STICKS											
Cinnamon Cake	1	450	30	60	7	35	310	42	1	4	3 carb, 5 fat
Glazed Cake	1	490	29	53	7	35	310	51	1	4	3 1/2 carb, 5 fat
Glazed Chocolate	1	470	29	56	7	0	490	49	2	4	3 carb, 5 fat
Jelly	1	530	29	49	7	35	320	61	1	4	4 carb, 5 fat
Plain Cake	1	420	29	62	7	35	310	35	1	4	2 carb, 6 fat
Powdered Cake	1	450	29	58	7	35	310	42	1	4	3 carb, 5 fat
YEAST DOUGHNUTS											
✓Apple Crumb	1	230	10	39	3	0	270	34	1	3	2 carb, 1 1/2 fat
✓Apple N' Spice	1	200	8	36	1.5	0	270	29	1	3	2 carb, 1 fat
✓Bavarian Kreme	1	210	9	39	2	0	270	30	1	3	2 carb, 1 fat
✓Black Raspberry	1	210	8	34	1.5	0	280	32	1	3	2 carb, 1 fat

✔Blueberry Crumb	1	240	10	38	3	0	260	36	1	3	2 carb, 2 fat
✔Boston Kreme	1	240	9	34	2	0	280	36	1	3	2 carb, 2 fat
✔Chocolate Frosted	1	200	9	41	2	0	260	29	1	3	2 carb, 1 fat
✔Chocolate Kreme Filled	1	270	13	43	3	0	260	35	1	3	2 carb, 2 1/2 fat
✔French Cruller	1	150	8	48	2	20	105	17	1	2	1 carb, 2 fat
✔Glazed	1	180	8	40	1.5	0	250	25	1	3	1 1/2 carb, 1 1/2 fat
✔Jelly Filled	1	210	8	34	1.5	0	280	32	1	3	2 carb, 2 fat
✔Lemon Burst	1	300	14	42	5	0	300	35	3	3	2 carb, 3 fat
✔Maple Frosted	1	210	9	39	2	0	260	30	1	3	2 carb, 2 fat
✔Strawberry	1	210	8	34	1.5	0	260	32	1	3	2 carb, 2 fat
✔Strawberry Frosted	1	210	9	39	2	0	260	30	1	3	2 carb, 2 fat
✔Sugar Raised	1	170	8	42	1.5	0	250	22	1	3	1 1/2 carb, 1 1/2 fat
✔Vanilla Kreme Filled	1	270	13	43	3	0	250	36	1	3	2 carb, 2 fat

✔ = Healthiest Bets

Einstein Bros Bagels

❖ Einstein Bros Bagels provided nutrition information for its menu items for this book; the information is not on its Web site at www.einsteinbros.com.

Light 'n Lean Choice

Dark Pumpernickel Bagel with 2 T Sun-Dried Tomato & Basil Cream Cheese
Cappuccino, regular nonfat *(12 oz)*

Calories	440	Sodium (mg)	925
Fat (g)	7	Carbohydrate (g)	79
% calories from fat	14	Fiber (g)	3
Saturated fat (g)	3.5	Protein (g)	18
Cholesterol (mg)	20		

Exchanges: 4 starch, 1 fat-free milk, 1 fat

Healthy 'n Hearty Choice

Low-Fat Minestrone Soup *(cup/7 oz)*
Albacore Tuna on Artisan Wheat Bread

Calories	520	Sodium (mg)	1,460
Fat (g)	13	Carbohydrate (g)	70
% calories from fat	23	Fiber (g)	7
Saturated fat (g)	1	Protein (g)	34
Cholesterol (mg)	1		

Exchanges: 4 1/2 starch, 3 lean meat

Einstein Bros Bagels

	Amount	Cal.	Fat (g)	% Cal. Fat	Sat. Fat (g)	Chol. (mg)	Sod. (mg)	Carb. (g)	Fiber (g)	Pro. (g)	Servings/Exchanges
ASSEMBLED SANDWICHES											
✓Albacore Tuna on Artisan Wheat	1	400	9	20	1	35	520	49	5	30	3 starch, 3 lean meat, 1 fat
Black Forest Ham on Challah	1	620	23	33	8	125	2040	65	3	37	4 starch, 3 lean meat, 4 fat
Calipso Chicken Salad	1	460	9	18	1	40	1100	72	3	26	4 starch, 2 lean meat, 1 fat
Club Mex on Challah	1	620	27	39	10	130	1660	56	3	42	3 1/2 starch, 4 medium-fat meat, 1 fat
Cobbie on Challah	1	600	27	41	10	115	1620	57	5	40	3 1/2 starch, 4 lean meat, 2 fat

✓ = Healthiest Bets

(*Continued*)

ASSEMBLED SANDWICHES (*Continued*)	Amount	Cal.	Fat (g)	% Cal. Fat	Sat. Fat (g)	Chol. (mg)	Sod. (mg)	Carb. (g)	Fiber (g)	Pro. (g)	Servings/Exchanges
Einstein Club on Rustic White	1	660	26	35	6	85	1350	55	4	37	3 1/2 starch, 4 lean meat, 3 1/2 fat
✓Harvest Chicken Salad on Challah	1	400	9	20	1	35	520	49	5	30	3 starch, 3 lean meat
Mediterranean Hummus & Feta on Ciabatta	1	450	10	20	3.5	15	1110	77	5	17	4 1/2 starch, 1 veg, 1 lean meat, 1/2 fat
New York Lox & Bagel	1	660	27	37	19	85	1150	79	3	26	5 starch, 2 high-fat meat, 1 fat
Roasted Turkey on Artisan Wheat	1	610	28	41	10	100	1350	51	5	42	3 1/2 starch, 3 lean meat, 3 fat
Tasty Turkey on Asiago Bread	1	630	18	26	11	95	1600	83	3	39	5 1/2 starch, 3 lean meat, 1 fat
Turkey Cranberry Chutney w/ side of chutney	1	600	13	20	1.5	50	1050	83	4	35	5 1/2 starch, 3 lean meat, 1/2 fat

✓Veg Out on Sesame Seed Bagel	1	500	13	23	7	30	690	82	4	17	5 starch, 1 veg, 1 lean meat, 1 fat
BAGEL DOGS											
Asiago Chicago	1	740	34	41	15	80	1360	78	2	29	5 starch, 3 high-fat meat, 1 fat
Chicago (onion/no cheese)	1	680	30	40	12	70	1220	78	2	25	5 starch, 3 high-fat meat
Chicago Chili Cheese	1	810	38	42	17	105	1550	83	4	33	5 1/2 starch, 3 high-fat meat, 1 1/2 fat
Chicago w/ everything	1	730	34	42	12	70	1850	80	3	26	5 starch, 3 high-fat meat, 1 fat
BAGELS											
✓Asiago Cheese	1	360	3	8	1.5	5	570	70	2	13	4 1/2 starch, 1/2 fat
✓Chocolate Chip	1	370	3	7	2	0	500	76	3	11	4 1/2 starch, 1/2 fat
✓Chopped Garlic	1	380	3	7	1	0	680	79	4	13	5 starch, 1/2 fat

✓ = Healthiest Bets

(Continued)

BAGELS (*Continued*)	**Amount**	**Cal.**	**Fat (g)**	**% Cal. Fat**	**Sat. Fat (g)**	**Chol. (mg)**	**Sod. (mg)**	**Carb. (g)**	**Fiber (g)**	**Pro. (g)**	**Servings/Exchanges**
✔Chopped Onion	1	330	1	3	0	0	500	71	2	11	4 1/2 starch
✔Cinnamon Raisin Swirl	1	350	1	3	0	0	490	78	2	11	5 starch
✔Cinnamon Sugar	1	330	1	3	0	0	490	74	2	10	5 starch
Cinnamon Sugar Chicago Style	1	500	21	38	4.5	0	730	72	2	11	4 1/2 starch, 3 fat
✔Cranberry	1	350	1	3	0	0	490	78	3	10	5 starch
✔Dark Pumpernickel	1	320	1	3	0	0	730	68	3	11	4 1/2 starch
✔Egg	1	340	3	8	1	385	510	69	2	11	4 1/2 starch, 1/2 fat
Everything	1	340	2	5	0	0	820	75	2	13	5 starch
✔Honey Whole Wheat	1	320	1	3	0	0	470	71	3	10	4 1/2 starch
✔Lower Carb 9 Grain	1	210	4	17	10	0	650	28	10	25	2 starch, 2 lean meat

Lower Carb 9 Grain w/ Plain Cream Cheese	1	310	13	38	7	30	730	29	10	27	2 starch, 2 lean meat, 1 1/2 fat
✓Mango	1	360	1	3	0	0	490	80	2	10	5 starch
✓Marble Rye	1	340	2	5	0	0	690	73	3	11	4 1/2 starch
✓Nutty Banana	1	360	3	8	1	0	510	74	2	11	4 1/2 starch
✓Plain Bagel	1	320	1	3	0	0	520	71	2	11	4 1/2 starch
✓Poppy Dip'd Bagel	1	350	2	5	0	0	680	74	2	12	4 1/2 starch
✓Potato	1	350	5	13	1	0	590	69	2	10	4 1/2 starch
✓Power	1	410	2	4	0.5	0	310	81	4	13	5 starch
✓Power w/ Peanut Butter	1	750	34	41	6	0	780	92	7	27	6 starch, 2 high-fat meat, 2 fat
✓Pumpkin	1	310	2	6	0	0	590	66	3	11	4 starch
Salt	1	330	1	3	0	0	1790	73	2	11	4 1/2 starch
✓Sesame Dip'd	1	380	5	12	1	0	680	75	3	11	5 starch

✓ = Healthiest Bets

(*Continued*)

BAGELS (*Continued*)	Amount	Cal.	Fat (g)	% Cal. Fat	Sat. Fat (g)	Chol. (mg)	Sod. (mg)	Carb. (g)	Fiber (g)	Pro. (g)	Servings/Exchanges
✓Sun-Dried Tomato	1	320	1	3	0	0	520	69	3	11	4 1/2 starch
✓Wild Blueberry	1	350	1	3	0	0	510	77	3	11	5 starch
COFFEE EXTRAS											
Almond Syrup	2 T	90	0	0	0	0	0	23	0	0	1 carb
Blackberry	2 T	77	0	0	0	0	0	19	0	0	1 carb
Hazelnut Syrup	2 T	80	0	0	0	0	0	19	0	0	1 carb
Light Whipped Cream	2 T	30	2	60	1.5	10	0	2	0	0	1/2 fat
Raspberry Syrup	2 T	80	0	0	0	0	0	20	0	0	1 carb
✓Reduced Fat Topping	2 T	20	2	90	1	0	5	2	0	0	free
✓Sugar Free Caramel Syrup	2 T	0	0	0	0	0	0	0	0		free
✓Sugar Free Vanilla Syrup	2 T	0	0	0	0	0	0	0	0		free
Vanilla Syrup	2 T	80	0	0	0	0	0	19	0	0	1 carb

CONDIMENTS											
✓Ancho Lime Mayonnaise	1 T	50	5	90	1	5	160	1	0	0	1 fat
Ancho Lime Salsa	1/4 cup	20	1	45	0	0	670	3	0	0	free
✓Deli Mustard	1 t	4	0	0	0	0	65	0	0	0	free
✓French Dijon Mustard	1 t	10	0	0	0	0	130	0	0	0	free
✓Gorgonzola Mayonnaise	1 T	50	5	90	2.5	1	120	1	0	1	1 fat
✓Grained Dijon Mustard	1 t	5	0	0	0	0	105	0	0	0	free
✓Honey Mustard	1 t	15	0	0	0	0	45	2	0	0	free
Whole Kosher Pickle	1	5	0	0	0	0	650	1	1	0	free
✓Yellow Mustard	1 t	0	0	0	0	80	0	0	0		free
HALF SALADS											
Asiago Caesar	1	330	26	71	5	20	295	13	2	8	3 veg, 1 medium-fat meat, 4 fat
Asiago Chicken Caesar	1	375	27	65	5.5	45	925	13	1	17	3 veg, 2 lean meat, 4 fat

✓ = Healthiest Bets

(Continued)

HALF SALADS (*Continued*)	Amount	Cal.	Fat (g)	% Cal. Fat	Sat. Fat (g)	Chol. (mg)	Sod. (mg)	Carb. (g)	Fiber (g)	Pro. (g)	Servings/Exchanges
Bros Bistro	1	405	35	78	6.5	13	265	19	2	8	3 veg, 1 medium-fat meat, 6 fat
✓Chicken Chipotle	1	315	20	57	4.5	40	705	19	4	16	3 veg, 2 lean meat, 3 fat
✓Harvest Cobb	1	280	18	58	4	40	655	16	4	16	3 veg, 2 medium-fat meat, 1 fat
✓Jamaican Jerk	1	170	5	26	35	48	325	22	2	12	3 veg, 2 lean meat
LOWER CARB 9-GRAIN BAGEL SANDWICHES											
Bagel Dog	1	560	33	53	13	70	1370	35	10	39	2 starch, 5 medium-fat meat, 1 fat
Denver Omelet Panini	1	650	32	44	14	460	1730	35	10	60	2 starch, 8 medium-fat meat, 1 fat
Frittata Egg	1	470	22	42	10	415	970	31	10	45	2 starch, 4 medium-fat meat

Frittata Egg & Bacon	1	720	45	56	19	155	1320	32	10	53	2 starch, 4 medium-fat meat, 2 high-fat meat, 1 1/2 fat
Frittata Egg w/ Black Forest Ham	1	550	24	39	11	445	1560	33	10	56	2 starch, 7 lean meat
Frittata Egg w/ Turkey Sausage	1	550	26	43	11	445	1300	31	10	56	2 starch, 7 lean meat
Tasty Turkey	1	490	19	35	10	92	1550	40	11	51	2 1/2 starch, 6 lean meat
Turkey Deli	1	330	6	16	1.5	45	1550	32	11	48	2 starch, 3 lean meat
NAKED EGGS											
Denver Omelet	1 order	440	29	59	13	460	1080	7	2	35	5 medium-fat meat, 1 fat
✔Plain	1 order	270	19	63	9	415	310	3	0	20	3 medium-fat meat, 1 fat
Santa Fe	1 order	400	27	61	14	460	900	7	0	32	4 medium-fat meat, 2 fat
w/ Black Forest Ham	1 order	340	20	53	10	445	900	5	0	30	4 medium-fat meat, 1 fat

✔ = Healthiest Bets

(*Continued*)

NAKED EGGS (*Continued*)	Amount	Cal.	Fat (g)	% Cal. Fat	Sat. Fat (g)	Chol. (mg)	Sod. (mg)	Carb. (g)	Fiber (g)	Pro. (g)	Servings/Exchanges
w/ Sausage	1 order	340	22	58	10	445	650	3	0	31	2 medium-fat meat, 2 high-fat meat
w/ Thick Cut Bacon	1 order	520	41	71	18	455	660	4	0	28	2 medium-fat meat, 2 high-fat meat, 4 fat
PANINI SANDWICHES											
Cali Club	1	990	56	51	19	130	2500	71	4	54	4 1/2 starch, 6 medium-fat meat, 4 fat
Ham & Cheese	1	640	23	32	10	100	2090	68	2	41	4 1/2 starch, 4 medium-fat meat
Italian Chicken	1	690	27	35	10	95	1460	68	3	47	4 1/2 starch, 5 lean meat, 1 1/2 fat
SALAD DRESSINGS & SPREADS											
Butter & Margarine Blend	1 T	60	7	100	1.5	0	75	0	0	0	1 1/2 fat

Caesar Dressing	2 T	150	16	96	2.5	10	360	0	0	1	3 fat
Chipotle Vinaigrette	2 T	110	10	82	1.5	0	440	5	0	0	2 fat
Cranberry Chutney	2 T	80	1	11	0	0	20	16	0	0	1 starch
Creamy Peanut Butter	2 T	190	15	71	2	0	140	8	2	7	1 high-fat meat, 2 fat
Feta & Pinenut Spread	2 T	60	5	75	3	15	150	2	0	3	1 1/2 fat
Grape Spread	2 T	75	0	0	0	0	3	19	0	0	1 carb
Honey Butter	1 T	90	8	80	4	15	35	4	0	0	2 fat
Hummus	4 T	110	7	57	0.5	0	390	9	2	3	1/2 starch, 1 1/2 fat
Mango Ginger Vinaigrette	2 T	60	2	30	0	15	105	11	0	0	1/2 starch, 1/2 fat
Orange Pomegranate Vinaigrette	2 T	80	7	79	1	0	220	3	0	0	1 1/2 fat
Peppercorn Spread	2 T	100	10	90	3	20	220	2	0	1	2 fat
Raspberry Vinaigrette	2 T	160	14	79	2	0	80	8	0	0	3 fat

✔ = Healthiest Bets

(*Continued*)

SALAD DRESSINGS & SPREADS (*Continued*)	Amount	Cal.	Fat (g)	% Cal. Fat	Sat. Fat (g)	Chol. (mg)	Sod. (mg)	Carb. (g)	Fiber (g)	Pro. (g)	Servings/Exchanges
Spicy Roasted Tomato Spread	2 T	140	14	90	2	15	240	3	1	0	3 fat
Strawberry Spread	2 T	75	0	0	0	0	17	19	0	0	1 carb
Thousand Island	2 T	110	9	74	20	10	210	5	0	0	2 fat
SALAD EXTRAS & SIDES											
✓Bagel Croutons	1/4 cup	25	1	36	0	0	75	4	0	1	1/2 starch
Candied Walnuts	1 oz	180	15	75	1.5	0	85	7	1	5	1/2 carb, 1 high-fat meat, 1 fat
Cranberry Almond Cous Cous	4 oz	180	9	45	1	0	250	23	3	4	1 1/2 starch, 1 high-fat meat
Lahvash Flatbread	2 oz	190	7	33	2	5	520	26	2	7	1 1/2 starch, 1 1/2 fat
✓Roasted Corn Salad	3 oz	90	3	30	0	0	150	13	4	2	1 starch
Traditional Potato Salad	1/2 cup	290	21	65	3	15	600	21	2	3	1 1/2 starch, 4 fat

SALADS											
Asiago Caesar	1	660	53	72	11	40	590	25	3	15	1 starch, 2 veg, 2 high-fat meat, 7 fat
Asiago Chicken Caesar	1	740	54	66	11	90	1400	25	3	33	1 starch, 2 veg, 4 medium-fat meat, 8 fat
Bros Bistro	1	810	69	77	13	25	530	37	4	15	1 1/2 starch, 3 veg, 2 high-fat meat, 9 fat
Chicken Chipotle	1	630	40	57	9	80	1410	38	7	31	1 1/2 starch, 3 veg, 4 lean meat, 5 fat
Harvest Cobb	1	560	35	56	8	80	1310	31	7	32	1 starch, 3 veg, 2 medium-fat meat, 2 high-fat meat, 5 fat
✔Jamaican Jerk Entrée	1	340	10	26	1	95	650	43	4	23	2 starch, 3 veg, 3 lean meat

✔ = Healthiest Bets

(Continued)

	Amount	Cal.	Fat (g)	% Cal. Fat	Sat. Fat (g)	Chol. (mg)	Sod. (mg)	Carb. (g)	Fiber (g)	Pro. (g)	Servings/Exchanges
SANDWICH FILLINGS											
American Cheese	1 slice	70	6	77	4	20	290	1	0	4	1 medium-fat meat
Cheddar Cheese	1 slice	80	7	79	4.5	20	130	0	0	5	1 medium-fat meat
Pepper Jack Cheese	1 slice	100	8	72	5	30	170	0	0	27	1 high-fat meat
✓Provolone Cheese	1 slice	70	3	39	0.5	15	180	0	0	5	1 high-fat meat
Smoked Salmon	2 oz	110	6	49	2	20	650	2	0	12	2 lean meat
Swiss Cheese	1 slice	80	6	68	3.5	20	55	1	0	6	1 medium-fat meat
Thick Cut Bacon	3.6 oz	420	10	21	15	35	588	2	0	13	2 high-fat meat, 5 fat
✓Turkey Sausage	1	70	4	51	1	30	190	0	0	9	1 medium-fat meat
SANDWICH FRITTATAS & PANINIS											
Denver Omelet Breakfast Panini	1	750	31	37	12	460	1760	70	2	46	4 1/2 starch, 5 medium-fat meat, 1 fat

Egg & Black Forest Ham Frittata	1	660	21	29	10	445	1420	76	2	41	5 starch, 3 lean meat, 1 medium-fat meat
Egg & Sausage Frittata	1	660	23	31	10	445	1170	74	2	42	5 starch, 3 lean meat, 1 medium-fat meat
Egg & Thick Cut Bacon Frittata	1	680	26	34	13	440	1090	75	2	38	5 starch, 1 medium-fat meat, 2 high-fat meat
Plain Egg Frittata	1	590	20	31	9	415	830	71	2	31	4 1/2 starch, 2 medium-fat meat, 1 fat
Santa Fe Egg Frittata	1	720	28	35	14	460	1420	78	2	43	5 starch, 4 medium-fat meat, 1/2 fat
Spinach & Bacon Breakfast Panini	1	930	49	47	2	190	1920	72	3	55	4 starch, 6 high-fat meat
SOUPS											
Broccoli & Sharp Cheddar	14 oz	540	35	58	18	90	1740	31	3	26	2 starch, 1 milk, 2 high-fat meat, 2 1/2 fat

✓ = Healthiest Bets

(*Continued*)

SOUPS (*Continued*)	Amount	Cal.	Fat (g)	% Cal. Fat	Sat. Fat (g)	Chol. (mg)	Sod. (mg)	Carb. (g)	Fiber (g)	Pro. (g)	Servings/Exchanges
Broccoli & Sharp Cheddar	7 oz	220	14	57	7	30	1040	12	1	10	1 starch, 1 milk, 1 high-fat meat
Butternut Squash Bisque	14 oz	660	27	37	16	85	1550	107	0	5	3 starch, 4 fat
Butternut Squash Bisque	7 oz	190	12	57	7	40	750	22	1	4	1 1/2 starch, 2 fat
Caribbean Crab Chowder	7 oz	220	14	57	12	25	790	14	1	6	1 starch, 1 lean meat, 2 fat
Caribbean Crab Chowder	14 oz	520	38	66	31	50	1550	30	4	14	2 starch, 2 lean meat, 5 1/2 fat
Chicken & Wild Rice	7 oz	240	7	26	1.5	20	1130	33	2	10	2 starch, 1 lean meat, 1 fat
Chicken & Wild Rice	14 oz	440	9	18	1.5	30	3360	67	5	24	4 starch, 2 lean meat, 1 fat
Chicken Noodle	7 oz	220	9	37	2.5	60	980	17	2	16	1 starch, 2 lean meat, 1 fat
Chicken Noodle	14 oz	510	21	37	6	135	2280	39	5	38	2 1/2 starch, 4 lean meat, 2 fat
Clam Chowda	7 oz	210	12	51	7	45	730	16	1	8	1/2 starch, 1 milk, 2 fat

Clam Chowda	14 oz	370	25	61	14	85	1120	25	1	13	2 milk, 4 fat
Low Fat Minestrone	7 oz	120	3.5	26	0	0	940	21	2	4	1 1/2 starch, 1/2 fat
Low Fat Minestrone	14 oz	360	10	25	1.5	0	2840	62	6	13	4 starch, 1 fat
Tomato Bisque	14 oz	440	23	47	8	35	3250	54	7	11	3 1/2 starch, 3 1/2 fat
Tomato Bisque	7 oz	190	12	57	6	30	870	22	2	6	1 1/2 starch, 1 1/2 fat
Tortilla Soup	7 oz	70	2	26	0	0	1150	14	2	2	1 starch
Tortilla Soup	14 oz	200	6	27	0	0	3570	32	4	4	2 starch, 1 fat
✓Turkey Chili	7 oz	180	6	30	1	30	730	30	4	16	2 starch, 1 lean meat
Turkey Chili	14 oz	330	11	30	2.5	45	2160	34	6	24	2 starch, 3 lean meat
SPECIALTY BREADS											
✓Artisan Wheat Bread	1 slice	120	2	15	0	0	360	22	2	6	1 1/2 starch
✓Challah Roll	1	300	5	15	1	40	270	55	2	11	3 1/2 starch
Ciabatta Bread	1 slice	310	3	9	0	0	680	63	2	11	4 starch

✓ = Healthiest Bets

(Continued)

SPECIALTY BREADS (*Continued*)	Amount	Cal.	Fat (g)	% Cal. Fat	Sat. Fat (g)	Chol. (mg)	Sod. (mg)	Carb. (g)	Fiber (g)	Pro. (g)	Servings/Exchanges
✓Lahvash Bread	1 slice	270	3	10	0.5	0	530	51	3	10	3 1/2 starch
✓Rustic White Bread	1 slice	140	0	0	0	0	330	28	1	5	2 starch
SPECIALTY COFFEES											
✓Café Latte	12 oz	140	5	32	3.5	20	140	13	0	9	1 milk, 1 fat
✓Café Latte, nonfat	12 oz	100	1	9	0	5	150	14	0	10	1 milk
✓Cappuccino	12 oz	90	4	40	2	15	95	9	0	6	1 milk, 1/2 fat
✓Cappuccino, nonfat	12 oz	60	0	0	0	5	95	9	0	6	1 milk
✓Chai, nonfat	12 oz	190	0	0	0	0	75	41	0	4	2 1/2 carb
Mocha	12 oz	230	6	23	4.5	15	135	34	0	8	1 carb, 1 milk, 1 fat
SPECIALTY COFFEES & OTHER BEVERAGES											
✓Chai	12 oz	210	2	9	1.5	10	75	41	0	4	2 1/2 carb, 1/2 fat
Hot Chocolate	12 oz	290	11	34	8	20	160	39	0	9	1 carb, 1 milk, 2 fat

Hot Chocolate, reduced fat	12 oz	260	7	24	6	5	160	39	0	9	1 carb, 1 milk, 1 fat
✓Iced Latte	16 oz	120	5	38	3	20	125	12	0	8	1 milk, 1 fat
✓Iced Latte, nonfat	12 oz	90	0	0	0	5	130	12	0	8	1 milk
Iced Mocha	16 oz	210	6	26	4	15	120	33	0	7	1 carb, 1 milk, 1 fat
Mocha Smoothie	16 oz	470	5	10	3	20	170	98	0	9	5 carb, 1 milk
SWEETS											
Apple Cinnamon Coffee Cake	1	570	24	38	4.5	5	240	87	0	5	5 1/2 carb, 3 fat
Banana Nut Muffin	1	640	32	45	4	80	430	81	2	10	5 carb, 4 1/2 fat
Blueberry Coffee Cake	1	600	24	36	4.5	5	250	94	0	5	6 carb, 2 fat
Blueberry Muffin	1	540	22	37	3.5	95	510	80	1	8	5 carb, 3 fat
Chocolate Chip Coffee Cake	1	660	29	40	8	5	230	96	2	7	6 1/2 carb, 3 fat

✓ = Healthiest Bets

(Continued)

SWEETS (*Continued*)	Amount	Cal.	Fat (g)	% Cal. Fat	Sat. Fat (g)	Chol. (mg)	Sod. (mg)	Carb. (g)	Fiber (g)	Pro. (g)	Servings/Exchanges
Cinnamon Twists	1	370	21	51	5	0	125	41	1	5	3 carb, 3 1/2 fat
Cinnamon Walnut Strudel	1	550	31	51	11	30	380	63	3	7	4 carb, 5 fat
Cranberry Orange Coffee Cake	1	620	25	36	5	10	250	97	2	6	6 1/2 carb, 2 fat
Heavenly Chocolate Chip Cookie	1	530	27	46	12	65	318	66	2	6	4 1/2 carb, 4 fat
Honey Roasted Peanut Butter Cookie	1	550	31	51	12	60	420	57	3	13	4 carb, 5 fat
Lemon Iced Pound Cake	1	510	28	49	5	5	280	62	1	3	4 carb, 4 fat
Marble Pound Cake	1	370	20	49	3.5	0	440	47	1	4	3 carb, 3 fat
Pumpkin Muffin w/ Cream Cheese Icing	1	500	23	41	5	10	510	67	1	7	4 1/2 carb, 4 1/2 fat

Trail Mix Cookie	1	480	19	36	8	75	300	70	4	8	4 1/2 carb, 3 fat
White Chocolate Pumpkin Walnut Cookie	1	439	24	49	3	34	577	52	2	6	3 1/2 carb, 3 1/2 fat
TOP SHELF BAGELS											
Roasted Red Pepper & Pesto	1	410	7	15	3.5	15	710	73	2	17	5 starch
Six-Cheese	1	390	6	14	3	15	650	71	1	16	4 1/2 starch, 1/2 fat
Spicy Nacho	1	450	9	18	5	20	890	77	3	17	5 carb, 1 fat
Spinach Florentine	1	410	7	15	4	20	620	72	3	17	4 1/2 starch, 1 fat
WHIPPED CREAM CHEESE											
Blueberry	2 T	70	5	64	3.5	15	50	6	0	1	1/2 carb, 1 fat
Cappuccino	2 T	70	5	64	3	15	50	5	0	1	1/2 carb, 1 fat
Garden Vegetable	2 T	60	5	75	3.5	15	100	3	0	1	1 fat

✓ = Healthiest Bets

(Continued)

WHIPPED CREAM CHEESE (*Continued*)	Amount	Cal.	Fat (g)	% Cal. Fat	Sat. Fat (g)	Chol. (mg)	Sod. (mg)	Carb. (g)	Fiber (g)	Pro. (g)	Servings/Exchanges
Honey Almond	2 T	70	5	64	3	15	45	6	0	1	1/2 carb, 1 fat
Jalapeno Salsa	2 T	60	5	75	3	15	110	3	0	1	1 fat
Maple Raisin Walnut	2 T	60	5	75	3.5	15	45	4	0	1	1 fat
Onion & Chive	2 T	70	6	77	4	20	60	3	0	1	1 fat
Plain	2 T	70	7	90	4.5	20	65	1	0	1	1 fat
Plain Reduced Fat	2 T	60	5	75	3.5	15	85	2	0	1	1 fat
Pumpkin	2 T	100	8	72	6	25	80	6	0	1	1 1/2 fat
Smoked Salmon	2 T	60	6	90	3.5	20	120	2	0	1	1 fat
Strawberry	2 T	70	2	26	3.5	15	50	5	0	1	1/2 carb, 1 fat
Sundried Tomato & Basil	2 T	60	5	75	3.5	15	100	2	0	1	1 fat

Jamba Juice

❖ Jamba Juice provides nutrition information on its Web site at www.jambajuice.com.

Light 'n Lean Choice

Pizza Protein Stick
Orange/Banana Juice *(1/2, 8 oz)*

Calories	330	Sodium (mg)	450
Fat (g)	6	Carbohydrate (g)	58
% calories from fat	16	Fiber (g)	3
Saturated fat (g)	1.5	Protein (g)	11
Cholesterol (mg)	5		

Exchanges: 2 starch, 2 fruit, 1 fat

Healthy 'n Hearty Choice

Grin 'n' Carrot Bread
Strawberry Wild Smoothie *(1/2, 8 oz)*

Calories	395	Sodium (mg)	307
Fat (g)	10	Carbohydrate (g)	71
% calories from fat	23	Fiber (g)	3
Saturated fat (g)	1	Protein (g)	9
Cholesterol (mg)	25		

Exchanges: 2 starch, 2 fruit, 2 fat

(Continued)

Jamba Juice

	Amount	Cal.	Fat (g)	% Cal. Fat	Sat. Fat (g)	Chol. (mg)	Sod. (mg)	Carb. (g)	Fiber (g)	Pro. (g)	Servings/Exchanges
BAKED GOODS											
Blueberry Cinnamon Swirl	1	320	6	17	1	40	380	55	3	10	3 1/2 carb, 1 fat
Cranberry Crumble	1	370	19	46	11	65	290	47	3	5	3 carb, 3 fat
BREADS											
Apple Cinnamon Pretzel	1	410	5	11	0	0	320	78	3	11	5 starch
✓Grin 'N' Carrot	1 slice	250	10	36	1	25	250	36	1	5	2 1/2 starch, 1 fat
Honey Berry Bran	1 slice	320	12	34	2	30	360	48	6	6	3 starch, 2 fat
Lemon Poppy Seed	1 slice	300	12	36	2	30	320	44	0	4	3 starch, 1 1/2 fat
✓Pizza Protein Stick	1 slice	230	6	23	1.5	5	450	33	2	9	2 starch, 1 1/2 fat
Sourdough Parmesan Pretzel	1	460	11	22	2	10	710	75	3	15	5 starch, 1 1/2 fat

ENLIGHTENED SMOOTHIES											
Berry Fulfilling	16 oz	160	1	6	0	5	230	33	4	7	2 carb
Blueberry Balance	16 oz	150	1	6	0	5	230	31	3	7	2 carb
Mango Mantra	16 oz	170	1	5	0	5	230	36	2	7	2 carb
Strawberry Nirvana	16 oz	160	0	0	0	5	230	34	3	6	2 carb
Tropical Awakening	16 oz	190	1	5	0	5	230	40	3	7	2 1/2 carb
JUICES											
Carrot	16 oz	100	1	9	0	0	250	23	0	3	4 veg
Lemonade	16 oz	300	0	0	0	0	10	75	0	1	5 carb
Orange	16 oz	220	1	4	0	0	0	52	0	3	4 fruit
Orange Carrot	16 oz	160	1	6	0	0	125	37	0	3	2 veg, 2 fruit
Orange/Banana	14 oz	200	1	5	0	0	0	49	2	3	3 fruit
Vibrant C	16 oz	210	0	0	0	0	0	50	1	2	1 starch, 2 fruit
Wheatgrass	1 oz	5	0	0	0	0	0	1	0	0	free

✓ = Healthiest Bets

(Continued)

	Amount	Cal.	Fat (g)	% Cal. Fat	Sat. Fat (g)	Chol. (mg)	Sod. (mg)	Carb. (g)	Fiber (g)	Pro. (g)	Servings/Exchanges
SMOOTHIES											
Aloha Pineapple	16 oz	330	1	3	0.5	5	20	75	3	6	5 carb
Banana Berry	16 oz	310	1	3	0	0	75	74	3	3	5 carb
Berry Lime Sublime	16 oz	300	1	3	0.5	5	25	70	3	2	4 1/2 carb
Bright Eyed and Blueberry	16 oz	280	1	3	0	5	90	55	3	14	3 1/2 carb
Caribbean Passion	16 oz	290	2	6	0.5	5	40	67	3	2	4 1/2 carb
Chocolate Moo'd	16 oz	500	6	11	4	20	260	102	2	12	6 1/2 carb
Citrus Squeeze	16 oz	310	2	6	0.5	5	25	72	3	3	4 1/2 carb
Cold Buster	16 oz	290	2	6	0.5	5	25	66	3	4	4 1/2 carb
Cranberry Craze	16 oz	280	0	0	0	0	30	63	3	5	4 carb
Jamba Power Boost	16 oz	280	1	3	0	0	40	67	8	6	4 1/2 carb
Kiwi Berry Burner	16 oz	310	0	0	0	0	75	73	3	2	5 carb

Mango-A-Go-Go	16 oz	330	2	5	0.5	5	40	77	2	2	5 carb
Orange Berry Blitz	16 oz	270	2	7	0.5	5	25	61	3	3	4 carb
Orange Dream Machine	16 oz	390	2	5	0.5	5	240	77	0	15	5 carb
Orange-A-Peel	16 oz	290	1	3	0	0	105	67	3	6	4 1/2 carb
Peach Pleasure	16 oz	310	2	6	0.5	5	40	72	3	2	4 1/2 carb
Peanut Butter Moo'd	16 oz	540	11	18	3	10	34	95	3	15	6 1/2 carb, 1 high-fat meat
Penya Kowlada	16 oz	460	5	10	3.5	5	120	100	3	6	6 1/2 carb
Protein Berry Pizzazz	16 oz	280	1	3	0	0	170	56	4	15	3 1/2 carb, 1 lean meat
Razzmatazz	16 oz	310	2	6	0.5	5	45	73	38	2	5 carb
Strawberry Wild	16 oz	290	0	0	0	0	115	69	3	4	4 1/2 carb
Sunrise Strawberry	16 oz	300	1	3	0	5	90	60	3	14	4 carb

Krispy Kreme Doughnuts

❖ Krispy Kreme Doughnuts provides nutrition information for all its menu items on its Web site at www.krispykreme.com.

Light 'n Lean Choice

2 Yeast Sugar-Free Mini Rings
8 oz Low-Fat Milk

Calories 246
Fat (g) 11
% calories from fat..40
Saturated fat (g) 4
Cholesterol (mg) 16
Sodium (mg) 221
Carbohydrate (g).........37
Fiber (g)......................1
Protein (g) 11

Exchanges: 1 1/2 carb, 1 fat-free milk, 1 fat

Healthy 'n Hearty Choice

1 Original Glazed Doughnut
8 oz Orange Juice

Calories 322
Fat (g) 12
% calories from fat..34
Saturated fat (g) 4
Cholesterol (mg) 5
Sodium (mg) 67
Carbohydrate (g).........49
Fiber (g)......................0
Protein (g) 4

Exchanges: 1 1/2 carb, 2 fruit, 2 fat

Krispy Kreme Doughnuts

	Amount	Cal.	Fat (g)	% Cal. Fat	Sat. Fat (g)	Chol. (mg)	Sod. (mg)	Carb. (g)	Fiber (g)	Pro. (g)	Servings/Exchanges
CAKE DOUGHNUTS											
Chocolate Iced	1	270	14	47	3	20	320	36	0	3	2 1/2 carb, 2 fat
Powdered	1	280	14	45	3	20	320	37	0	3	2 1/2 carb, 2 fat
Pumpkin Spice	1	340	18	48	4.5	20	310	42	0	3	3 carb, 2 1/2 fat
Traditional	1	230	13	51	3	20	320	25	0	3	1 1/2 carb, 2 1/2 fat
CRULLERS											
Chocolate Glazed	1	290	15	47	3.5	15	240	37	0	2	2 1/2 carb, 2 fat
Glazed	1	240	14	53	3.5	15	240	26	0	2	1 1/2 carb, 3 fat

✓ = Healthiest Bets

(*Continued*)

	Amount	Cal.	Fat (g)	% Cal. Fat	Sat. Fat (g)	Chol. (mg)	Sod. (mg)	Carb. (g)	Fiber (g)	Pro. (g)	Servings/Exchanges
DOUGHNUTS											
Caramel Kreme Crunch	1	350	19	49	5	5	170	43	0	4	3 carb, 3 fat
Chocolate Iced w/ Sprinkles	1	260	12	42	3	5	100	38	0	3	2 1/2 carb, 2 fat
Cinnamon Bun	1	260	16	55	4	5	125	28	0	3	2 carb, 2 1/2 fat
✓Cinnamon Twist	1	230	9	35	2.5	5	85	33	1	3	2 carb, 2 fat
Dulce De Leche	1	290	18	56	4.5	5	160	30	0	3	2 carb, 3 fat
Key Lime Pie	1	320	17	48	4.5	5	150	40	0	3	2 1/2 carb, 3 fat
New York Cheesecake	1	320	19	53	5	10	190	35	0	4	2 carb, 3 1/2 fat
Original Glazed	1	200	12	54	3	5	95	22	0	2	1 1/2 carb, 2 fat
Sugar	1	200	12	54	3	5	95	21	0	2	1 1/2 carb, 2 fat

FILLED DOUGHNUTS											
Chocolate Iced Custard	1	300	17	51	4	5	140	35	0	3	2 carb, 3 fat
Chocolate Iced Kreme	1	350	20	51	5	5	140	38	0	3	2 1/2 carb, 3 1/2 fat
Cinnamon Apple	1	290	16	50	4	5	150	32	0	3	2 carb, 3 fat
Glazed Kreme	1	340	20	53	5	5	140	38	0	3	2 1/2 carb, 3 1/2 fat
Glazed Lemon	1	290	16	50	4	5	135	35	0	3	2 1/2 carb, 2 1/2 fat
Powdered Blueberry	1	290	16	50	4	5	140	33	0	3	2 carb, 3 fat
FROZEN BLENDS											
Frozen Double Chocolate	12 oz	440	16	33	11	25	210	69	0	7	4 1/2 carb, 2 1/2 fat
Frozen Double Chocolate	16 oz	610	22	32	16	35	280	93	0	9	6 carb, 4 fat
Frozen Double Chocolate	20 oz	740	26	32	18	35	340	116	0	11	7 1/2 carb, 3 1/2 fat
Frozen Double Chocolate w/ Coffee	16 oz	600	22	33	15	35	280	93	0	8	6 carb, 4 fat

✔ = Healthiest Bets

(*Continued*)

FROZEN BLENDS (*Continued*)	Amount	Cal.	Fat (g)	% Cal. Fat	Sat. Fat (g)	Chol. (mg)	Sod. (mg)	Carb. (g)	Fiber (g)	Pro. (g)	Servings/Exchanges
Frozen Double Chocolate w/ Coffee	12 oz	440	16	33	10	25	210	69	0	6	4 1/2 carb, 2 1/2 fat
Frozen Double Chocolate w/ Coffee	20 oz	730	26	32	17	35	340	116	0	10	7 1/2 carb, 3 1/2 fat
Frozen Latte	20 oz	740	26	32	21	35	340	114	0	13	7 1/2 carb, 3 1/2 fat
Frozen Latte	16 oz	610	22	32	18	35	280	92	0	10	6 carb, 4 fat
Frozen Latte	12 oz	440	16	33	13	25	210	69	0	8	4 1/2 carb, 2 1/2 fat
Frozen Original Kreme	20 oz	730	24	30	20	35	330	117	0	10	7 1/2 carb, 3 1/2 fat
Frozen Original Kreme	16 oz	600	21	32	17	35	270	95	0	8	6 carb, 4 fat
Frozen Original Kreme	12 oz	440	15	31	12	25	200	70	0	6	4 1/2 carb, 2 1/2 fat
Frozen Raspberry	12 oz	430	13	27	10	25	160	74	0	5	5 carb, 2 fat

Frozen Raspberry	20 oz	710	22	28	17	35	270	123	0	8	8 carb, 3 fat
Frozen Raspberry	16 oz	590	19	29	15	35	230	99	0	6	6 1/2 carb, 2 1/2 fat
GLAZED DOUGHNUTS											
Blueberry	1	330	17	46	4	20	290	43	0	3	3 carb, 2 1/2 fat
Chocolate Cake	1	300	15	45	3.5	5	310	41	2	3	3 carb, 2 fat
Chocolate Iced	1	250	12	43	3	5	100	33	0	3	2 carb, 2 fat
Cinnamon	1	210	12	51	3	5	100	24	0	2	1 1/2 carb, 2 fat
Maple Iced	1	240	12	45	3	5	100	32	0	2	2 carb, 2 fat
Sour Cream	1	340	18	48	4.5	20	310	42	0	3	3 carb, 2 1/2 fat

Starbucks

❖ Starbucks provides nutrition information for most menu items on its Web site at www.starbucks.com.

Light 'n Lean Choice

Raspberry Scone *(1/2)*
Caffe Latte *(12 oz)*

Calories	340	Sodium (mg)	350
Fat (g)	9	Carbohydrate (g)	51
% calories from fat	24	Fiber (g)	1
Saturated fat (g)	4	Protein (g)	16
Cholesterol (mg)	30		

Exchanges: 2 1/2 starch, 1 fat-free milk, 1 fat

Healthy 'n Hearty Choice

Morning Sunrise Muffin
Coffee Frappuccino *(no whipped cream, 12 oz)*

Calories	440	Sodium (mg)	770
Fat (g)	13	Carbohydrate (g)	76
% calories from fat	27	Fiber (g)	4
Saturated fat (g)	5	Protein (g)	12
Cholesterol (mg)	35		

Exchanges: 3 starch, 1 1/2 carb, 2 fat

Starbucks

	Amount	Cal.	Fat (g)	% Cal. Fat	Sat. Fat (g)	Chol. (mg)	Sod. (mg)	Carb. (g)	Fiber (g)	Pro. (g)	Servings/Exchanges
BAGELS											
Cinnamon Raisin	1	440	1	2	0	0	570	96	3	13	6 1/2 starch
Sesame	1	440	3	6	0	0	630	92	6	16	6 starch
BISCOTTI											
Chocolate Hazelnut	1	110	5	41	2	25	80	15	1	2	1 starch, 1 fat
Vanilla Almond	1	110	5	41	1.5	25	75	15	1	2	1 starch, 1 fat
BROWNIES AND BARS											
Caramel Apple Bar	1	310	16	46	8	40	150	38	2	3	2 1/2 carb, 3 fat
Caramel Brownie	1	580	36	56	12	100	230	60	2	5	4 carb, 4 fat
Carrot Cake Bar	1	420	25	54	9	85	440	46	0	4	3 carb, 5 fat

✓ = Healthiest Bets

(Continued)

BROWNIES AND BARS (*Continued*)	Amount	Cal.	Fat (g)	% Cal. Fat	Sat. Fat (g)	Chol. (mg)	Sod. (mg)	Carb. (g)	Fiber (g)	Pro. (g)	Servings/Exchanges
Cranberry Bliss Bar	1	320	18	51	8	30	160	38	0	3	2 1/2 carb, 3 1/2 fat
Enrobed Espresso Brownie	1	430	25	52	16	75	140	48	3	5	3 carb, 5 fat
Espresso Brownie	1	370	21	51	13	85	115	43	2	4	3 carb, 4 fat
Lemon Bar	1	310	14	41	8	140	130	44	0	4	3 carb, 3 fat
Milk Chocolate Peanut Butter Brownie	1	460	29	57	9	50	170	45	2	6	3 carb, 6 fat
Oatmeal Cranberry Mountain	1	430	24	50	13	60	320	49	3	7	3 carb, 5 fat
Oreo Dream Bar	1	420	30	64	15	65	200	33	2	5	2 carb, 6 fat
Pecan Diamond	1	490	37	68	12	40	170	38	2	4	2 1/2 carb, 7 fat
Peppermint Brownie	1	440	27	55	11	55	135	48	2	4	3 carb, 5 1/2 fat
Raspberry Sammy	1	300	14	42	9	35	115	41	1	3	2 1/2 carb, 3 fat
Toffee Cream Cheese Chew	1	440	31	63	10	65	400	38	2	5	2 1/2 carb, 6 fat
Toffee Crunch Bar	1	430	21	44	8	50	420	56	1	4	3 1/2 carb, 4 fat

CAKES											
Apple Harvest Torte	1	350	15	39	3	0	140	53	4	3	3 1/2 carb, 3 fat
Apple Walnut Coffee	1	320	17	48	5	55	330	41	1	4	3 carb, 3 1/2 fat
Banana Pound	1	360	18	45	11	100	380	47	1	4	3 carb, 3 1/2 fat
Banana Pullman	1	400	17	38	5	65	320	57	2	5	4 carb, 3 1/2 fat
Blueberry Walnut Coffee	1	340	18	48	5	60	360	43	1	4	3 carb, 3 1/2 fat
Chocolate Big Baby Bundt	1	330	15	41	7	25	380	45	4	5	3 carb, 3 fat
Chocolate Pullman	1	380	17	40	7	55	270	54	2	5	3 1/2 carb, 3 1/2 fat
Cinnamon Walnut Coffee	1	360	18	45	5	65	390	46	1	4	3 carb, 3 1/2 fat
Classic Coffee	1	570	28	44	10	75	310	75	2	7	5 carb, 5 1/2 fat
Cranberry Walnut Pound	1	390	21	48	9	110	310	45	1	6	3 carb, 4 fat
Cranberry Walnut Pullman	1	360	15	38	4	25	240	53	2	5	3 1/2 carb, 3 fat
Crumb	1	670	32	43	15	115	360	89	1	8	6 carb, 6 fat

✔ = Healthiest Bets

(*Continued*)

CAKES (*Continued*)	Amount	Cal.	Fat (g)	% Cal. Fat	Sat. Fat (g)	Chol. (mg)	Sod. (mg)	Carb. (g)	Fiber (g)	Pro. (g)	Servings/Exchanges
Crumble Berry Coffee	1	520	26	45	10	75	350	69	2	6	4 1/2 carb, 5 fat
Hazelnut Coffee	1	630	35	50	14	125	460	74	2	9	5 carb, 7 fat
Holiday Gingerbread	1	480	16	30	8	100	410	81	1	5	5 carb, 3 fat
Iced Carrot Pound	1	540	13	22	2.5	35	320	101	3	5	6 1/2 carb, 2 1/2 fat
Iced Lemon Pound	1	500	23	41	12	145	390	69	0	6	4 1/2 carb, 4 1/2 fat
Key Lime Crumb	1	550	27	44	10	190	370	71	1	8	4 1/2 carb, 5 1/2 fat
Lemon Glazed Pullman	1	370	15	36	9	90	180	55	0	5	3 1/2 carb, 3 fat
Lemon Yogurt Bundt	1	350	13	33	4.5	55	250	56	0	4	3 1/2 carb, 2 1/2 fat
COOKIES											
Black and White	1	430	17	36	3	50	210	68	2	4	4 1/2 carb, 3 1/2 fat
✓Crisp Cinnamon Twist	1	60	2	30	0.5	0	25	9	0	0	1/2 carb, 1/2 fat
✓Dark Chocolate Graham	1	140	8	51	4.5	4	60	17	0	2	1 carb, 1 1/2 fat

Double Chocolate Chunk	1	430	21	44	7	15	350	58	3	5	3 1/2 carb, 4 fat
Home style Oatmeal Raisin	1	390	15	35	2	15	340	65	3	6	4 carb, 3 fat
✓Madeline	1	80	4	45	1.5	25	30	11	0	1	1 carb, 1/2 fat
✓Milk Chocolate Graham	1	140	8	51	4.5	4	60	17	0	2	1 carb, 1 1/2 fat
✓Shortbread	1	100	6	54	3	15	65	12	0	1	1 carb, 1 fat
White Chocolate Macadamia Nut	1	470	27	52	8	15	350	54	2	6	3 1/2 carb, 5 1/2 fat
CROISSANTS											
Almond Filled Croissant	1	330	18	49	7	30	230	39	2	6	2 1/2 carb, 3 1/2 fat
Butter Croissant w/ Apricot Glaze	1	320	17	48	1.5	25	280	37	1	5	2 1/2 carb, 3 1/2 fat
Cheese Filled Croissant	1	260	12	42	7	30	270	34	1	4	2 carb, 2 1/2 fat
Chocolate Filled Croissant	1	350	19	49	8	30	210	43	2	5	3 carb, 4 fat

✓ = Healthiest Bets

(Continued)

	Amount	Cal.	Fat (g)	% Cal. Fat	Sat. Fat (g)	Chol. (mg)	Sod. (mg)	Carb. (g)	Fiber (g)	Pro. (g)	Servings/Exchanges
DANISH AND ROLLS											
Apple w/ Mocha Swirls	1	370	19	46	1.5	25	330	44	2	5	3 carb, 4 fat
Caramel Pecan Sticky	1	730	40	49	7	40	860	75	7	10	5 carb, 8 fat
Cheese w/ Mocha Swirls	1	460	28	55	7	50	400	44	1	7	3 carb, 5 1/2 fat
Cinnamon	1	620	29	42	7	45	740	80	3	9	5 carb, 6 fat
Cinnamon Flavor Twist	1	320	17	48	1.5	25	280	37	1	5	2 1/2 carb, 3 1/2 fat
Raspberry w/ Mocha Swirls	1	370	19	46	1.5	25	380	45	1	5	3 carb, 4 fat
FRAPPUCCINO BLENDED COFFEES											
Caffe Vanilla w/ no whipped cream	12 oz	160	1	6	0	0	220	34	3	5	2 carb
Caffe Vanilla w/ whipped cream	12 oz	250	10	36	6	40	230	36	3	5	2 carb, 2 fat

✔Coffee Frappuccino w/ no whipped cream	12 oz	110	1	8	0	0	220	22	2	5	1 1/2 carb
Coffee Frappuccino w/ whipped cream	12 oz	200	10	45	6	40	230	23	2	5	1 1/2 carb, 2 fat
✔Mocha Frappuccino w/ no whipped cream	12 oz	140	2	13	0	0	220	28	3	5	2 carb
Mocha Frappuccino w/ whipped cream	12 oz	230	10	39	6	40	230	29	3	5	2 carb, 2 fat
ICED COFFEES											
✔Iced Caffe Americano	12 oz	10	0	0	0	0	10	2	0	1	free
✔Iced Caffe Latte	12 oz	70	0	0	0	4	105	11	0	7	1 milk
✔Iced Caffe Mocha w/ no whipped cream	12 oz	130	2	14	0	4	80	27	1	7	1 1/2 carb

✔ = Healthiest Bets

(Continued)

ICED COFFEES (*Continued*)	Amount	Cal.	Fat (g)	% Cal. Fat	Sat. Fat (g)	Chol. (mg)	Sod. (mg)	Carb. (g)	Fiber (g)	Pro. (g)	Servings/Exchanges
Iced Caffe Mocha w/ whipped cream	12 oz	230	10	39	6	40	85	28	1	7	2 carb, 2 fat
✓Iced Syrup Flavored Latte	12 oz	120	0	0	0	0	90	24	0	6	1 1/2 carb
✓Iced Vanilla Latte	12 oz	120	0	0	0	0	90	24	0	6	1/2 carb, 1 milk
Iced White Chocolate Mocha w/ whipped cream	12 oz	330	13	35	9	40	170	44	0	9	3 carb, 2 1/2 fat
Iced White Chocolate Mocha w/ no whipped cream	12 oz	240	4	15	3.5	4	170	42	0	9	3 carb, 1 fat
MUFFINS											
Blueberry	1	380	19	45	3.5	70	380	49	1	5	3 carb, 4 fat
Chocolate Cream Cheese	1	450	24	48	6	80	420	53	1	5	3 1/2 carb, 5 fat
Cranberry Orange	1	410	20	44	4	70	400	53	2	5	3 1/2 carb, 4 fat
Morning Sunrise	1	330	12	33	5	35	550	54	2	5	3 1/2 carb, 2 1/2 fat

SCONES											
Apricot Currant	1	450	17	34	8	60	360	67	3	7	3 1/2 carb, 3 1/2 fat
Blueberry	1	460	18	35	8	50	400	68	3	5	4 1/2 carb, 3 1/2 fat
Butterscotch Pecan	1	520	27	47	11	50	390	64	2	7	4 carb, 5 1/2 fat
Cinnamon Chip w/ Icing	1	510	23	41	10	50	480	71	2	6	4 1/2 carb, 4 1/2 fat
Maple Oat w/ Icing	1	490	22	40	9	45	430	69	2	7	4 1/2 carb, 4 1/2 fat
Raspberry	1	440	18	37	8	50	360	65	2	7	4 carb, 3 1/2 fat
SPECIALTY BEVERAGES											
Caramel Apple Cider w/ no whipped cream	12 oz	230	0	0	0	0	15	55	0	0	3 1/2 carb
Caramel Apple Cider w/ whipped cream	12 oz	320	8	23	5	35	25	59	0	0	4 carb, 1 1/2 fat
Hot Chocolate w/ no whipped cream	12 oz	190	2	9	0	5	170	35	1	13	1 1/2 carb, 1 milk

✓ = Healthiest Bets

(*Continued*)

SPECIALTY BEVERAGES (*Continued*)	Amount	Cal.	Fat (g)	% Cal. Fat	Sat. Fat (g)	Chol. (mg)	Sod. (mg)	Carb. (g)	Fiber (g)	Pro. (g)	Servings/Exchanges
Hot Chocolate w/ whipped cream	12 oz	270	9	30	5	35	170	36	1	13	1 1/2 carb, 1 milk, 2 fat
Pumpkin Spice Crème w/ no whipped cream	12 oz	220	0	0	0	5	220	40	0	13	1 1/2 carb, 1 milk
Pumpkin Spice Crème w/ whipped cream	12 oz	300	8	24	5	40	220	42	0	13	1 1/2 carb, 1 milk, 1 1/2 fat
Steamed Apple Cider	12 oz	180	0	0	0	0	15	45	0	0	3 carb
Vanilla Crème w/ no whipped cream	12 oz	180	0	0	0	4	170	32	0	11	1 carb, 1 milk
Vanilla Crème w/ whipped cream	12 oz	260	8	28	5	35	170	33	0	11	1 carb, 1 milk, 1 1/2 fat
White Hot Chocolate w/ no whipped cream	12 oz	300	5	15	3.5	10	250	51	0	15	2 1/2 carb, 1 milk, 1/2 fat

White Hot Chocolate w/ whipped cream	12 oz	380	12	28	8	40	260	52	0	15	2 1/2 carb, 1 milk, 2 1/2 fat
SPECIALTY COFFEES											
✓Café Mistro/Café Au Lait	12 oz	60	0	0	0	4	90	9	0	6	1 milk
✓Caffe Americano	12 oz	10	0	0	0	0	0	2	0	1	free
✓Caffe Latte	12 oz	120	0	0	0	5	170	18	0	12	1 1/2 milk
Caffe Mocha w/ whipped cream	12 oz	260	9	31	5	35	140	34	1	11	1 1/2 carb, 1 milk, 2 fat
Caffe Mocha w/ no whipped cream	12 oz	170	2	11	0	5	135	33	1	11	1 1/2 carb, 1 milk
✓Cappuccino	12 oz	80	0	0	0	4	100	11	0	7	1 milk
Caramel Mocha w/ no whipped cream	12 oz	230	2	8	0	5	125	48	1	11	2 1/2 carb, 1 milk
Caramel Mocha w/ whipped cream	12 oz	320	9	25	5	35	130	49	1	11	2 1/2 carb, 1 milk, 2 fat

✓ = Healthiest Bets

(*Continued*)

SPECIALTY COFFEES (*Continued*)	Amount	Cal.	Fat (g)	% Cal. Fat	Sat. Fat (g)	Chol. (mg)	Sod. (mg)	Carb. (g)	Fiber (g)	Pro. (g)	Servings/Exchanges
Syrup Flavored Latte	12 oz	170	0	0	0	4	150	31	0	11	1 carb, 1 milk
Toffee Nut Latte w/ no whipped cream	12 oz	180	0	0	0	5	270	32	0	11	1 carb, 1 milk
Toffee Nut Latte w/ whipped cream	12 oz	270	8	27	5	40	280	35	0	11	1 carb, 1 milk, 1 1/2 fat
Vanilla Latte	12 oz	170	0	0	0	4	150	31	0	11	1 carb, 1 milk
White Chocolate Mocha w/ no whipped cream	12 oz	260	4	14	3	5	210	45	0	12	2 carb, 1 milk, 1 fat
White Chocolate Mocha w/ whipped cream	12 oz	340	11	29	8	40	220	46	0	12	2 carb, 1 milk, 2 fat

Tim Hortons

❖ Tim Hortons provides nutrition information for all its menu items on its Web site at www.timhortons.com.

Light 'n Lean Choice

Multigrain Bagel
1/2 Package Light Plain Cream Cheese *(1 1/2 T)*

Calories	345	Sodium (mg)	755
Fat (g)	7	Carbohydrate (g)	60
% calories from fat	18	Fiber (g)	6
Saturated fat (g)	3	Protein (g)	14
Cholesterol (mg)	10		

Exchanges: 4 starch, 1 fat

Healthy 'n Hearty Choice

Minestrone Soup *(10 oz)*
Chicken and Roasted Red Peppers Sandwich

Calories	462	Sodium (mg)	1,775
Fat (g)	6	Carbohydrate (g)	78
% calories from fat	12	Fiber (g)	5
Saturated fat (g)	1.5	Protein (g)	26
Cholesterol (mg)	30		

Exchanges: 4 1/2 starch, 1 veg, 2 lean meat

(*Continued*)

Tim Hortons

	Amount	Cal.	Fat (g)	% Cal. Fat	Sat. Fat (g)	Chol. (mg)	Sod. (mg)	Carb. (g)	Fiber (g)	Pro. (g)	Servings/Exchanges
BAGELS											
✓Blueberry	1	300	2	6	0	0	520	59	3	11	4 starch
✓Cinnamon Raisin	1	300	2	6	0	0	390	58	4	11	4 starch
✓Everything	1	300	2	6	0	0	560	57	3	12	4 starch
✓Multigrain	1	300	3	9	0	0	655	58	6	12	4 starch
✓Onion	1	295	2	6	0	0	530	58	3	11	4 starch
✓Plain	1	290	2	6	0	0	600	57	3	11	4 starch
✓Poppy Seed	1	300	3	9	0	0	500	58	4	11	4 starch
✓Sesame Seed	1	300	3	9	0	0	570	57	4	11	4 starch
✓Whole Wheat & Honey	1	300	2	6	0	0	590	59	6	11	4 starch

BAKED GOODS											
Butter Croissant	1	330	19	52	5	0	270	36	2	6	2 1/2 starch, 4 fat
Cheese Croissant	1	360	22	55	7	15	340	34	2	9	2 starch, 4 1/2 fat
Cherry Cheese Danish	1	320	14	39	4.5	15	200	43	0	5	3 carb, 3 fat
Maple Pecan Danish	1	380	20	47	3.5	10	450	48	1	4	3 carb, 4 fat
✓Plain Tea Biscuit	1	220	6	25	2	0	590	36	1	5	2 1/2 starch, 1 fat
✓Raisin Tea Biscuit	1	230	6	23	2	0	630	36	1	5	2 1/2 starch, 1 fat
Southern Country Raspberry Biscuit	1	470	19	36	5	0	1050	68	2	7	4 1/2 starch, 4 fat
BEVERAGES											
Café Mocha	10 oz	150	6	36	4.5	0	135	23	1	1	1 1/2 carb, 1 fat
French Vanilla Cappuccino	10 oz	240	9	34	1.5	0	210	39	0	4	2 1/2 carb, 2 fat
Fruit Punch	10 oz	150	0	0	0	0	10	38	0	0	2 1/2 carb

✓ = Healthiest Bets

(*Continued*)

BEVERAGES (Continued)	Amount	Cal.	Fat (g)	% Cal. Fat	Sat. Fat (g)	Chol. (mg)	Sod. (mg)	Carb. (g)	Fiber (g)	Pro. (g)	Servings/Exchanges
Hot Chocolate	10 oz	220	6	25	2	0	350	44	0	2	3 carb, 1 fat
Iced Cappuccino	12 oz	300	14	42	9	55	55	39	0	3	2 1/2 carb, 3 fat
Peach Drink	12 oz	140	0	0	0	0	47	37	0	0	2 1/2 carb
COOKIES											
✓Chocolate Chip	1	155	7	41	2.5	21	140	21	1	2	2 1/2 carb, 1 1/2 fat
✓Double Chocolate Fudge	1	160	7	39	3	15	140	22	1	2	1 1/2 carb, 1 1/2 fat
✓M&M w/ Chocolate Chips	1	160	7	39	2.5	5	125	21	0	1	1 1/2 carb, 1 1/2 fat
✓Oatmeal Raisin	1	150	6	36	1.5	15	140	33	2	2	2 carb, 1 fat
✓Peanut Butter	1	165	9	49	3	20	190	18	1	3	1 carb, 2 fat
✓Peanut Butter Chocolate Chunk	1	170	9	48	3	15	150	19	1	3	1 carb, 2 fat

CREAM CHEESE											
Garden Vegetable Light	3 T	90	6	60	3.5	20	160	4	0	3	1 1/2 fat
Plain	3 T	140	14	90	10	45	140	1	0	3	3 fat
Plain Light	3 T	90	7	70	5	20	200	3	0	4	2 fat
Strawberry	3 T	150	12	72	8	35	150	7	0	1	1/2 carb, 1 1/2 fat
DONUTS											
Angel Cream	1	300	12	36	3.5	0	270	45	1	5	3 carb, 2 1/2 fat
✓Apple Fritter	1	310	9	26	2	0	280	50	2	6	3 1/2 carb, 2 fat
✓Blueberry	1	220	5	20	1.5	0	250	37	1	4	2 1/2 carb, 1 fat
✓Boston Cream	1	220	6	25	1.5	0	280	37	1	4	2 1/2 carb, 1 fat
✓Canadian Maple	1	240	6	23	1.5	0	300	41	1	4	3 carb, 1 fat
✓Chocolate Dip	1	200	7	32	1.5	0	230	30	1	4	2 carb, 1 1/2 fat

✓ = Healthiest Bets

(Continued)

DONUTS (Continued)	Amount	Cal.	Fat (g)	% Cal. Fat	Sat. Fat (g)	Chol. (mg)	Sod. (mg)	Carb. (g)	Fiber (g)	Pro. (g)	Servings/Exchanges
✔Chocolate Glazed	1	240	8	30	1.5	5	360	40	2	4	3 carb, 1 1/2 fat
✔Dutchie	1	230	6	23	1.5	0	230	40	2	4	3 carb, 1 fat
✔Honey Dip	1	200	6	27	1.5	0	230	33	1	4	2 carb, 1 fat
Honey Stick	1	280	13	42	2.5	20	290	38	1	3	2 1/2 carb, 2 1/2 fat
✔Maple Dip	1	200	7	32	1.5	0	230	31	1	4	2 carb, 1 1/2 fat
✔Old Fashion Glazed	1	240	7	26	1.5	10	280	42	1	3	3 carb, 1 1/2 fat
✔Old Fashion Plain	1	180	7	35	1.5	10	280	27	1	3	2 carb, 1 1/2 fat
Sour Cream Plain	1	250	15	54	3.5	10	190	27	1	3	2 carb, 3 fat
✔Strawberry	1	210	5	21	1.5	0	290	36	1	4	2 1/2 carb, 1 fat
✔Sugar Twist	1	210	7	30	1.5	0	260	34	1	5	2 carb, 1 1/2 fat
Walnut Crunch	1	350	20	51	4.5	5	350	39	1	4	2 1/2 carb, 4 fat

MUFFINS											
Blueberry	1	340	11	29	2	25	460	55	3	5	3 1/2 starch, 2 fat
Blueberry Bran	1	350	12	31	2	10	710	54	6	5	3 1/2 starch, 2 1/2 fat
Carrot Whole Wheat	1	440	23	47	3.5	25	560	52	4	5	3 1/2 starch, 4 1/2 fat
Chocolate Chip Plain	1	440	16	33	5	15	410	68	3	6	4 1/2 starch, 3 fat
Cranberry Blueberry Bran	1	340	12	32	2	10	700	53	6	5	3 1/2 starch, 2 1/2 fat
Cranberry Fruit	1	360	12	30	2.5	25	460	59	3	5	4 starch, 2 1/2 fat
Fruit Explosion	1	360	11	28	2	25	460	61	3	5	4 starch, 2 fat
Low Fat Blueberry	1	300	2	6	0	0	690	65	7	5	4 starch
Raisin Bran	1	390	12	28	2	10	630	65	5	5	4 starch, 2 1/2 fat
Strawberry Sensation	1	380	12	28	2.5	25	460	61	3	5	4 starch, 2 1/2 fat
SOUP AND CHILI											
Beef Noodle	10 oz	135	2	13%	0.5	15	979	23	1	7	1 1/2 starch

✔ = Healthiest Bets

(Continued)

SOUP AND CHILI (Continued)	Amount	Cal.	Fat (g)	% Cal. Fat	Sat. Fat (g)	Chol. (mg)	Sod. (mg)	Carb. (g)	Fiber (g)	Pro. (g)	Servings/Exchanges
✓Cauliflower & Cheese	10 oz	180	8	40	3.5	0	847	24	1	3	1 1/2 starch, 1 1/2 fat
✓Chicken Gumbo	10 oz	125	2	14	1	5	868	24	1	4	1 1/2 starch
Chicken Stew	10 oz	240	13	49	3	40	970	14	0	15	1 starch, 1 lean meat, 2 fat
Chili	10 oz	300	16	48	6	50	920	18	5	21	1 starch, 2 high-fat meat
✓Clam Chowder	10 oz	184	4	20	2	5	970	31	1	5	1 starch, 1 milk, 1/2 fat
Cream Broccoli	10 oz	191	7	33	3.5	5	1086	30	1	3	2 starch, 1 1/2 fat
✓Cream of Asparagus	10 oz	175	7	36	3	0	749	25	1	3	1 1/2 starch, 1 1/2 fat
✓Cream of Mushroom	10 oz	185	9	44	3.5	0	814	23	1	2	1 1/2 starch, 2 fat
✓Cream of Turkey Vegetable	10 oz	156	6	35	3	5	953	22	1	3	1 1/2 starch, 1 fat
✓Hearty Vegetable	10 oz	123	1	7	0	0	963	27	2	3	1 1/2 starch, 1 veg
Italian Florentine	10 oz	163	4	22	1.5	10	1033	26	1	5	1 1/2 starch, 1 fat

✓Minestrone	10 oz	122	2	15	0.5	0	775	24	2	4	1 1/2 starch
Potato Bacon	10 oz	182	6	30	2.5	0	1005	29	1	3	2 starch, 1 fat
✓Split Pea w/ Ham	10 oz	149	3	18	0.5	0	949	27	5	6	2 starch, 1/2 fat
✓'Tim's Own' Chicken Noodle	10 oz	114	3	24	1	15	806	18	1	4	1 starch, 1 fat
Tomato Florentine	10 oz	97	2	19	0.5	10	1262	18	1	3	1 starch, 1/2 fat
Tomato Parmesan	10 oz	220	6	25	4	0	1770	40	1	2	2 1/2 starch, 1 fat
✓Turkey & Wild Rice	10 oz	123	2	15	0.5	0	983	24	1	3	1 1/2 starch
✓Vegetable Beef Barley	10 oz	113	2	16	0.5	5	967	21	2	5	1 1/2 starch
TIMBITS											
✓Banana Cream	1	60	2	30	0	0	65	9	0	1	1/2 carb, 1/2 fat
✓Blueberry	1	60	2	30	0	0	55	11	0	1	1/2 carb, 1/2 fat
✓Chocolate Glazed	1	60	2	30	0	0	100	10	0	1	1/2 carb, 1/2 fat

✓ = Healthiest Bets

(Continued)

TIMBITS (Continued)	Amount	Cal.	Fat (g)	% Cal. Fat	Sat. Fat (g)	Chol. (mg)	Sod. (mg)	Carb. (g)	Fiber (g)	Pro. (g)	Servings/Exchanges
✓Dutchie	1	50	2	36	0	0	50	10	0	1	1/2 carb, 1/2 fat
✓Honey Dip	1	60	2	30	0	0	50	10	0	1	1/2 carb, 1/2 fat
✓Lemon	1	60	2	30	0	0	55	11	0	1	1/2 carb, 1/2 fat
✓Old Fashion Plain	1	50	2	36	0	0	80	8	0	1	1/2 carb, 1/2 fat
✓Strawberry	1	60	2	30	0	0	70	10	0	1	1/2 carb, 1/2 fat
"TIM'S OWN" SANDWICHES											
Albacore Tuna Salad	1	450	19	38	3	45	1050	50	3	21	3 1/2 starch, 2 lean meat, 2 fat
B.L.T.	1	490	24	44	6	35	800	50	2	17	3 1/2 starch, 1 high-fat meat, 3 fat
Black Forest Ham & Swiss w/ honey mustard	1	420	8	17	4	40	1760	61	2	25	4 starch, 2 lean meat

Black Forest Ham & Swiss w/ Tim's Own Dressing	1	420	12	26	4.5	45	1920	55	2	25	3 1/2 starch, 2 lean meat
Chicken & Roasted Red Pepper	1	340	4	11	1	30	1000	54	3	22	3 1/2 starch, 2 lean meat
Chunky Chicken Salad	1	490	23	42	4	65	710	49	3	23	3 starch, 2 lean meat, 3 fat
✓Egg Salad	1	450	20	40	4	265	740	48	2	16	3 starch, 1 medium-fat meat, 3 fat
✓Garden Vegetable	1	340	8	21	4	20	680	58	3	13	3 1/2 starch, 1 lean meat, 1/2 fat
Harvest Turkey Breast	1	350	5	13	1	25	1620	54	2	22	3 1/2 starch, 1 medium-fat meat
Turkey Bacon Club	1	440	8	16	2.5	25	1730	63	2	30	4 starch, 2 lean meat, 1/2 fat

✓ = Healthiest Bets

Burgers, Fries, and More

RESTAURANTS

Burger King
Carl's Jr.
Dairy Queen/Brazier
Hardee's
Jack in the Box
McDonald's
Sonic, America's Drive-In
Wendy's

NUTRITION PROS

- Small portions are plentiful as long as you know and use the right words, such as regular, small, junior, and single.
- There's no waiting for food. You order and then eat.
- No foods greet you at the table. What you order is what you eat. This puts you in the driver's seat.
- You can get a few grams of fiber from multigrain buns and baked potatoes. Granted, they aren't available often.
- It's easy to add to your five-a-day (fruits and vegetables) with an entrée or a side salad. Because of health concerns, these restaurants have added several entrée salads. Be careful to limit the addition of high-fat toppings, such as cheese, fried chicken, fried noodles, and nuts. Also pour the salad dressing gingerly.

- Salad dressing is served on the side. There's no need for a special request.
- More fruits and vegetables are creeping into menus in response to health concerns—baby carrots, apple slices, and more.
- Healthier cold drinks flow freely: low-fat (1%) or fat-free milk, fruit juice, water, unsweetened ice tea, diet soft drinks.
- Low-fat and low-calorie or fat-free salad dressings are now common. Keep in mind that these salad dressings are not calorie free. They can also be high in sodium.
- Healthier dessert options include low-fat frozen yogurt in a cone or dish or low-fat milkshakes.
- Honesty is their policy. Full disclosure of nutrition information is there for the asking.
- You know the menu well. You can plan what to order before you walk in the door.

NUTRITION CONS

- Many menu items are high in fat. Cheese, cheese sauce, bacon, special sauce, and mayonnaise add fat.
- Large portions are all too frequent: large, jumbo, double, and triple are a few words to watch out for.
- Sodium can skyrocket from the salt on french fries, in special sauces, and in salad dressings.
- Chicken and fish start off healthy, but they are often buried in a crisp, golden, high-fat coating.

Healthy Tips

★ Zero in on the words regular, junior, small, or single. These mean small portions.
★ Try lower-calorie ketchup, mustard, or barbecue sauce as an option to higher-fat mayonnaise or special sauce.
★ Walk in rather than drive through. If you eat and drive, you hardly realize food has passed your lips.
★ Order less food to start. Remember, you can go back and get more in a flash.
★ Want fries? Go ahead, but split a small or medium order.

- Some of the salad toppings and salad dressings can undo the healthiness of entrée salads.
- Biscuits are loaded with fat to begin with. Tuck sausage, bacon, egg, and/or cheese in the middle and you've just downed your fat grams for the day in one fell swoop.
- Fruit is hard to find.
- French fries or onion rings—deep fried of course—are still the traditional side.
- The meal deals can push you to eat larger portions because you can buy more food for less. Don't get caught up in this unhealthy mentality.

Get It Your Way

★ Avoid the busy times. This way you'll get your food your way with a smile on the order taker's face.

★ Be ready to wait. Fast-food restaurants are not set up for special requests.

★ Ask for simple changes: leave off the special sauce or mayonnaise; hold the pickles, bacon, or cheese; or hold the salt on the french fries.

Burger King

❖ Burger King provides nutrition information for all its menu items on its Web site at www.burgerking.com.

Light 'n Lean Choice

Chili
Fire-Grilled Chicken Caesar Salad
Tomato Balsamic Vinaigrette *(1/2 serving, 2 T)*

Calories	435	Sodium (mg)	2320
Fat (g)	20	Carbohydrate (g)	31
% calories from fat	41	Fiber (g)	6
Saturated fat (g)	6.5	Protein (g)	38
Cholesterol (mg)	74		

Exchanges: 1 starch, 2 veg, 4 lean meat, 2 fat

Healthy 'n Hearty Choice

Kids Meal
Cheeseburger
French Fries *(small)*
Strawberry Applesauce

Calories	670	Sodium (mg)	1010
Fat (g)	8	Carbohydrate (g)	83
% calories from fat	38	Fiber (g)	3
Saturated fat (g)	11	Protein (g)	22
Cholesterol (mg)	50		

Exchanges: 4 1/2 starch, 1 fruit, 2 medium-fat meat, 2 fat

(*Continued*)

Burger King

	Amount	Cal.	Fat (g)	% Cal. Fat	Sat. Fat (g)	Chol. (mg)	Sod. (mg)	Carb. (g)	Fiber (g)	Pro. (g)	Servings/Exchanges
BREAKFAST											
Croissan'wich w/ Bacon, Egg & Cheese	1	360	22	55	8	195	950	25	0	15	1 1/2 starch, 2 medium-fat meat, 2 fat
✓Croissan'wich w/ Egg & Cheese	1	320	19	53	7	185	730	24	0	12	1 1/2 starch, 1 medium-fat meat, 3 fat
Croissan'wich w/ Ham, Egg & Cheese	1	360	20	50	8	200	1500	25	0	18	1 1/2 starch, 2 medium-fat meat, 2 fat
Croissan'wich w/ Sausage and Cheese	1	420	31	66	11	45	840	23	0	14	1 1/2 starch, 2 high-fat meat, 5 fat
Croissan'wich w/ Sausage, Egg & Cheese	1	520	39	68	14	210	1090	24	1	19	1 1/2 starch, 2 high-fat meat, 5 fat

Double Croissan'wich w/ Bacon, Egg & Cheese	1	430	26	54	11	220	1360	27	0	19	1 1/2 starch, 2 medium-fat, 2 fat
Double Croissan'wich w/ Ham, Bacon, Egg & Cheese	1	420	25	54	10	225	1910	27	0	23	1 1/2 starch, 2 medium-fat meat, 2 fat
Double Croissan'wich w/ Ham, Egg & Cheese	1	420	23	49	9	235	2450	27	0	26	1 1/2 starch, 2 medium-fat meat, 2 fat
Double Croissan'wich w/ Ham, Sausage, Egg & Cheese	1	580	41	64	15	245	2040	27	1	27	1 1/2 starch, 2 medium-fat meat, 2 fat
Double Croissan'wich w/ Sausage, Bacon, Egg & Cheese	1	590	43	66	16	240	1490	27	1	24	1 1/2 starch, 2 medium-fat meat, 2 fat
Double Croissan'wich w/ Sausage, Egg & Cheese	1	750	60	72	21	260	1630	26	2	28	1 1/2 starch, 2 medium-fat meat, 2 fat

✓ = Healthiest Bets

(*Continued*)

BREAKFAST (*Continued*)	Amount	Cal.	Fat (g)	% Cal. Fat	Sat. Fat (g)	Chol. (mg)	Sod. (mg)	Carb. (g)	Fiber (g)	Pro. (g)	Servings/Exchanges
French Toast Sticks	5 sticks	390	20	46	4.5	0	440	46	2	6	3 starch, 3 1/2 fat
Hash Brown Rounds, large	1 serving	390	25	58	7	0	760	38	4	3	2 1/2 starch, 4 fat
Hash Brown Rounds, small	1 serving	230	15	59	4	0	450	23	2	2	1 1/2 starch, 3 fat
BURGERS											
Bacon Cheeseburger	1	390	20	46	9	60	990	31	1	22	2 starch, 2 medium-fat meat, 2 fat
Bacon Double Cheeseburger	1	570	34	54	17	110	1250	32	2	35	2 starch, 4 medium-fat meat, 3 fat
BK Veggie Burger w/out mayo	1	300	7	21	1.5	0	870	46	4	14	3 starch, 1 lean meat, 1/2 fat
✓Cheeseburger	1	350	17	44	8	50	770	31	1	19	2 starch, 2 medium-fat meat, 1 fat

Double Cheeseburger	1	530	31	53	15	100	1030	32	2	32	2 starch, 4 medium-fat meat, 1 1/2 fat
Double Hamburger	1	440	23	47	10	75	600	30	1	28	2 starch, 3 medium-fat meat, 1 1/2 fat
✓Hamburger	1	310	13	38	5	40	550	30	1	17	2 starch, 2 medium-fat meat, 1/2 fat
Original Whopper w/out mayo	1	540	24	40	10	75	900	52	4	30	3 1/2 starch, 3 medium-fat meat, 1 1/2 fat
Original Double Whopper w/ cheese w/out mayo	1	900	51	51	24	170	1410	53	4	56	3 1/2 starch, 4 high-fat meat, 1 fat
Original Double Whopper w/out mayo	1	810	44	49	19	150	980	52	4	52	3 1/2 starch, 6 medium-fat meat, 3 fat
✓Original Whopper Jr. w/ cheese w/out mayo	1	350	17	44	8	50	700	32	2	19	2 starch, 2 medium-fat meat, 1 fat
✓Original Whopper Jr. w/out mayo	1	310	13	38	5	40	490	31	2	17	2 starch, 2 medium-fat meat, 1/2 fat

✓ = Healthiest Bets

(*Continued*)

BURGERS (*Continued*)	Amount	Cal.	Fat (g)	% Cal. Fat	Sat. Fat (g)	Chol. (mg)	Sod. (mg)	Carb. (g)	Fiber (g)	Pro. (g)	Servings/Exchanges
Original Whopper w/ cheese w/out mayo	1	640	31	44	15	95	1330	53	4	35	3 1/2 starch, 4 medium-fat meat, 1 1/2 fat
The Angus Bacon and Cheese	1	710	33	42	15	215	1990	64	3	41	4 starch, 4 medium-fat meat, 4 fat
The Angus Steak Burger	1	570	22	35	8	180	1270	62	3	33	4 starch, 3 medium-fat meat, 1 1/2 fat
CHICKEN & FISH											
✓BK Fish Fillet Sandwich w/out mayo	1	360	13	33	5	40	700	42	2	18	3 starch, 2 lean meat, 1/2 fat
✓Chicken Tenders	4 pieces	170	9	48	2.5	25	420	10	0	11	1/2 starch, 1 lean meat, 2 fat
✓Chicken Tenders	6 pieces	250	14	50	4	35	630	15	0	16	1 starch, 2 lean meat, 1 1/2 fat

Chicken Tenders	8 pieces	340	19	50	5	50	840	20	0	22	1 starch, 3 lean meat, 2 fat
✓Chicken Tenders	5 pieces	210	12	51	3.5	30	530	13	0	14	1 starch, 2 lean meat, 1/2 fat
Chicken Whopper Sandwich on small bun w/out mayo	1	320	7	20	1.5	60	1130	31	3	35	2 starch, 4 lean meat
Chicken Whopper Sandwich w/out mayo	1	410	7	15	2	60	1280	48	4	38	3 starch, 4 lean meat
Original Chicken Sandwich w/out mayo	1	460	17	33	4.5	55	1190	52	3	25	3 1/2 starch, 2 lean meat, 2 fat
Tender Crisp Chicken Sandwich w/out mayo	1	570	21	33	3.5	40	1540	70	6	26	4 1/2 starch, 2 lean meat, 3 fat
DESSERTS											
Dutch Apple Pie	1	340	14	37	3	0	470	52	1	2	3 carb, 3 fat
Hershey's Sundae Pie	1	300	18	54	10	10	190	31	1	3	2 carb, 3 1/2 fat

✓ = Healthiest Bets

(*Continued*)

DESSERTS (*Continued*)	Amount	Cal.	Fat (g)	% Cal. Fat	Sat. Fat (g)	Chol. (mg)	Sod. (mg)	Carb. (g)	Fiber (g)	Pro. (g)	Servings/Exchanges
Nestle Toll House Chocolate Chip Cookies	2	440	16	33	5	20	360	68	0	5	4 1/2 carb, 3 fat
DIPPING SAUCES											
Barbeque	2 T	35	0	0	0	0	390	9	0	0	1/2 carb
Honey Flavor	2 T	90	0	0	0	0	0	23	0	0	1 1/2 carb
Honey Mustard	2 T	90	6	60	1	10	150	9	0	0	1/2 carb
Ranch	2 T	140	15	96	2.5	5	95	1	0	1	3 fat
✓Sweet and Sour	2 T	40	0	0	0	0	65	10	0	0	1/2 carb
Zesty Onion	2 T	150	15	90	2.5	15	210	3	0	0	3 fat
MILK SHAKES											
Chocolate	small	410	13	29	8	50	300	65	0	7	4 carb, 2 1/2 fat
Chocolate	large	850	27	29	17	105	620	133	2	15	9 carb, 5 1/2 fat

Chocolate	medium	600	18	27	11	70	470	97	2	10	6 1/2 carb, 3 1/2 fat
Strawberry	small	410	13	29	8	50	220	64	0	7	4 carb, 2 1/2 fat
Strawberry	medium	590	17	26	11	70	300	96	0	9	6 1/2 carb, 3 1/2 fat
Strawberry	large	840	26	28	17	105	450	131	0	14	9 carb, 5 fat
Vanilla	large	800	29	33	19	120	480	113	0	16	7 1/2 carb, 6 fat
Vanilla	medium	540	20	33	13	80	320	76	0	11	5 carb, 4 fat
Vanilla	small	400	15	34	9	60	240	57	0	8	3 1/2 carb, 3 fat
SALAD DRESSINGS & TOPPINGS											
Creamy Garlic Caesar	4 T	130	11	76	2	20	710	7	0	2	1/2 starch, 2 fat
Fat Free Honey Mustard	4 T	70	0	0	0	0	230	18	0	0	1 starch
Garden Ranch	4 T	120	10	75	1.5	20	610	7	0	0	1/2 starch, 2 fat
Garlic Parmesan Toast	1 serving	70	3	39	0	0	120	9	0	2	1/2 starch, 1/2 fat
✔Hidden Valley Fat Free Ranch	3 T	35	0	0	0	0	370	7	0	0	1/2 starch

✔ = Healthiest Bets

(*Continued*)

SALAD DRESSINGS & TOPPINGS (*Continued*)	Amount	Cal.	Fat (g)	% Cal. Fat	Sat. Fat (g)	Chol. (mg)	Sod. (mg)	Carb. (g)	Fiber (g)	Pro. (g)	Servings/Exchanges
Sweet Onion Vinaigrette	4 T	100	8	72	1	0	960	8	0	0	1/2 starch, 1 1/2 fat
Tomato Balsamic Vinaigrette	4 T	110	9	74	1	0	760	9	0	0	1/2 starch, 1 fat
SALADS											
✓Fire-Grilled Chicken Caesar Salad w/out dressing or toast	1	190	7	33	3	50	900	9	1	25	1/2 carb, 3 lean meat
✓Fire-Grilled Chicken Garden Salad w/out dressing or toast	1	210	7	30	3	50	910	12	2	26	1 starch, 3 lean meat, 1 fat
✓Fire-Grilled Shrimp Caesar Salad w/out dressing or toast	1	180	10	50	3	120	880	9	2	20	1/2 starch, 3 lean meat

✔Fire-Grilled Shrimp Garden Salad w/out dressing or toast	1	200	10	45	3	120	900	13	3	21	1 starch, 3 lean meat
✔Side Garden Salad w/out dressing or toast	1	20	0	0	0	0	15	4	0	1	1 veg
Tender Crisp Caesar Salad w/out dressing or toast	1	390	22	51	5	40	1160	25	4	24	1/2 starch, 3 lean meat
Tender Crisp Garden Salad w/out dressing or toast	1	410	22	48	5	40	1170	28	5	25	1/2 starch, 3 lean meat
SIDE ORDERS											
Bacon for Whopper Sandwiches	4 strips	50	4	72	1.5	10	290	0	0	4	1 fat

✔ = Healthiest Bets

(*Continued*)

SIDE ORDERS (*Continued*)	Amount	Cal.	Fat (g)	% Cal. Fat	Sat. Fat (g)	Chol. (mg)	Sod. (mg)	Carb. (g)	Fiber (g)	Pro. (g)	Servings/Exchanges
Bacon for Whopper Sandwiches	3 strips	40	3	68	1	10	210	0	0	3	1 fat
Chili	1 order	190	8	38	3	25	1040	17	5	13	1 starch, 2 lean meat
French Fries, king salted	1 order	600	30	45	8	0	1070	76	6	7	5 starch, 6 fat
French Fries, king unsalted	1 order	600	30	45	8	0	620	76	6	7	5 starch, 6 fat
French Fries, large salted	1 order	500	25	45	7	0	880	63	5	6	4 starch, 5 fat
French Fries, large unsalted	1 order	500	25	45	7	0	510	63	5	6	4 starch, 5 fat
French Fries, medium salted	1 order	360	18	45	5	0	640	46	4	4	3 starch, 3 1/2 fat
French Fries, medium unsalted	1 order	360	18	45	5	0	380	46	4	4	3 starch, 3 1/2 fat

French Fries, small salted	1 order	230	11	43	3	0	410	29	2	3	2 starch, 2 fat
French Fries, small unsalted	1 order	230	11	43	3	0	240	29	2	3	2 starch, 2 fat
Mott's Strawberry Flavored Apple Sauce	4 oz	90	0	0	0	0	0	23	0	0	1 1/2 fruit
Onion Rings, king	1 order	550	27	44	7	5	800	70	5	8	4 1/2 starch, 5 1/2 fat
Onion Rings, large	1 order	480	23	43	6	0	690	60	5	7	4 starch, 4 1/2 fat
Onion Rings, medium	1 order	320	16	45	4	0	460	40	3	4	2 1/2 starch, 3 fat
✓Onion Rings, small	1 order	180	9	45	2	0	260	22	2	2	1 1/2 starch, 2 fat
Shredded Cheddar Cheese	1 order	90	7	70	4.5	20	130	0	0	5	1 high-fat meat

✓ = Healthiest Bets

Carl's Jr.

❖ Carl's Jr. provides nutrition information for all its menu items on its Web site at www.carlsjr.com.

Light 'n Lean Choice

Charbroiled BBQ Chicken Sandwich
Garden Salad-To-Go
Fat-Free French Salad Dressing *(2 T)*

Calories	550	Sodium (mg)	1,640
Fat (g)	7	Carbohydrate (g)	60
% calories from fat	11	Fiber (g)	6
Saturated fat (g)	3	Protein (g)	38
Cholesterol (mg)	65		

Exchanges: 4 starch, 1 veg, 4 lean meat

Healthy 'n Hearty Choice

Hamburger
French Fries *(medium, 1/2 serving)*
Garden Salad-to-Go
House Dressing *(2 T, 1/2 serving)*

Calories	740	Sodium (mg)	1070
Fat (g)	34	Carbohydrate (g)	73
% calories from fat	41	Fiber (g)	6
Saturated fat (g)	11	Protein (g)	22
Cholesterol (mg)	50		

Exchanges: 4 1/2 starch, 1 veg, 2 medium-fat meat, 3 fat

Carl's Jr.

	Amount	Cal.	Fat (g)	% Cal. Fat	Sat. Fat (g)	Chol. (mg)	Sod. (mg)	Carb. (g)	Fiber (g)	Pro. (g)	Servings/Exchanges
BAKED POTATOES											
Bacon and Cheese	1	620	29	42	8	40	1160	71	7	22	4 1/2 starch, 2 high-fat meat, 1 1/2 fat
Broccoli and Cheese	1	510	21	37	5	15	940	71	7	12	4 1/2 starch, 4 fat
✓Plain Potato with Margarine	1	380	12	28	2	0	140	63	7	7	4 starch, 2 1/2 fat
✓Plain Potato without Margarine	1	280	0	0	0	0	30	63	7	7	4 starch
✓Potato w/ Sour Cream and Chives	1	410	14	31	4	10	190	65	7	9	4 starch, 3 fat

✓ = Healthiest Bets

(*Continued*)

	Amount	Cal.	Fat (g)	% Cal. Fat	Sat. Fat (g)	Chol. (mg)	Sod. (mg)	Carb. (g)	Fiber (g)	Pro. (g)	Servings/Exchanges
BREAKFAST											
Breakfast Burrito	1	560	32	51	11	495	980	37	1	29	2 1/2 starch, 3 medium-fat meat, 3 1/2 fat
Breakfast Quesadilla	1	390	18	42	5	285	920	38	2	17	2 1/2 starch, 2 medium-fat meat, 1 fat
Croissant Sunrise Sandwich no meat	1	360	21	53	8	245	470	28	0	13	2 starch, 1 lean meat, 2 1/2 fat
Croissant Sunrise Sandwich with Bacon	1	410	25	55	9	225	610	29	0	16	2 starch, 2 high-fat meat, 1 fat
Croissant Sunrise Sandwich with Sausage	1	550	40	65	14	285	970	31	0	21	2 starch, 2 high-fat meat, 4 fat
French Toast Dips, no syrup	9 pieces	670	30	40	9	5	650	88	1	15	6 starch, 4 1/2 fat

French Toast Dips, no syrup	6 pieces	450	20	40	6	5	570	59	0	10	4 starch, 3 fat
Scrambled Egg - Bacon	1	760	42	50	11	500	1140	69	5	23	4 1/2 starch, 2 medium-fat meat, 4 fat
Scrambled Egg - Sausage	1	900	56	56	15	525	1480	72	5	27	4 1/2 starch, 1 medium-fat meat, 2 high-fat meat, 6 fat
Sourdough Sandwich with Bacon	1	470	24	46	11	305	680	39	2	25	2 1/2 starch, 1 medium-fat meat, 2 high-fat meat
Sourdough Sandwich with Ham	1	460	20	39	9	270	950	40	2	28	3 starch, 3 medium-fat meat
Sourdough Sandwich with Sausage	1	610	37	55	16	290	1040	39	2	26	2 1/2 starch, 1 medium-fat meat, 2 high-fat meat, 3 fat
Sourdough Sandwich, no meat	1	410	19	42	9	255	510	39	2	21	2 1/2 starch, 2 medium-fat meat, 1 1/2 fat

✔ = Healthiest Bets

(*Continued*)

	Amount	Cal.	Fat (g)	% Cal. Fat	Sat. Fat (g)	Chol. (mg)	Sod. (mg)	Carb. (g)	Fiber (g)	Pro. (g)	Servings/Exchanges
DESSERTS											
Chocolate Cake	1	300	12	36	3	30	350	48	1	3	3 carb, 2 fat
Chocolate Chip Cookie	1	350	18	46	7	20	330	46	1	3	3 carb, 3 fat
✓Strawberry Swirl Cheesecake	1	290	17	53	9	65	230	30	0	6	2 carb, 3 fat
DIPPING SAUCE CUPS											
BBQ Sauce	2 T	50	0	0	0	0	270	11	0	1	1/2 carb
✓Buffalo Wing Sauce	2 T	0	0		0	0	30	0	0	0	free
Honey Sauce	2 T	90	0	0	0	0	0	22	0	0	1 1/2 carb
House Sauce	2 T	110	11	90	2	10	220	2	0	0	2 fat
Mustard Sauce	2 T	50	0	0	0	0	210	11	0	0	1/2 carb
✓Sweet 'n' Sour Sauce	2 T	50	0	0	0	0	80	12	0	0	1/2 carb

SALAD DRESSING											
1000 Island	4 T	250	24	86	4	25	450	7	0	1	1/2 carb, 5 fat
Blue Cheese	4 T	320	35	98	6	25	370	1	0	2	7 fat
Buffalo Ranch	4 T	330	35	95	5	25	720	2	0	1	7 fat
Fat Free French	4 T	60	0	0	0	0	680	16	0	0	1 starch
Fat Free Italian	4 T	15	0	0	0	0	770	4	0	0	free
House	4 T	220	22	90	4	20	440	3	0	1	4 1/2 fat
SALADS WITHOUT DRESSING											
Buffalo Ranch Chicken	1	380	16	38	3	35	1180	42	6	19	2 starch, 3 veg, 1 medium-fat meat, 1 1/2 fat
Charbroiled Chicken To-Go	1	330	7	19	4	75	880	17	5	34	3 veg, 5 lean meat
Croutons	1	70	3	39	0	0	170	8	0	1	1/2 starch, 1/2 fat
✓Garden To-Go	1	120	3	23	2	5	230	5	2	3	1 veg, 1 fat

✓ = Healthiest Bets

(*Continued*)

	Amount	Cal.	Fat (g)	% Cal. Fat	Sat. Fat (g)	Chol. (mg)	Sod. (mg)	Carb. (g)	Fiber (g)	Pro. (g)	Servings/Exchanges
SANDWICHES/BURGERS											
Carl's Bacon Swiss Crispy Chicken	1	750	28	34	11	80	1900	91	3	31	6 starch, 2 lean meat, 3 1/2 fat
Carl's Catch Fish	1	560	27	43	7	80	990	58	2	19	4 starch, 2 medium-fat meat, 3 1/2 fat
Carl's Ranch Crispy Chicken	1	660	31	42	7	70	1180	72	3	24	4 1/2 starch, 2 medium-fat meat, 3 1/2 fat
Carl's Western Bacon Crispy Chicken	1	760	38	45	11	90	1550	72	3	31	4 1/2 starch, 3 medium-fat meat, 4 fat
Charbroiled BBQ Chicken	1	370	4	10	1	60	1070	47	4	35	3 starch, 3 lean meat
Charbroiled Chicken Club	1	550	23	38	7	95	1330	43	4	42	3 starch, 5 lean meat, 1 fat
Charbroiled Santa Fe Chicken	1	610	32	47	8	100	1440	43	4	38	3 starch, 4 lean meat, 4 fat

Chili Burger	1	690	35	46	15	110	1400	57	5	39	4 starch, 4 lean meat, 3 1/2 fat
Double Sourdough Bacon Cheese	1	920	59	58	24	170	1020	45	2	52	3 starch, 6 high-fat meat, 2 fat
Double Western Bacon Cheeseburger	1	920	50	49	21	155	1730	65	2	51	4 starch, 6 high-fat meat
Famous Star Hamburger	1	590	32	49	9	70	910	50	3	24	3 starch, 3 high-fat meat, 1 fat
Famous StarHamburger with Cheese	1	650	37	51	12	85	1170	51	3	28	3 1/2 starch, 3 high-fat meat, 1 1/2 fat
✔Hamburger	1	280	9	29	4	35	480	36	1	14	2 starch, 2 lean meat, 1/2 fat
Sourdough Bacon Cheeseburger	1	550	29	47	14	85	500	41	2	31	3 starch, 3 high-fat meat
Spicy Chicken	1	480	26	49	5	40	1220	48	2	14	3 starch, 2 medium-fat meat, 2 fat

✔ = Healthiest Bets

(Continued)

SANDWICHES/BURGERS (*Continued*)	Amount	Cal.	Fat (g)	% Cal. Fat	Sat. Fat (g)	Chol. (mg)	Sod. (mg)	Carb. (g)	Fiber (g)	Pro. (g)	Servings/Exchanges
Super Star Double Cheese	1	920	57	56	21	160	1490	53	3	48	3 1/2 starch, 5 high-fat meat, 3 fat
Super Star Hamburger	1	790	47	54	14	130	980	52	3	41	3 1/2 starch, 5 high-fat meat
The Six Dollar Burger	1	1000	62	56	25	135	1680	72	6	39	4 1/2 starch, 4 high-fat meat, 5 1/2 fat
The Western Bacon Six Dollar Burger	1	1060	81	69	27	135	2180	79	2	45	5 starch, 4 high-fat meat, 6 fat
Western Bacon Cheeseburger	1	660	30	41	12	85	1410	64	2	32	4 starch, 3 medium-fat meat, 2 1/2 fat
SHAKES											
Chocolate, medium	32 oz	820	16	18	10	70	550	148	0	22	9 1/2 carb, 3 fat
Chocolate, small	21 oz	540	11	18	7	45	360	98	0	15	6 1/2 carb, 2 fat

Strawberry, medium	32 oz	750	15	18	10	65	490	133	0	20	8 1/2 carb, 3 fat
Strawberry, small	21 oz	520	11	19	7	45	340	93	0	14	6 carb, 2 fat
Vanilla, medium	32 oz	700	16	21	11	70	520	115	0	22	7 1/2 carb, 3 fat
Vanilla, small	21 oz	470	11	21	7	45	350	77	0	15	5 carb, 2 fat
SIDES											
American Cheese	1 order	60	5	75	4	15	260	1	0	3	1 medium-fat meat
✓Bacon, 2 slices	1 order	45	4	80	2	10	150	0	0	3	1 1/2 fat
Chicken Breast Strips, 3 pieces	1 order	380	21	50	4	55	1360	27	1	22	1 1/2 starch, 3 medium-fat meat, 1/2 fat
Chicken Breast Strips, 5 pieces	1 order	630	34	49	6	90	2260	45	2	37	3 starch, 4 medium-fat meat, 1 1/2 fat
Chicken Stars, 6 pieces	1 order	270	17	57	5	40	500	15	0	14	1 starch, 2 medium-fat meat, 1 fat
Chicken Stars, 9 pieces	1 order	410	26	57	7	60	780	23	1	21	1 1/2 starch, 3 medium-fat meat, 1 1/2 fat

✓ = Healthiest Bets

(*Continued*)

SIDES (*Continued*)	Amount	Cal.	Fat (g)	% Cal. Fat	Sat. Fat (g)	Chol. (mg)	Sod. (mg)	Carb. (g)	Fiber (g)	Pro. (g)	Servings/Exchanges
Chili Cheese Fries	1 order	920	51	50	16	65	1030	69	9	29	4 1/2 starch, 2 high-fat meat, 7 fat
Criss Cut Fries	1 order	410	24	53	5	0	950	43	4	5	3 starch, 5 fat
French Fries, kids	1 order	250	12	43	3	0	150	32	3	4	2 starch, 2 fat
French Fries, large	1 order	620	29	42	8	0	380	80	7	10	5 1/2 starch, 3 fat
French Fries, medium	1 order	460	22	43	5	0	280	59	5	7	4 starch, 4 fat
French Fries, small	1 order	290	14	43	3	0	170	37	3	5	2 1/2 starch, 3 fat
Hash Brown Nuggets	1 order	330	21	57	5	0	470	32	3	3	2 starch, 4 fat
Onion Rings	1 order	440	22	45	5	0	700	53	3	7	3 1/2 starch, 4 fat
✓Swiss Style Cheese	1 order	50	4	72	3	15	230	0	0	4	1 medium-fat meat
Zucchini	1 order	320	19	53	5	0	880	31	2	6	1 1/2 starch, 1 veg, 4 fat

✓ = Healthiest Bets

Dairy Queen/Brazier

❖ Dairy Queen/Brazier provides nutrition information for all its menu items on its Web site at www.dairyqueen.com.

Light 'n Lean Choice

DQ Homestyle Cheeseburger
Vanilla Cone *(small)*

Calories	570	Sodium (mg)	965
Fat (g)	24	Carbohydrate (g)	67
% calories from fat	38	Fiber (g)	2
Saturated fat (g)	13	Protein (g)	26
Cholesterol (mg)	75		

Exchanges: 2 starch, 2 1/2 carb, 3 medium-fat meat

Healthy 'n Hearty Choice

Grilled Chicken Sandwich
1/2 French Fries *(small)*
DQ Chocolate Soft Serve *(1/2 cup)*

Calories	640	Sodium (mg)	1,425
Fat (g)	27	Carbohydrate (g)	70
% calories from fat	38	Fiber (g)	4
Saturated fat (g)	7.5	Protein (g)	28
Cholesterol (mg)	70		

Exchanges: 3 1/2 starch, 1 1/2 carb, 3 lean meat, 2 fat

(*Continued*)

Dairy Queen/Brazier

	Amount	Cal.	Fat (g)	% Cal. Fat	Sat. Fat (g)	Chol. (mg)	Sod. (mg)	Carb. (g)	Fiber (g)	Pro. (g)	Servings/Exchanges
BLIZZARD TREATS											
Oreo Cookie Blizzard, large	1	1010	37	33	18	70	770	148	2	18	10 carb, 5 fat
Oreo Cookie Blizzard, medium	1	700	26	33	12	45	560	103	1	13	7 carb, 3 1/2 fat
Oreo Cookie Blizzard, small	1	570	21	33	10	40	430	83	0	11	5 1/2 carb, 3 fat
BURGERS											
DQ Home style Bacon Double Cheeseburger	1	610	36	53	18	130	1380	31	2	41	2 carb, 5 medium-fat meat, 1 1/2 fat
DQ Home Style Cheeseburger	1	340	17	45	8	55	850	29	2	20	2 starch, 2 high-fat meat

DQ Home style Double Cheeseburger	1	540	31	52	16	115	1130	30	2	35	2 starch, 4 medium-fat meat, 2 fat
DQ Home style Hamburger	1	290	12	37	5	45	630	29	2	17	2 starch, 2 medium-fat meat
DQ Ultimate Burger	1	670	43	58	19	135	1210	29	2	40	2 starch, 5 medium-fat meat, 3 fat
CONES											
Chocolate Cone, medium	1	340	11	29	7	30	160	53	0	8	3 1/2 carb, 2 fat
Chocolate Cone, small	1	240	8	30	5	20	115	37	0	6	2 1/2 carb, 1 1/2 fat
Dipped Cone, large	1	710	36	46	17	45	250	85	0	12	5 1/2 carb, 6 fat
Dipped Cone, medium	1	490	24	44	13	30	190	59	1	8	4 carb, 4 fat
Dipped Cone, small	1	340	17	45	9	20	130	42	1	6	3 carb, 2 fat
✔DQ Chocolate Soft Serve	1/2 cup	150	5	30	3.5	15	75	22	0	4	1 1/2 carb, 1 fat

✔ = Healthiest Bets

(*Continued*)

CONES (*Continued*)	Amount	Cal.	Fat (g)	% Cal. Fat	Sat. Fat (g)	Chol. (mg)	Sod. (mg)	Carb. (g)	Fiber (g)	Pro. (g)	Servings/Exchanges
✓DQ Vanilla Soft Serve 1/2 cup	1/2 cup	140	5	32	3	15	70	22	0	3	1 1/2 carb, 1 fat
Vanilla Cone, large	1	480	15	28	9	45	230	76	0	11	5 carb, 3 fat
Vanilla Cone, medium	1	330	9	25	6	30	160	53	0	8	3 1/2 carb, 2 fat
Vanilla Cone, small	1	230	7	27	4.5	20	115	38	0	6	2 1/2 carb, 1 1/2 fat
FRIES/ONION RINGS											
French Fries, large	1	480	19	36	4	0	1140	72	5	5	4 1/2 starch, 4 fat
French Fries, medium	1	380	15	36	3	0	800	56	4	4	3 1/2 starch, 3 fat
French Fries, small	1	300	12	36	2.5	0	700	45	3	3	3 starch, 2 1/2 fat
Onion Rings	1	470	30	57	6	0	740	45	3	6	2 1/2 starch, 6 fat
FROZEN CAKE											
8″ Round Frozen Cake	1/8 of cake	370	13	32	8	25	280	56	0	7	4 carb, 2 1/2 fat

HOT DOGS											
Chili 'n' Cheese Dog	1	330	21	57	9	45	1090	22	2	14	1 1/2 starch, 2 high-fat meat, 2 fat
✓Hot Dog	1	240	14	53	5	25	730	19	4	9	1 carb, 1 high-fat meat, 1 fat
Super Dog	1	580	37	57	13	75	1710	39	2	20	2 1/2 starch, 2 high-fat meat, 4 fat
Super Dog Chili 'n' Cheese	1	710	47	60	18	105	2270	42	3	27	3 starch, 3 high-fat meat 6 fat
NOVELTIES											
Buster Bar	1	450	28	56	12	15	280	41	2	10	3 carb, 5 1/2 fat
✓Chocolate Dilly Bar	1	210	13	56	7	10	75	21	0	3	5 carb, 2 1/2 fat
✓DQ Fudge Bar - no sugar added	1	50	0	0	0	0	70	13	0	4	1 carb
DQ Sandwich	1	200	6	27	3	10	140	31	1	4	2 carb, 1 fat

✓ = Healthiest Bets

(Continued)

NOVELTIES (*Continued*)	Amount	Cal.	Fat (g)	% Cal. Fat	Sat. Fat (g)	Chol. (mg)	Sod. (mg)	Carb. (g)	Fiber (g)	Pro. (g)	Servings/Exchanges
✓DQ Vanilla Orange Bar - no sugar added	1	60	0	0	0	0	40	17	0	2	1 carb
✓Lemon DQ freez'r, 1/2 cup	1	80	0	0	0	0	10	20	0	0	1 carb
✓Starkiss	1	80	0	0	0	0	10	21	0	0	1 1/2 carb
SALAD DRESSING											
DQ Blue Cheese	4 T	210	20	86	4	5	700	4	0	2	4 fat
DQ Honey Mustard	4 T	260	21	73	3.5	20	370	18	0	1	1 carb, 4 fat
DQ Ranch	4 T	310	33	96	5	25	390	3	0	1	6 1/2 fat
Fat Free Red French	3 T	40	0	0	0	0	330	10	0	0	1/2 carb
Fat Free Buttermilk Ranch	3 T	35	0	0	0	0	440	6	0	1	1/2 carb

✔Fat Free Honey Mustard	3 T	50	0	0	0	0	160	13	0	0	1 carb
Fat Free Italian	3 T	10	0	0	0	0	390	3	0	0	free
Fat Free Ranch	3 T	60	0	0	0	0	410	13	1	1	1 carb
Fat Free Thousand Island	3 T	60	0	0	0	0	400	16	0	0	1 carb
Reduced Calorie Buttermilk	3 T	140	13	84	2	15	390	5	0	0	3 fat
Wish-bone Fat Free Italian	3 T	25	0	0	0	0	520	6	0	0	1/2 carb
SALADS											
✔Crispy Chicken - no dressing	1	350	20	51	6	40	620	21	6	21	1/2 starch, 2 veg, 3 medium-fat meat, 1 fat
Grilled Chicken - no dressing	1	240	10	38	5	65	950	12	4	26	2 veg, 3 lean meat, 1 fat
✔Side	1	60	3	45	1.5	5	60	6	2	3	1 veg, 1/2 fat

✔ = Healthiest Bets

(*Continued*)

	Amount	Cal.	Fat (g)	% Cal. Fat	Sat. Fat (g)	Chol. (mg)	Sod. (mg)	Carb. (g)	Fiber (g)	Pro. (g)	Servings/Exchanges
SANDWICHES/BASKETS											
✓BBQ Beef	1	300	9	27	3.5	35	610	37	2	16	2 carb, 2 medium-fat meat
✓BBQ Pork	1	280	8	26	2	55	790	36	2	17	2 carb, 2 medium-fat meat
Breaded Chicken	1	510	27	48	4	40	1070	47	4	19	3 carb, 2 medium-fat meat 3 fat
Chicken Strip	1	1000	50	45	13	55	2510	102	5	35	6 1/2 carb, 5 medium-fat meat, 2 1/2 fat
Grilled Chicken	1	340	16	42	2.5	55	1000	26	2	22	1 1/2 starch, 3 medium-fat meat
SHAKES AND MALTS											
Chocolate Malt, large	1	1320	35	24	22	110	670	222	2	29	15 carb, 7 fat
Chocolate Malt, medium	1	870	22	23	14	70	450	153	2	20	10 carb, 4 1/2 fat

Chocolate Malt, small	1	640	16	23	11	55	340	111	1	15	7 1/2 carb, 3 fat
Chocolate Shake, small	1	560	15	24	10	50	280	93	1	13	6 carb, 3 fat
Misty Slush, medium	1	290	0	0	0	0	30	74	0	0	5 carb
Misty Slush, small	1	220	0	0	0	0	20	56	0	0	3 1/2 carb
SUNDAES											
Banana Split	1	510	12	21	8	30	180	96	3	8	6 carb, 2 fat
Brownie Earthquake	1	740	27	33	16	50	350	112	0	10	7 1/2 starch, 3 1/2 fat
Chocolate Sundae, large	1	580	15	23	10	45	260	100	1	11	6 1/2 carb, 2 fat
Chocolate Sundae, medium	1	400	10	23	6	30	210	71	0	8	4 1/2 carb, 1 1/2 fat
Chocolate Sundae, small	1	280	7	23	4.5	20	140	49	0	5	3 carb, 1 1/2 fat
Peanut Buster Parfait	1	730	31	38	17	35	400	99	3	8	6 1/2 carb, 3 fat
Pecan Praline Parfait	1	720	29	36	11	30	610	105	1	9	7 carb, 4 fat

✓ = Healthiest Bets

(Continued)

SUNDAES (*Continued*)	Amount	Cal.	Fat (g)	% Cal. Fat	Sat. Fat (g)	Chol. (mg)	Sod. (mg)	Carb. (g)	Fiber (g)	Pro. (g)	Servings/Exchanges
Strawberry Shortcake	1	430	14	29	9	60	360	70	1	7	4 1/2 carb, 2 fat
Strawberry Sundae, large	1	500	15	27	9	45	230	83	0	10	5 1/2 carb, 2 fat
Strawberry Sundae, medium	1	340	9	24	6	30	160	58	0	7	4 carb, 1 fat
Strawberry Sundae, small	1	240	7	26	4.5	20	110	40	0	5	2 1/2 carb, 1 fat
Triple Chocolate Utopia	1	770	39	46	17	55	390	96	5	12	6 1/2 carb, 6 fat

Hardee's

❖ Hardee's provides nutrition information for all its menu items on its Web site at www.hardees.com.

Light 'n Lean Choice

Regular Roast Beef Sandwich
1/2 French Fries *(regular)*

Calories	530	Sodium (mg)	980
Fat (g)	15	Carbohydrate (g)	54
% calories from fat	42	Fiber (g)	4
Saturated fat (g)	11	Protein (g)	22
Cholesterol (mg)	40		

Exchanges: 3 1/2 starch, 2 medium-fat meat, 2 fat

Healthy 'n Hearty Choice

Hot Ham 'n' Cheese Sandwich
Mashed Potatoes with Chicken Gravy
Chocolate Shake, Hand-Dipped *(1/2)*

Calories	657	Sodium (mg)	1,485
Fat (g)	30	Carbohydrate (g)	80
% calories from fat	41	Fiber (g)	2
Saturated fat (g)	15	Protein (g)	26
Cholesterol (mg)	89		

Exchanges: 3 starch, 2 carb, 2 medium-fat meat, 2 fat

(*Continued*)

Hardee's

	Amount	Cal.	Fat (g)	% Cal. Fat	Sat. Fat (g)	Chol. (mg)	Sod. (mg)	Carb. (g)	Fiber (g)	Pro. (g)	Servings/Exchanges
BREAKFAST											
Big Country Platter - Bacon	1	980	56	51	13	435	2080	90	3	28	6 starch, 2 high-fat meat, 6 1/2 fat
Big Country Platter - Breakfast Ham	1	970	52	48	12	455	2450	90	3	34	6 starch, 3 high-fat meat, 2 fat
Big Country Platter - Chicken	1	1140	61	48	13	480	2580	105	4	44	7 starch, 3 high-fat meat, 4 fat
Big Country Platter - Country Ham	1	970	53	49	12	460	2600	90	3	33	6 starch, 3 high-fat meat, 4 1/2 fat
Big Country Platter - Country Steak	1	1150	68	53	16	455	2260	98	4	36	6 1/2 starch, 3 high-fat meat, 7 1/2 fat
Big Country Platter - Sausage	1	1060	64	54	15	455	2140	91	4	30	6 starch, 3 high-fat meat, 6 fat

Frisco Sandwich	1	410	17	37	7	245	870	39	2	27	2 1/2 starch, 2 high-fat meat
Loaded Biscuit 'n' Gravy Bowl	1	770	54	63	15	245	1950	49	0	20	3 starch, 2 high-fat meat, 7 fat
Low Carb Breakfast Bowl	1	620	50	73	21	325	1380	6	2	36	1/2 starch, 5 high-fat meat, 2 fat
Pancakes - 3	1 serving	300	5	15	1	25	830	55	2	8	3 1/2 starch
✓Tortilla Scrambler	1	230	13	51	6	30	520	18	0	9	1 starch, 1 high-fat meat, 1 fat
BREAKFAST BISCUITS											
Bacon	1	430	28	59	7	10	1110	35	0	8	2 starch, 1 high-fat meat, 1 1/2 fat
Bacon, Egg and Cheese	1	560	38	61	11	225	1360	37	0	16	2 1/2 starch, 2 high-fat meat, 3 1/2 fat
Biscuit 'n' Gravy	1	530	34	58	8	10	1550	47	0	8	3 starch, 4 fat

✓ = Healthiest Bets

(*Continued*)

BREAKFAST BISCUITS (*Continued*)	Amount	Cal.	Fat (g)	% Cal. Fat	Sat. Fat (g)	Chol. (mg)	Sod. (mg)	Carb. (g)	Fiber (g)	Pro. (g)	Servings/Exchanges
Chicken Fillet	1	600	34	51	7	55	1680	50	1	24	3 1/2 starch, 2 high-fat meat, 2 1/2 fat
Country Ham	1	440	26	53	6	35	1710	36	0	14	2 starch, 2 high-fat meat, 2 fat
Country Steak	1	620	41	60	11	35	1360	44	0	16	3 starch, 1 high-fat meat, 6 fat
Ham, Egg and Cheese	1	560	35	56	10	245	1800	37	0	23	2 1/2 starch, 3 high-fat meat, 1 1/2 fat
Loaded Omelet	1	640	44	62	15	245	1510	37	0	21	2 1/2 starch, 2 high-fat meat, 5 1/2 fat
Sausage	1	530	38	65	10	30	1240	36	0	11	2 1/2 starch, 1 high-fat meat, 5 fat
Sausage and Egg	1	610	44	65	11	235	1290	36	0	17	2 1/2 starch, 2 high-fat meat, 4 1/2 fat

Scratch	1	370	23	56	5	0	890	35	0	5	2 starch, 4 1/2 fat
Smoked Sausage	1	620	46	67	15	40	1680	37	0	15	2 1/2 starch, 2 high-fat meat, 5 fat
BREAKFAST CROISSANT											
Sunrise with Bacon	1	450	29	58	12	240	900	28	0	19	2 starch, 2 high-fat meat, 2 fat
Sunrise with Ham	1	430	26	54	10	250	1050	28	0	23	2 starch, 2 medium-fat meat, 2 1/2 fat
Sunrise with Sausage Patty	1	550	38	62	15	265	1030	29	0	22	2 starch, 2 high-fat meat, 4 fat
BREAKFAST SIDES											
American Cheese Slice (small)	1	50	4	72	3	10	200	1	0	2	1 medium-fat meat
✔Bacon (1.5 strips)	1 serving	60	5	75	2	5	220	0	0	2	1 1/2 fat
Biscuit Gravy	4 oz	160	11	62	3	10	660	12	0	3	1 starch, 2 fat

✔ = Healthiest Bets

(*Continued*)

BREAKFAST SIDES (*Continued*)	Amount	Cal.	Fat (g)	% Cal. Fat	Sat. Fat (g)	Chol. (mg)	Sod. (mg)	Carb. (g)	Fiber (g)	Pro. (g)	Servings/Exchanges
Breakfast Ham	1 serving	60	3	45	1	30	660	1	0	10	1 lean meat
✔Butter Blend Packet	1	25	3	100	1	0	45	0	0	0	1/2 fat
Chicken Fillet	1 serving	230	11	43	2	55	790	15	1	19	1 starch, 2 medium-fat meat
Cinnamon N Raisin Biscuit	1 serving	280	12	39	3	0	650	40	0	3	2 1/2 starch, 2 fat
Country Ham	1 serving	60	3	45	2	35	810	1	0	9	1 lean meat
Country Steak	1 serving	240	18	68	5	30	470	9	0	11	2 high-fat meat, 1 fat
Croissant	1 serving	210	10	43	4	5	200	26	0	4	1 1/2 starch, 2 1/2 fat
Folded Egg	1	80	6	68	2	205	50	1	0	6	1 medium-fat meat
✔Grape Jam	1 T	10	0	0	0	0	0	2	0	0	free
✔Grits	4 oz	110	5	41	1	0	480	16	0	2	1 starch, 1 fat
Hash Rounds - large	1 serving	460	29	57	6	0	650	45	4	5	3 starch, 5 fat

Hash Rounds - medium	1 serving	350	22	57	5	0	490	34	3	4	2 starch, 4 1/2 fat
Hash Rounds - small	1 serving	260	16	55	4	0	360	25	2	3	1 1/2 starch, 3 fat
Pancake Syrup	2 T	90	0	0	0	0	0	21	0	0	1 starch
Sausage Patty	1 serving	150	14	84	5	30	350	1	0	6	1 high-fat meat, 1 fat
Scrambled Egg	1	160	12	68	3	405	100	1	0	12	2 medium-fat meat
Smoked Sausage	1 serving	250	23	83	10	40	790	2	0	9	1 high-fat meat, 3 1/2 fat
✓Strawberry Jam	1 serving	35	0	0	0	0	0	9	0	0	1/2 carb
✓Swiss Cheese Slice	1	50	4	72	3	15	230	0	0	4	1 medium-fat meat
DESSERTS											
Apple Turnover	1	290	15	47	5	5	350	36	1	2	2 carb, 3 fat
Chocolate Chip Cookie	1	290	11	34	5	20	270	44	0	4	3 carb, 1 fat
DIPPING SAUCE CUPS											
BBQ Sauce	2 T	45	0	0	0	0	250	10	0	1	1/2 carb
Honey Mustard	2 T	110	9	74	2	10	220	6	0	0	1/2 carb, 1 1/2 fat

✓ = Healthiest Bets

(*Continued*)

DIPPING SAUCE CUPS (*Continued*)	Amount	Cal.	Fat (g)	% Cal. Fat	Sat. Fat (g)	Chol. (mg)	Sod. (mg)	Carb. (g)	Fiber (g)	Pro. (g)	Servings/Exchanges
✓Horseradish Packet	2 T	25	2	72	0	5	35	1	0	0	1/2 fat
✓Hot Sauce Packet	2 T	0	0		0	0	210	0	0	0	free
✓Ketchup Packet	1	10	0	0	0	0	105	2	0	0	free
Mayonnaise Packet	1	90	9	90	1.5	5	70	1	0	0	2 fat
Ranch Dressing	2 T	160	16	90	3	15	240	2	0	0	3 fat
✓Sweet N Sour	2 T	45	0	0	0	0	85	11	0	0	1/2 carb
FRIED CHICKEN & SIDES											
Fried Chicken Breast	1	370	15	36	4	75	1190	29	0	29	2 starch, 4 lean meat
✓Fried Chicken Leg	1	170	7	37	2	45	570	15	0	13	1 starch, 2 lean meat
Fried Chicken Thigh	1	330	15	41	4	60	1000	30	0	19	2 starch, 2 lean meat
✓Fried Chicken Wing	1	200	8	36	2	30	740	23	0	10	1 1/2 starch, 1 lean meat, 1/2 fat

INDIVIDUAL ITEMS											
✓American Cheese	1 slice	60	5	75	4	5	260	1	0	3	1 medium-fat meat
Au Jus Sauce	1 serving	10	0	0	0	0	320	2	0	0	free
✓Bacon 1 1/2 Strips	1 serving	60	5	75	2	5	220	0	0	2	1 1/2 fat
✓Grilled Onions	1 serving	35	3	77	3	0	0	2	0	0	1/2 fat
✓Swiss Cheese	1 slice	50	4	72	3	15	230	0	0	4	1 medium-fat meat
SANDWICHES											
1/2 lb Grilled Sourdough Thickburger	1	1040	73	63	30	155	1420	49	3	45	3 starch, 5 high-fat meat, 6 1/2 fat
1/2 lb Six Dollar Burger	1	1060	72	61	30	150	1860	60	3	40	4 starch, 5 high-fat meat, 5 1/2 fat
1/3 lb Bacon Cheese Thickburger	1	910	63	62	24	115	1490	50	3	33	3 starch, 4 high-fat meat, 4 fat
1/3 lb Cheeseburger	1	680	39	52	19	90	1450	52	2	29	3 1/2 starch, 3 high-fat meat, 2 fat

✓ = Healthiest Bets

(Continued)

SANDWICHES (*Continued*)	Amount	Cal.	Fat (g)	% Cal. Fat	Sat. Fat (g)	Chol. (mg)	Sod. (mg)	Carb. (g)	Fiber (g)	Pro. (g)	Servings/Exchanges
1/3 lb Chili Cheese Thickburger	1	870	54	56	26	135	1840	55	4	41	3 1/2 starch, 4 high-fat meat, 4 1/2 fat
1/3 lb Low Carb Thickburger	1	420	32	69	12	115	1010	5	2	30	4 high-fat meat
1/3 lb Mushroom 'n' Swiss Thickburger	1	720	42	53	21	100	1570	48	2	35	3 starch, 4 high-fat meat, 2 fat
1/3 lb Thickburger	1	850	57	60	22	105	1470	54	3	30	3 1/2 starch, 3 high-fat meat, 6 fat
2/3 lb Double Bacon Cheese Thickburger	1	1300	96	66	40	205	2110	51	3	55	3 1/2 starch, 6 high-fat meat, 9 1/2 fat
2/3 lb Double Thickburger	1	1230	90	66	38	195	2090	53	3	52	3 1/2 starch, 6 high-fat meat, 8 fat
3 Piece Chicken Strips	1 serving	380	21	50	4	55	1360	27	1	22	2 starch, 3 lean meat, 1 fat
5 Piece Chicken Strips	1 serving	630	34	49	6	90	2260	45	2	37	3 starch, 4 lean meat, 4 fat

Big Chicken Sandwich	1	770	36	42	8	95	2000	73	4	39	5 starch, 4 lean meat, 3 1/2 fat
Big Hot Ham 'n' Cheese	1	435	20	41	10	74	2009	40	2	36	2 1/2 starch, 4 medium-fat meat
Big Roast Beef	1	470	23	44	10	60	1290	38	2	29	2 1/2 starch, 3 medium-fat meat, 1 fat
Charbroiled Chicken Sandwich	1	590	26	40	7	80	1180	53	4	36	3 1/2 starch, 4 lean meat, 2 fat
Hot Dog	1	420	30	64	12	55	1200	22	1	16	1 1/2 starch, 2 high-fat meat, 2 fat
Hot Ham 'n' Cheese	1	287	13	41	6	37	1110	30	2	20	2 starch, 2 medium-fat meat
Kids Meal - Chicken Strips (no sauce)	1	500	25	45	5	35	1050	50	3	19	3 1/2 starch, 2 lean meat, 2 1/2 fat
Kids Meal - Slammer	1	720	35	44	13	70	740	71	4	30	4 1/2 starch, 3 high-fat meat, 2 fat

✔ = Healthiest Bets

(*Continued*)

SANDWICHES (*Continued*)	Amount	Cal.	Fat (g)	% Cal. Fat	Sat. Fat (g)	Chol. (mg)	Sod. (mg)	Carb. (g)	Fiber (g)	Pro. (g)	Servings/Exchanges
Low Carb Charbroiled Chicken Club	1	420	24	51	7	95	1230	11	2	41	1 starch, 5 lean meat, 2 fat
Regular Roast Beef	1	330	16	44	7	40	860	29	2	19	2 starch, 2 medium-fat meat, 1/2 fat
✔Slammer	1	240	12	45	5	35	3030	19	0	13	1 starch, 2 medium-fat meat
✔Slammer with Cheese	1	280	16	51	8	45	500	20	0	15	1 starch, 2 medium-fat meat, 1 fat
Spicy Chicken Sandwich	1	470	26	50	5	40	1220	46	2	14	3 starch, 2 lean meat, 2 1/2 fat
SHAKES											
Chocolate hand-dipped	16 oz	510	27	48	18	105	230	61	0	11	4 carb, 4 1/2 fat
Chocolate soft-serve	16 oz	710	7	9	5	20	550	137	12	27	9 carb

Strawberry hand-dipped	16 oz	480	27	51	15	105	230	58	0	11	3 1/2 carb, 4 1/2 fat
Strawberry soft-serve	16 oz	720	14	18	8	40	430	128	0	22	8 1/2 carb, 1 fat
Vanilla hand-dipped	16 oz	480	27	51	18	120	240	52	0	14	3 1/2 carb, 4 1/2 fat
Vanilla soft-serve	16 oz	650	17	24	10	50	510	98	0	27	6 1/2 carb, 3 fat
SIDES											
✔Chicken Gravy	1	20	1	45	0	0	220	3	0	0	1/2 starch
Chili Cheese Fries	1	700	39	50	13	50	780	67	7	22	4 1/2 starch, 1 high-fat meat, 5 1/2 fat
Cole Slaw (large = 3 servings)	1 serving	170	10	53	2	10	140	20	2	1	1 starch, 1 veg, 1 1/2 fat
Cole Slaw (small = 1 serving)	1	170	10	53	2	10	140	20	2	1	1 starch, 1 veg, 1 1/2 fat
Crispy Curls, large	1	480	23	43	6	0	1190	60	5	6	4 starch, 4 fat

✔ = Healthiest Bets

(*Continued*)

SIDES (*Continued*)	Amount	Cal.	Fat (g)	% Cal. Fat	Sat. Fat (g)	Chol. (mg)	Sod. (mg)	Carb. (g)	Fiber (g)	Pro. (g)	Servings/Exchanges
Crispy Curls, medium	1	410	20	44	5	0	1020	52	4	5	3 1/2 starch, 3 fat
Crispy Curls, small	1	340	17	45	4	0	840	43	4	4	3 starch, 2 fat
French Fries, kids	1	250	12	43	3	0	150	32	3	4	2 starch, 2 fat
French Fries, large	1	610	28	41	6	0	370	78	6	10	5 starch, 5 fat
French Fries, medium	1	520	24	42	5	0	320	67	5	8	4 1/2 starch, 4 fat
French Fries, small	1	390	19	44	4	0	240	51	4	6	3 1/2 starch, 3 fat
Mashed Potatoes (large = 3 servings)	1 serving	90	2	20	0	0	410	17	0	1	1 starch
✔Mashed Potatoes (small = 1 serving)	1	90	2	20	0	0	410	17	0	1	1 starch

✔ = Healthiest Bets

Jack in the Box

❖ Jack in the Box provides nutrition information for all its menu items on its Web site at www.jackinthebox.com.

Light 'n Lean Choice

Hamburger
Side Salad with Low-Fat Balsamic Vinaigrette
(2 T, 1/2 serving)

Calories	485	Sodium (mg)	1,180
Fat (g)	24	Carbohydrate (g)	48
% calories from fat	44	Fiber (g)	0
Saturated fat (g)	7.5	Protein (g)	22
Cholesterol (mg)	55		

Exchanges: 2 starch, 1 veg, 2 medium-fat meat, 1 1/2 fat

Healthy 'n Hearty Choice

Chicken Fajita Pita
Natural-Cut Fries *(1/2 medium)*
Side Salad with Low-Fat Balsamic Vinaigrette
(2 T, 1/2 serving)

Calories	670	Sodium (mg)	1,970
Fat (g)	28	Carbohydrate (g)	74
% calories from fat	38	Fiber (g)	2
Saturated fat (g)	8.5	Protein (g)	30
Cholesterol (mg)	75		

Exchanges: 4 starch, 2 veg, 3 lean meat, 3 fat

(*Continued*)

Jack in the Box

	Amount	Cal.	Fat (g)	% Cal. Fat	Sat. Fat (g)	Chol. (mg)	Sod. (mg)	Carb. (g)	Fiber (g)	Pro. (g)	Servings/Exchanges
BURGERS											
Bacon Cheeseburger	1	780	50	58	18.5	90	1545	50	2	33	3 1/2 starch, 3 high-fat meat, 4 fat
Bacon Ultimate Cheeseburger	1	1025	71	62	29	135	1985	53	2	46	3 1/2 starch, 5 high-fat meat, 5 1/2 fat
✓Hamburger	1	310	14	41	5	45	590	30	0	17	2 starch, 2 medium-fat meat
Hamburger Deluxe	1	370	21	51	6	50	545	32	0	17	2 starch, 2 high-fat meat
Hamburger Deluxe with Cheese	1	460	28	55	10	75	915	34	0	21	2 starch, 3 high-fat meat
✓Hamburger with Cheese	1	355	18	46	7	55	770	31	0	19	2 starch, 2 high-fat meat

Jumbo Jack	1	600	35	53	12	45	935	52	2	20	3 1/2 starch, 2 high-fat meat, 3 fat
Jumbo Jack with Cheese	1	695	42	54	16	70	1305	55	2	24	3 1/2 starch, 3 high-fat meat, 2 1/2 fat
Junior Bacon Cheeseburger	1	525	36	62	9.5	70	880	32	0	21	2 starch, 2 high-fat meat, 3 1/2 fat
Sourdough Jack	1	715	51	64	18	75	1165	36	2	26	2 1/2 starch, 3 high-fat meat, 5 fat
Ultimate Cheeseburger	1	945	65	62	27	120	1525	52	2	39	3 1/2 starch, 4 high-fat meat, 6 fat
CHICKEN AND FISH											
Chicken Breast Strips	8 oz	630	38	54	8	90	1470	39	3	35	2 1/2 starch, 4 medium-fat meat, 3 fat
Chicken Cordon Blue Sandwich	1	555	28	45	8.5	100	1335	33	2	40	2 starch, 5 medium-fat meat
Chicken Fajita Pita	1	315	9	26	4	65	1080	33	0	22	2 starch, 2 lean meat, 1 fat

✓ = Healthiest Bets

(*Continued*)

CHICKEN AND FISH (*Continued*)	Amount	Cal.	Fat (g)	% Cal. Fat	Sat. Fat (g)	Chol. (mg)	Sod. (mg)	Carb. (g)	Fiber (g)	Pro. (g)	Servings/Exchanges
Chicken Sandwich	1	390	21	48	4	35	730	39	1	15	2 1/2 starch, 1 medium-fat meat, 2 1/2 fat
Chicken Sandwich with Cheese	1	430	24	50	6	45	880	40	1	17	2 1/2 starch, 2 high-fat meat, 1 fat
Fish and Chips	1	840	56	60	11	55	1600	69	4	16	4 1/2 starch, 2 medium-fat meat, 7 1/2 fat
Jack's Spicy Chicken	1	615	31	45	5.5	50	4090	62	3	24	4 starch, 3 medium-fat meat, 1 1/2 fat
Jack's Spicy Chicken with Cheese	1	695	37	48	9.5	70	1400	63	3	29	4 starch, 3 medium-fat meat, 3 1/2 fat
Sourdough Grilled Chicken Club	1	505	27	48	6.5	75	1220	35	2	29	2 1/2 starch, 3 medium-fat meat, 2 fat
Southwest Pita	1	260	5	17	1	40	880	35	4	20	2 1/2 starch, 1 lean meat

DESSERTS											
Cheesecake	1	310	16	46	9	55	220	34	0	7	2 starch, 3 1/2 fat
Double Fudge Cake	1	310	11	32	3	25	270	49	4	3	3 starch, 2 fat
FRIES & RINGS											
Natural Cut Fries - large	1	530	25	42	6	0	870	69	5	8	4 1/2 starch, 4 fat
Natural Cut Fries - medium	1	360	17	43	4	0	590	47	4	5	3 starch, 3 fat
Natural Cut Fries - small	1	270	12	40	3	0	440	35	3	4	2 starch, 2 1/2 fat
Onion Rings	1	500	30	54	6	0	420	51	3	6	3 1/2 starch, 5 fat
Seasoned Curly Fries - large	1	550	31	51	6	0	1200	60	6	8	4 starch, 5 fat
Seasoned Curly Fries - medium	1	400	23	52	5	0	890	45	5	6	3 starch, 3 1/2 fat
Seasoned Curly Fries - small	1	270	15	50	3	0	590	30	3	4	2 starch, 1 fat

✓ = Healthiest Bets

(Continued)

	Amount	Cal.	Fat (g)	% Cal. Fat	Sat. Fat (g)	Chol. (mg)	Sod. (mg)	Carb. (g)	Fiber (g)	Pro. (g)	Servings/Exchanges
SALADS											
Asian Chicken	1	595	33	50	4.5	25	1315	58	8	20	3 starch, 3 veg, 2 lean meat, 3 1/2 fat
Chicken Club	1	825	62	68	12.5	95	2065	34	5	34	1 starch, 3 veg, 3 lean meat, 1 high-fat meat, 9 fat
Greek	1	690	50	65	10.5	45	2625	32	3	24	1 starch, 3 veg, 3 high-fat meat, 5 fat
Side	1	155	8	46	2.5	10	290	16	0	5	3 veg, 2 fat
Southwest Chicken	1	735	44	54	10	95	2155	46	4	27	2 starch, 3 veg, 3 lean meat, 7 1/2 fat
SANDWICHES											
Deli Trio Pannido	1	645	34	47	8.5	95	2530	53	2	30	3 1/2 starch, 2 medium-fat meat, 5 fat

Ham & Turkey Pannido	1	610	29	43	7	110	1785	54	2	36	3 1/2 starch, 4 lean meat, 2 1/2 fat
Ultimate Club	1	630	29	41	9	105	1985	52	2	36	3 1/2 starch, 4 medium-fat meat, 5 fat
Zesty Turkey Pannido	1	740	44	54	10.5	135	1880	51	2	40	3 1/2 starch, 4 lean meat, 5 1/2 fat

SAUCES AND DRESSINGS

Barbeque Dipping Sauce	2 T	45	0	0	0	0	330	11	0	0	1/2 high-fat meat
Buttermilk House Dipping Sauce	2 T	130	13	90	2	10	210	3	0	0	3 fat
Creamy Caesar Dressing	4 1/2 T	310	30	87	6	35	800	6	0	3	1/2 starch, 6 fat
Frank's Red Hot Buffalo Dipping Sauce	2 T	10	0	0	0	0	840	2	0	0	free
Lite Ranch Dressing	4 1/2 T	190	18	85	3	25	700	3	0	1	4 fat

✔ = Healthiest Bets

(*Continued*)

SAUCES AND DRESSINGS (*Continued*)	Amount	Cal.	Fat (g)	% Cal. Fat	Sat. Fat (g)	Chol. (mg)	Sod. (mg)	Carb. (g)	Fiber (g)	Pro. (g)	Servings/Exchanges
Low - Fat Herb Mayo Sauce	1 T	15	1	60	0	0	110	1	0	0	free
Low Fat Balsamic Dressing	4 1/2 T	40	2	45	0	0	600	6	0	0	1/2 starch
Mayo - Onion Sauce	1 T	60	7	100	1	5	60	1	0	0	1 1/2 fat
Ranch Dressing	4 1/2 T	390	41	95	6	30	590	4	0	1	9 fat
Soy Sauce	1 T	5	0	0	0	0	480	1	0	0	free
Sweet & Sour Dipping Sauce	2 T	45	0	0	0	0	160	11	0	0	1 starch
Taco Sauce	3 T	0	0		0	0	80	0	0	0	free
Tartar Dipping Sauce	3 T	210	22	94	3.5	20	370	2	0	0	4 1/2 fat

SHAKES											
Chocolate Ice Cream	small	660	29	40	18	110	270	89	1	11	6 carb, 4 fat
Chocolate Ice Cream	large	1310	57	39	36	225	540	178	2	23	12 carb, 7 1/2 fat
Chocolate Ice Cream	medium	850	38	40	24	150	340	111	1	15	7 carb, 5 fat
Creamy Caramel Ice Cream	large	1330	59	40	37	235	570	173	1	22	11 1/2 carb, 9 fat
Creamy Caramel Ice Cream	small	670	30	40	19	115	290	87	0	11	5 1/2 carb, 4 1/2 fat
Creamy Caramel Ice Cream	medium	860	40	42	25	155	360	109	0	15	7 carb, 7 fat
Oreo Cookie Ice Cream	large	1350	66	44	37	225	700	161	2	22	1 1/2 carb, 11 fat
Oreo Cookie Ice Cream	medium	870	43	44	25	150	420	103	1	15	7 carb, 7 fat
Oreo Cookie Ice Cream	small	670	33	44	19	110	350	81	1	11	5 carb, 6 fat

✓ = Healthiest Bets

(Continued)

SHAKES (*Continued*)	Amount	Cal.	Fat (g)	% Cal. Fat	Sat. Fat (g)	Chol. (mg)	Sod. (mg)	Carb. (g)	Fiber (g)	Pro. (g)	Servings/Exchanges
Strawberry Banana Ice Cream	medium	900	38	38	24	150	300	122	0	14	8 carb, 6 fat
Strawberry Banana Ice Cream	large	1410	56	36	35	225	450	199	0	21	13 carb, 8 fat
Strawberry Banana Ice Cream	small	700	28	36	18	110	230	100	0	10	6 1/2 carb, 4 fat
Strawberry Ice Cream	medium	830	38	41	24	150	300	106	0	14	7 carb, 6 fat
Strawberry Ice Cream	small	640	28	39	18	110	220	84	0	10	5 1/2 carb, 4 1/2 fat
Strawberry Ice Cream	large	1270	56	40	35	225	440	167	0	21	11 carb, 9 fat
Vanilla Ice Cream	medium	750	38	46	24	150	290	85	0	14	5 1/2 carb, 6 fat
Vanilla Ice Cream	small	570	29	46	18	115	220	65	0	11	4 carb, 5 fat
Vanilla Ice Cream	large	1140	58	46	36	230	440	129	0	22	8 1/2 carb, 10 fat

TACOS AND SNACKS

Bacon Cheddar Potato Wedges	8.5 oz	620	41	60	15	55	1300	45	5	18	3 starch, 2 high-fat meat, 3 fat
Egg Roll	1	175	6	31	2	5	470	26	2	5	1 1/2 starch, 1 fat
Egg Rolls	3	445	19	38	6	15	1080	55	6	14	3 1/2 starch, 3 1/2 fat
✓Monster Taco	1	240	14	53	5	20	390	20	3	8	1 starch, 1 high-fat meat, 1 1/2 fat
Stuffed Jalapenos	3	230	13	51	6	20	690	22	2	7	1 1/2 starch, 2 1/2 fat
Stuffed Jalapenos	7	530	30	51	13	45	1600	51	4	15	3 1/2 starch, 5 1/2 fat
✓Taco	1	160	8	45	3	15	270	15	2	5	1 starch, 2 fat

✓ = Healthiest Bets; n/a = not available

McDonald's

❖ McDonald's provides nutrition information for all its menu items on its Web site at www.mcdonalds.com.

Light 'n Lean Choice

Grilled Chicken California Cobb Salad
Newman's Own Cobb Dressing *(2 T, 1/2 serving)*
Fruit 'n Yogurt Parfait with Granola

Calories.......................490
Fat (g) 17
% calories from fat..31
Saturated fat (g) 7
Cholesterol (mg) 155
Sodium (mg) 1,365
Carbohydrate (g).........44
Fiber (g).....................3
Protein (g) 38

Exchanges: 2 veg, 2 carb, 4 lean meat, 1 fat

Healthy 'n Hearty Choice

Hamburger
French Fries *(1/2 medium)*
Side Salad
Low-Fat Balsamic Vinaigrette Dressing
(2 T, 1/2 serving)

Calories.......................550
Fat (g) 23
% calories from fat..38
Saturated fat (g) 6
Cholesterol (mg) 30
Sodium (mg) 1,220
Carbohydrate (g).........71
Fiber (g).....................6
Protein (g) 16

Exchanges: 2 starch, 1 veg, 1 medium fat, 3 fat

McDonald's

	Amount	Cal.	Fat (g)	% Cal. Fat	Sat. Fat (g)	Chol. (mg)	Sod. (mg)	Carb. (g)	Fiber (g)	Pro. (g)	Servings/Exchanges
BREAKFAST											
Bacon, Egg & Cheese Biscuit	1	460	28	55	9	245	1370	32	1	21	2 starch, 3 high-fat meat
Bacon, Egg & Cheese McGriddles	1	440	21	43	7	240	1270	43	1	19	3 starch, 1 high-fat meat, 2 fat
Big Breakfast	1	700	47	60	13	455	1430	45	3	24	3 starch, 3 high-fat meat, 4 fat
Biscuit	1	240	11	41	2.5	0	640	30	1	4	2 starch, 2 fat
Cinnamon Roll	1	340	15	40	5	35	250	52	3	5	3 1/2 starch, 1 1/2 fat
Deluxe Breakfast	1	1190	61	46	15	470	1990	130	3	30	8 1/2 starch, 3 high-fat meat, 5 1/2 fat

✔ = Healthiest Bets

(*Continued*)

BREAKFAST (*Continued*)	Amount	Cal.	Fat (g)	% Cal. Fat	Sat. Fat (g)	Chol. (mg)	Sod. (mg)	Carb. (g)	Fiber (g)	Pro. (g)	Servings/Exchanges
Egg McMuffin	1	300	12	36	5	235	840	29	2	18	2 starch, 2 medium-fat meat
✓English Muffin	1	150	2	12	0.5	0	260	27	2	5	2 starch
Ham, Egg & Cheese Bagel	1	550	23	38	8	255	1500	28	2	26	2 starch, 3 high-fat meat, 2 fat
✓Hash Browns	1 order	130	8	55	1.5	0	330	14	1	1	1 starch, 1 1/2 fat
Hotcakes (margarine and syrup)	1 order	600	17	26	3	20	770	104	0	9	5 starch, 2 carb, 3 fat
Hotcakes and Sausage	1 order	780	33	38	9	50	1060	104	0	15	7 starch, 2 high-fat meat 3 fat
✓Plain Bagel	1	260	1	3	0	0	520	54	2	9	3 1/2 starch
Sausage	1 order	170	16	85	5	35	290	0	0	6	1 high-fat meat, 1 1/2 fat
Sausage Biscuit	1	410	28	61	8	35	930	30	1	10	2 starch, 1 high-fat meat, 4 fat

Sausage Biscuit w/ Egg	1	490	33	61	10	245	1010	31	1	16	2 starch, 2 high-fat meat, 3 fat
✓Sausage Burrito	1	290	16	50	6	170	680	24	2	13	1 1/2 starch, 1 high-fat meat, 1 1/2 fat
Sausage McGriddles	1	420	23	49	7	35	970	42	1	11	3 starch, 1 high-fat meat, 3 fat
Sausage McMuffin	1	370	23	56	9	50	790	28	2	14	2 starch, 1 high-fat meat, fat
Sausage McMuffin w/ Egg	1	450	28	56	10	260	930	29	2	20	2 starch, 2 high-fat meat, 2 fat
Sausage, Egg & Cheese McGriddles	1	550	33	54	11	260	1290	43	1	20	3 starch, 2 high-fat meat, 3 fat
✓Scrambled Eggs	2	160	11	62	3.5	425	170	1	0	13	2 medium-fat meat
Spanish Omelet Bagel	1	710	40	51	15	275	1520	59	3	27	4 starch, 3 medium-fat meat, 5 fat

✓ = Healthiest Bets

(*Continued*)

BREAKFAST (*Continued*)	Amount	Cal.	Fat (g)	% Cal. Fat	Sat. Fat (g)	Chol. (mg)	Sod. (mg)	Carb. (g)	Fiber (g)	Pro. (g)	Servings/Exchanges
Steak, Egg & Cheese Bagel	1	640	31	44	12	265	1540	57	2	31	4 starch, 4 medium-fat meat, 2 fat
CHICKEN MCNUGGETS											
Chicken McNuggets (10 piece)	1 order	420	24	51	5	60	1120	26	0	25	1 1/2 starch, 3 lean meat, 3 fat
Chicken McNuggets (20 piece)	1 order	840	49	53	11	125	2240	51	0	50	3 1/2 starch, 6 lean meat, 5 fat
Chicken McNuggets (4 piece)	1 order	170	10	53	2	25	450	10	0	10	1/2 starch, 1 lean meat, 1 1/2 fat
Chicken McNuggets (6 piece)	1 order	250	15	54	3	35	670	15	0	15	1 starch, 2 lean meat, 2 fat
CHICKEN MCNUGGETS SAUCES											
Barbeque	2 T	45	0	0	0	0	250	10	0	0	1/2 starch
✓Honey	1 T	45	0	0	0	0	0	12	0	0	1 carb

✔Honey Mustard	2 T	50	5	90	0.5	10	95	3	0	0	1 fat
Hot Mustard	2 T	60	4	60	0	5	240	7	0	0	1/2 carb, 1/2 fat
✔Light Mayonnaise	1 pkg	45	5	100	0.5	10	100	0	0	0	1 fat
✔Sweet 'N Sour	2 T	50	0	0	0	0	140	11	0	0	1/2 carb
Creamy Ranch	5 T	200	21	95	3.5	10	300	3	0	0	0 lean meat, 0 medium-fat meat, 0 high-fat meat, 4 fat
✔Spicy Buffalo	5 T	60	6	90	1	0	910	1	1	0	0 lean meat, 0 medium-fat meat, 0 high-fat meat, 1 fat
✔Tangy Honey Mustard	5 T	70	2	26	0	0	160	13	1	1	1 carb, 0 lean meat, 0 medium-fat meat, 0 high-fat meat
DESSERTS/SHAKES											
Apple Dippers	1 pkg	35	0	0	0	0	0	8	0	0	1/2 carb

✔ = Healthiest Bets

(Continued)

DESSERTS/SHAKES (*Continued*)	Amount	Cal.	Fat (g)	% Cal. Fat	Sat. Fat (g)	Chol. (mg)	Sod. (mg)	Carb. (g)	Fiber (g)	Pro. (g)	Servings/Exchanges
Apple Dippers w/ low fat Caramel Dip	3.2 oz	100	1	9	0.5	5	35	22	0	0	1 1/2 starch
Baked Apple Pie	1	260	13	45	3.5	0	200	34	0	3	1 starch, 1 fruit, 2 1/2 fat
✓Chocolate Chip Cookie	1	160	8	45	2	5	125	22	0	2	1 1/2 carb, 2 fat
Chocolate Triple Thick Shake	12 oz	430	12	25	8	50	210	70	1	11	4 1/2 carb, 2 fat
Chocolate Triple Thick Shake	16 oz	580	17	26	11	65	280	94	1	15	6 carb, 3 fat
Chocolate Triple Thick Shake	21 oz	750	22	26	14	90	360	123	2	19	8 carb, 4 fat
Chocolate Triple Thick Shake	32 oz	1150	33	26	22	135	550	187	3	30	12 1/2 carb, 6 fat
✓Fruit 'n Yogurt Parfait	5.3 oz	160	2	11	1	5	85	30	0	4	2 carb

✓Fruit 'n Yogurt Parfait w/out granola	5.0 oz	130	2	14	1	5	55	25	0	4	1 1/2 carb
Hot Caramel Sundae	6.4 oz	360	10	25	6	35	180	61	0	7	4 carb, 2 fat
Hot Fudge Sundae	6.3 oz	340	12	32	9	30	170	52	1	8	3 1/2 carb, 2 1/2 fat
✓Kiddie Cone	1.0 oz	45	1.5	30	1	5	20	7	0	1	1/2 carb
Low Fat Caramel Dip	2 T	70	1	13	0.5	5	35	14	0	0	1 carb
M&M McFlurry	12 oz	630	23	33	15	75	210	90	1	16	6 carb, 4 1/2 fat
M&M McFlurry	17.8 oz	910	33	33	22	105	300	131	2	23	8 1/2 carb, 6 fat
McDonaldland Chocolate Chip Cookies	2 oz	280	14	45	8	40	170	37	1	3	2 1/2 carb, 3 fat
McDonaldland Cookies	2.0 oz	230	8	31	2	0	250	38	1	3	2 1/2 carb, 1 1/2 fat
Nuts for Sundaes	.3 oz	40	4	90	0	0	55	2	0	2	1 fat
✓Oatmeal Raisin Cookie	1	150	6	36	1	5	100	23	1	2	1 1/2 carb, 1 fat
Oreo McFlurry	16 oz	820	29	32	17	100	420	119	1	22	8 carb, 5 fat

✓ = Healthiest Bets

(*Continued*)

DESSERTS/SHAKES (*Continued*)	Amount	Cal.	Fat (g)	% Cal. Fat	Sat. Fat (g)	Chol. (mg)	Sod. (mg)	Carb. (g)	Fiber (g)	Pro. (g)	Servings/Exchanges
Oreo McFlurry	11.9 oz	570	20	32	12	70	280	82	0	15	5 1/2 carb, 4 fat
Strawberry Sundae	6.3 oz	290	7	22	5	30	95	50	0	7	3 1/2 carb, 1 fat
Strawberry Triple Thick Shake	32 oz	1120	32	26	22	135	380	178	2	28	12 carb, 6 fat
Strawberry Triple Thick Shake	21 oz	730	21	26	14	90	250	116	1	19	7 1/2 carb, 4 fat
Strawberry Triple Thick Shake	16 oz	560	16	26	11	65	190	89	0	14	6 carb, 3 fat
Strawberry Triple Thick Shake	12 oz	420	12	26	8	50	140	67	0	11	4 1/2 carb, 2 fat
✓Sugar Cookie	1	140	6	39	1	10	120	20	0	2	1 1/2 carb, 1 fat
✓Vanilla Reduced Fat Ice Cream Cone	3.2 oz	150	5	30	3	20	75	23	0	4	1 1/2 carb, 1 fat

Vanilla Triple Thick Shake	16 oz	570	16	25	11	65	400	89	0	14	6 carb, 3 fat
Vanilla Triple Thick Shake	32 oz	1140	32	25	22	135	810	178	0	28	12 carb, 6 fat
Vanilla Triple Thick Shake	21 oz	750	21	25	14	90	530	116	0	18	7 1/2 carb, 4 fat
Vanilla Triple Thick Shake	12 oz	430	12	25	8	50	300	67	0	11	4 1/2 carb, 2 fat
FRENCH FRIES											
Large French Fries	1 order	540	26	43	4.5	0	350	68	6	8	4 1/2 starch, 5 fat
McValue French Fries	1 order	320	16	45	2.5	0	210	40	4	5	3 starch, 3 fat
Medium French Fries	1 order	450	22	44	4	0	290	57	5	6	4 starch, 4 fat
✓Small French Fries	1 order	210	10	43	1.5	0	135	26	2	3	1 1/2 starch, 2 fat
Super Size French Fries	1 order	610	29	43	5	0	390	77	7	9	5 starch, 6 fat

✓ = Healthiest Bets

(*Continued*)

	Amount	Cal.	Fat (g)	% Cal. Fat	Sat. Fat (g)	Chol. (mg)	Sod. (mg)	Carb. (g)	Fiber (g)	Pro. (g)	Servings/Exchanges
SALAD DRESSING											
Newman's Own Cobb Dressing	4 T	120	9	68	1.5	10	440	9	0	1	1/2 carb, 2 fat
Newman's Own Creamy Caesar Dressing	2 oz	190	18	85	3.5	20	500	4	0	2	4 fat
Newman's Own Low Fat Balsamic Vinaigrette	3 T	40	3	68	0	0	730	4	0	0	1 fat
Newman's Own Ranch Dressing	4 T	290	30	93	4.5	20	530	4	0	1	6 fat
SALADS											
✓Bacon Ranch w/out Chicken	1	130	8	55	4	25	280	7	3	10	1 veg, 1 high-fat meat
✓Butter Garlic Croutons	.5 oz	50	2	36	0	0	140	8	0	1	1/2 starch

✓Caesar w/out Chicken	1	90	4	40	2.5	10	170	7	3	7	1 veg, 1 medium-fat meat
✓California Cobb w/out Chicken	1	150	9	54	4.5	85	410	7	3	11	1 veg, 1 medium-fat meat, 1 fat
Crispy Chicken Bacon Ranch	1	350	19	49	6	65	1000	20	3	26	1 starch, 1 veg, 3 lean meat, 2 fat
Crispy Chicken Caesar	1	310	16	46	4.5	50	890	20	3	23	1 starch, 1 veg, 3 lean meat, 1 fat
Crispy Chicken California Cobb	1	370	21	51	6	125	1130	20	3	27	1 starch, 1 veg, 3 lean meat, 2 fat
Grilled Chicken Bacon Ranch	1	250	10	36	4.5	85	930	9	3	31	1 veg, 4 lean meat
Grilled Chicken Caesar	1	200	6	27	3	70	820	9	3	29	1 veg, 3 lean meat
Grilled Chicken California Cobb	1	270	11	37	5	145	1060	9	3	33	1 veg, 4 lean meat, 1 fat
✓Side	1	15	0	0	0	0	10	3	1	1	free

✓ = Healthiest Bets

(*Continued*)

	Amount	Cal.	Fat (g)	% Cal. Fat	Sat. Fat (g)	Chol. (mg)	Sod. (mg)	Carb. (g)	Fiber (g)	Pro. (g)	Servings/Exchanges
SANDWICHES											
Big Mac	1	600	33	50	11	85	1050	50	4	25	3 1/2 starch, 2 medium-fat meat, 4 fat
Big N' Tasty	1	540	32	53	10	80	780	38	3	24	2 1/2 starch, 2 medium-fat meat, 2 fat
Big N' Tasty w/ Cheese	1	590	36	55	12	95	1020	39	3	27	2 1/2 starch, 3 medium-fat meat, 4 fat
✓Cheeseburger	1	330	14	38	6	45	790	36	2	15	2 1/2 starch, 1 medium-fat meat, 1 1/2 fat
Chicken McGrill	1	400	16	36	3	70	1020	37	3	27	2 1/2 starch, 3 lean meat, 1 fat
Crispy Chicken	1	510	26	46	4.5	50	1090	47	3	22	3 starch, 2 lean meat, 4 fat

Double Cheeseburger	1	490	26	48	12	85	1220	38	2	25	2 1/2 starch, 2 medium-fat meat, 3 fat
Double Quarter Pounder w/ Cheese	1	770	47	55	20	165	1440	39	3	46	2 1/2 starch, 5 medium-fat meat, 4 fat
✓Filet-O-Fish	1	410	20	44	4	45	660	41	1	15	3 starch, 1 lean meat, 3 fat
✓Hamburger	1	280	10	32	4	30	560	36	2	12	2 1/2 starch, 1 medium-fat meat, 1 fat
Hot n' Spicy McChicken	1	450	26	52	5	45	820	40	1	15	2 1/2 starch, 1 lean meat, 4 1/2 fat
McChicken	1	430	23	48	4.5	45	930	41	3	14	3 starch, 1 lean meat, 3 1/2 fat
Quarter Pounder	1	430	21	44	8	70	770	38	3	23	2 1/2 starch, 2 medium-fat meat, 2 fat
Quarter Pounder w/ Cheese	1	540	29	48	13	95	1240	39	3	29	2 1/2 starch, 3 medium-fat meat, 3 fat

✓ = Healthiest Bets

Sonic, America's Drive-In

❖ Sonic, America's Drive-In, provides nutrition information for all its menu items on its Web site at www.sonicdrivein.com.

Light 'n Lean Choice

Jr. Burger
1/2 Large Tater Tots
1 Low-Fat Milk *(8 oz)*

Calories	637	Sodium (mg)	2,080
Fat (g)	33	Carbohydrate (g)	59
% calories from fat	46	Fiber (g)	3
Saturated fat (g)	10	Protein (g)	22
Cholesterol (mg)	57		

Exchanges: 3 starch, 1 fat-free milk, 2 medium-fat meat, 3 fat

Healthy 'n Hearty Choice

Grilled Chicken Wrap *(without ranch dressing)*
1/2 Onion Rings
1/2 Vanilla Shake

Calories	785	Sodium (mg)	1,157
Fat (g)	24	Carbohydrate (g)	87
% calories from fat	28	Fiber (g)	5
Saturated fat (g)	12	Protein (g)	38
Cholesterol (mg)	88		

Exchanges: 4 1/2 starch, 1 veg, 1 carb, 4 lean meat, 2 fat

Sonic, America's Drive-In

	Amount	Cal.	Fat (g)	% Cal. Fat	Sat. Fat (g)	Chol. (mg)	Sod. (mg)	Carb. (g)	Fiber (g)	Pro. (g)	Servings/Exchanges
ADD-INS											
Blue Coconut Syrup	2 T	65	0	0	0	0	23	16	0	0	1 carb
Cherry Syrup	2 T	64	0	0	0	0	0	16	0	0	1 carb
Chocolate Cone Coat	2 T	143	8	50	7	0	40	16	1	1	1 carb, 1 1/2 fat
Full Flavor Chocolate Syrup	2 T	74	0	0	0	0	52	18	0	0	1 carb
Grape Syrup	2 T	63	0	0	0	0	19	16	0	0	1 carb
Hot Fudge Topping	2 T	101	4	36	3	0	39	16	0	1	1 carb, 1 fat
✓Maraschino Cherry	1	10	0	0	0	0	0	3	0	0	free
Pineapple Topping	2 T	108	0	0	0	0	27	28	0	0	2 carb

✓ = Healthiest Bets

(Continued)

ADD-INS (*Continued*)	Amount	Cal.	Fat (g)	% Cal. Fat	Sat. Fat (g)	Chol. (mg)	Sod. (mg)	Carb. (g)	Fiber (g)	Pro. (g)	Servings/Exchanges
✓Strawberry Topping	3 T	38	0	0	0	0	0	10	1	0	1/2 carb
Vanilla Syrup	2 T	61	0	0	0	0	0	15	0	0	1 carb
Watermelon Syrup	2 T	71	0	0	0	0	28	18	0	0	1 carb
ADD-ONS											
Bacon	1 serving	80	7	79	3	15	330	0	0	5	1 high-fat meat
Cheese	1 serving	70	6	77	4	15	350	1	0	4	1 medium-fat meat
Fat Free Golden Italian Dressing	4 T	50	0	0	0	0	600	13	0	0	1 carb
French Dressing	4 T	240	20	75	3	0	650	14	0	0	1 carb, 4 fat
Honey Mustard Dressing	4 T	110	9	74	1	10	300	9	0	0	1/2 carb, 2 fat
Jalapenos-Nacho sliced	1 serving	5	0	0	0	0	302	1	1	0	free
Light Original Ranch Dressing	4 T	120	7	53	1	15	740	14	0	1	1 carb, 1 1/2 fat

Marinara Sauce	2 T	15	0	0	0	0	260	3	0	0	free
Original Ranch Dressing	4 T	260	28	97	5	20	490	0	0	0	2 1/2 fat
Ranch Dressing	2 T	147	16	98	2	5	215	2	0	0	3 fat
Robuston Creamy Caesar Dressing	4 T	180	17	85	3	15	520	4	0	1	3 1/2 fat
Shredded Cheddar Cheese	2 T	104	9	78	6	28	491	1	0	6	1 high-fat meat
✓Slaw	2 T	45	3	60	0	0	45	4	1	0	1 veg, 1/2 fat
✓Sonic Chili	2 T	52	4	69	2	8	59	1	0	2	1 fat
✓Sonic Green Chiles	2 T	10	0	0	0	0	24	3	0	0	free
Sonic Hickory Barbeque Sauce	4 T	41	0	0	0	0	429	10	0	0	1/2 carb
Southwest Ranch Dressing	4 T	120	7	53	1	15	770	15	0	1	1 carb, 1 1/2 fat
Sweet Pickle Relish	2 T	40	0	0	0	0	248	11	0	0	1/2 carb

✓ = Healthiest Bets

(Continued)

ADD-ONS (*Continued*)	Amount	Cal.	Fat (g)	% Cal. Fat	Sat. Fat (g)	Chol. (mg)	Sod. (mg)	Carb. (g)	Fiber (g)	Pro. (g)	Servings/Exchanges
Thousand Island Dressing	2 T	150	15	90	2	10	170	3	0	0	3 fat
Thousand Island Dressing	4 T	260	25	87	4	30	590	9	0	1	1/2 carb, 5 fat
BREAKFAST											
Breakfast Burrito	1 order	731	47	58	22	167	1535	29	47	19	2 starch, 2 high-fat meat, 7 fat
✓Pancake on a Stick	1 order	240	14	53	7	30	520	22	0	7	1 1/2 starch, 3 fat
Sonic Bacon Egg & Cheese Toaster	1 order	500	29	52	11	156	1698	28	40	96	2 starch, 3 high-fat meat
Sonic Ham Egg & Cheese Toaster	1 order	436	19	39	7	174	2079	33	41	60	2 starch, 2 high-fat meat, 1 fat
Sonic Sausage Egg & Cheese Toaster	1 order	570	36	57	14	126	1038	24	44	123	1 1/2 starch, 4 high-fat meat, 1 fat
Sonic Sunrise	large	368	0	0	0	0	72	100	0	0	6 1/2 carb

Sonic Sunrise	regular	224	0	0	0	0	41	60	0	0	4 carb
Sunshine Smoothie	large	447	9	18	9	23	204	80	3	6	5 carb, 1 1/2 fat
✓Sunshine Smoothie	regular	336	6	16	6	15	136	58	2	4	4 carb, 1 fat
BURGERS											
Bacon Cheeseburger	1	727	49	61	13	67	1433	44	2	23	3 starch, 2 high-fat meat, 6 fat
Jr. Burger	1	353	21	54	6	45	1294	27	1	14	2 starch, 1 high-fat meat, 2 1/2 fat
No. 1 Sonic Burger	1	577	36	56	7	37	753	43	2	14	3 starch, 1 high-fat meat, 5 fat
No. 1 Sonic Cheeseburger	1	647	42	58	11	52	1103	44	2	18	3 starch, 2 high-fat meat, 4 1/2 fat
✓No. 2 Sonic Burger	1	481	25	47	5	29	761	43	2	14	3 starch, 1 high-fat meat, 3 fat
No. 2 Sonic Cheeseburger	1	551	31	51	9	44	1111	44	2	18	3 starch, 2 high-fat meat, 2 1/2 fat

✓ = Healthiest Bets

(Continued)

BURGERS (*Continued*)	Amount	Cal.	Fat (g)	% Cal. Fat	Sat. Fat (g)	Chol. (mg)	Sod. (mg)	Carb. (g)	Fiber (g)	Pro. (g)	Servings/Exchanges
Supersonic No. 1	1	929	66	64	19	96	1476	45	2	28	3 starch, 3 high-fat meat, 8 fat
Supersonic No. 2	1	839	55	59	17	88	1571	46	3	28	3 starch, 3 high-fat meat, 6 1/2 fat
CHICKEN											
Breaded Chicken Sandwich	1	582	23	36	4	53	427	66	2	28	4 1/2 starch, 2 lean meat, 3 fat
Chicken Strip Dinner	1	749	32	38	5	47	1973	86	5	32	5 1/2 starch, 2 lean meat, 5 fat
Chicken Strip Snack	1	272	13	43	2	35	760	22	0	19	1 1/2 starch, 2 lean meat, 1 1/2 fat
Grilled Chicken Sandwich	1	343	13	34	2	70	829	31	2	27	2 starch, 3 lean meat, 1 fat

CONEYS											
✓Corn Dog	1	262	17	58	5	15	480	23	1	6	1 1/2 starch, 1 high-fat meat, 1 1/2 fat
Extra Long Cheese Coney	1	666	42	57	17	87	1648	47	2	23	3 starch, 2 high-fat meat, 5 fat
Extra Long Coney Plain	1	483	27	50	10	50	1162	44	1	14	3 starch, 1 high-fat meat, 4 fat
Regular Cheese Coney	1	366	24	59	10	52	962	24	1	13	1 1/2 starch, 2 high-fat meat, 1 1/2 fat
✓Regular Coney Plain	1	262	16	55	5	30	657	22	1	8	1 1/2 starch, 1 high-fat meat, 1 1/2 fat
FAMOUS SLUSHES											
Large Blue Coconut Slush	1	521	0	0	0	0	27	134	0	0	9 carb
Large Cherry Slush	1	517	0	0	0	0	17	134	0	0	9 carb
Large Grape Slush	1	520	0	0	0	0	24	134	0	0	9 carb

✓ = Healthiest Bets

(Continued)

FAMOUS SLUSHES (*Continued*)	Amount	Cal.	Fat (g)	% Cal. Fat	Sat. Fat (g)	Chol. (mg)	Sod. (mg)	Carb. (g)	Fiber (g)	Pro. (g)	Servings/Exchanges
Large Lemon Berry Slush	1	519	0	0	0	0	14	134	1	0	9 carb
Large Lemon Slush	1	491	0	0	0	0	14	127	0	0	8 1/2 carb
Large Lime Slush	1	497	0	0	0	0	13	129	1	0	8 1/2 carb
Large Orange Slush	1	519	0	0	0	0	10	134	0	0	9 carb
Large Strawberry Slush	1	531	0	0	0	0	10	137	1	0	9 carb
Large Watermelon Slush	1	526	0	0	0	0	31	136	0	0	9 carb
Regular Blue Coconut Slush	1	329	0	0	0	0	18	83	0	0	5 1/2 carb
Regular Cherry Slush	1	327	0	0	0	0	11	83	0	0	5 1/2 carb
Regular Grape Slush	1	329	0	0	0	0	16	83	0	0	5 1/2 carb
Regular Lemon Berry Slush	1	331	0	0	0	0	11	86	1	0	5 1/2 carb

Regular Lemon Slush	1	313	0	0	0	0	11	81	0	0	5 carb
Regular Lime Slush	1	319	0	0	0	0	9	83	1	0	5 1/2 carb
Regular Orange Slush	1	328	0	0	0	0	6	85	0	0	5 1/2 carb
Regular Strawberry Slush	1	334	0	0	0	0	6	86	1	0	5 1/2 carb
Regular Watermelon Slush	1	332	0	0	0	0	21	82	0	0	5 1/2 carb
Rte 44 Blue Coconut Slush	1	718	0	0	0	0	37	185	0	0	12 carb
Rte 44 Cherry Slush	1	713	0	0	0	0	24	184	0	0	12 carb
Rte 44 Grape Slush	1	717	0	0	0	0	33	185	0	0	12 carb
Rte 44 Lemon Berry Slush	1	710	0	0	0	0	20	184	1	0	12 carb
Rte 44 Lemon Slush	1	673	0	0	0	0	20	175	1	0	11 1/2 carb
Rte 44 Lime Slush	1	680	0	0	0	0	17	177	2	0	11 1/2 carb
Rte 44 Orange Slush	1	714	0	0	0	0	14	184	0	0	12 carb
Rte 44 Strawberry Slush	1	728	0	0	0	0	14	188	1	1	12 carb

✔ = Healthiest Bets

(Continued)

FAMOUS SLUSHES (*Continued*)	Amount	Cal.	Fat (g)	% Cal. Fat	Sat. Fat (g)	Chol. (mg)	Sod. (mg)	Carb. (g)	Fiber (g)	Pro. (g)	Servings/Exchanges
Rte 44 Watermelon Slush	1	724	0	0	0	0	42	187	0	0	12 carb
Small Blue Coconut Slush	1	224	0	0	0	0	10	58	0	0	4 carb
Small Cherry Slush	1	223	0	0	0	0	7	58	0	0	4 carb
Small Grape Slush	1	224	0	0	0	0	9	58	0	0	4 carb
Small Lemon Berry Slush	1	233	0	0	0	0	9	60	0	0	4 carb
Small Lemon Slush	1	224	0	0	0	0	9	58	0	0	4 carb
Small Lime Slush	1	225	0	0	0	0	7	59	1	0	4 carb
Small Orange Slush	1	223	0	0	0	0	5	58	0	0	4 carb
Small Strawberry Slush	1	227	0	0	0	0	5	59	0	0	4 carb
Small Watermelon Slush	1	225	0	0	0	0	12	58	0	0	4 carb
Wacky Pack Blue Coconut Slush	1	194	0	0	0	0	10	50	0	0	3 1/2 carb

Wacky Pack Cherry Slush	1	193	0	0	0	0	6	50	0	0	3 1/2 carb
Wacky Pack Grape Slush	1	194	0	0	0	0	9	50	0	0	3 1/2 carb
Wacky Pack Lemon Berry Slush	1	194	0	0	0	0	8	50	0	0	3 1/2 carb
Wacky Pack Lemon Slush	1	194	0	0	0	0	8	50	0	0	3 1/2 carb
Wacky Pack Lime Slush	1	195	0	0	0	0	7	51	1	0	3 1/2 carb
Wacky Pack Orange Slush	1	193	0	0	0	0	4	50	0	0	3 1/2 carb
Wacky Pack Strawberry Slush	1	188	0	0	0	0	4	48	0	0	3 carb
Wacky Pack Watermelon Slush	1	196	0	0	0	0	11	51	0	0	3 1/2 carb
FAVES & CRAVES SIDE ORDERS											
Ched 'R' Peppers	1 order	256	12	42	5	28	1056	29	4	8	2 starch, 2 1/2 fat

✔ = Healthiest Bets

(Continued)

FAVES & CRAVES SIDE ORDERS (*Continued*)	Amount	Cal.	Fat (g)	% Cal. Fat	Sat. Fat (g)	Chol. (mg)	Sod. (mg)	Carb. (g)	Fiber (g)	Pro. (g)	Servings/Exchanges
Fritos Chili Pie	1 order	611	44	65	13	53	816	36	3	18	2 1/2 starch, 1 high-fat meat, 7 fat
Large Cheese Fries	1 order	322	19	53	6	15	1108	31	5	7	2 starch, 4 fat
Large Cheese Tots	1 order	435	27	56	8	15	1708	41	4	4	3 starch, 5 1/2 fat
Large Chili Cheese Fries	1 order	357	22	55	7	2	1062	32	5	8	2 starch, 4 1/2 fat
Large Chili Cheese Tots	1 order	547	36	59	11	37	1844	43	5	9	3 starch, 7 fat
Large French Fries	1 order	252	13	46	2	0	758	30	5	3	2 starch, 2 1/2 fat
Large Onion Rings	1 order	507	7	12	1	0	486	102	10	12	7 starch, 1 1/2 fat
Large Tater Tots	1 order	365	21	52	4	0	1358	40	4	0	3 starch, 4 fat
Mozzarella Sticks	1 order	382	19	45	11	50	1300	35	0	20	2 starch, 2 high-fat meat, 1/2 fat
Regular Cheese Fries	1 order	265	17	58	6	15	998	23	4	6	1 1/2 starch, 3 1/2 fat

Regular Cheese Tater Tots	1 order	329	22	60	7	15	1396	28	3	4	2 starch, 4 1/2 fat
Regular Chili Cheese Fries	1 order	299	19	57	6	22	952	24	4	8	1 1/2 starch, 4 fat
Regular Chili Cheese Tater Tots	1 order	363	25	62	7	22	1350	28	3	5	2 starch, 5 fat
Regular French Fries	1 order	195	11	51	2	0	648	22	4	2	1 1/2 starch, 2 fat
✓Regular Onion Rings	1 order	331	5	14	1	0	311	66	7	8	4 1/2 starch, 1 fat
Regular Tater Tots	1 order	259	16	56	3	0	1046	27	3	0	2 starch, 3 fat
Super Sonic Fries	1 order	358	18	45	3	0	963	44	7	5	3 starch, 3 1/2 fat
Super Sonic Onion Rings	1 order	706	10	13	1	1	788	141	11	16	9 1/2 starch, 2 fat
Super Sonic Tots	1 order	485	28	52	5	0	1670	53	5	0	3 1/2 starch, 5 1/2 fat
FROZEN FAVORITES DESSERTS											
add malt to any shake	2 T	104	1	9	0	0	23	22	0	4	1 1/2 starch
Banana Shake	regular	508	18	32	18	45	363	46	1	10	3 carb, 3 1/2 fat

✓ = Healthiest Bets

(Continued)

FROZEN FAVORITES DESSERTS (*Continued*)	Amount	Cal.	Fat (g)	% Cal. Fat	Sat. Fat (g)	Chol. (mg)	Sod. (mg)	Carb. (g)	Fiber (g)	Pro. (g)	Servings/Exchanges
Banana Shake	large	713	25	32	24	60	485	70	3	13	4 1/2 carb, 5 fat
Banana Split	1	467	11	21	10	23	224	75	3	6	5 carb, 2 fat
Blended Float Drink	large	553	17	28	17	43	373	62	0	9	4 carb, 3 1/2 fat
Blended Float Drink	regular	386	12	28	12	30	260	44	0	6	3 carb, 2 1/2 fat
Chocolate Covered Fruit Shake	large	825	35	38	33	61	534	73	1	13	5 carb, 7 fat
Chocolate Covered Fruit Shake	regular	587	24	37	23	46	393	51	1	10	3 1/2 carb, 5 fat
Chocolate Covered Peanut Butter Shake	regular	678	34	45	25	46	469	50	1	12	3 1/2 carb, 7 fat
Chocolate Covered Peanut Butter Shake	large	1007	54	48	36	61	687	72	2	17	4 1/2 carb, 11 fat
Chocolate Shake	regular	564	18	29	18	45	440	58	0	10	4 carb, 3 1/2 fat

Chocolate Shake	large	752	25	30	24	60	587	77	0	13	5 carb, 5 fat
Chocolate Sundae	1	362	11	27	11	26	270	41	0	6	3 carb, 2 fat
Cream Pie Shake	regular	721	26	32	21	47	474	79	1	11	5 carb, 5 fat
Cream Pie Shake	large	1004	35	31	27	63	636	116	1	15	7 1/2 carb, 7 fat
Dish of Vanilla	1	265	11	37	11	26	212	19	0	5	1 carb, 2 fat
Hot Fudge Sundae	1	392	15	34	15	27	225	40	0	6	3 carb, 3 fat
Ice Cream Cone	1	285	11	35	11	26	223	23	0	6	1 1/2 carb, 2 fat
Pineapple Shake	regular	615	18	26	18	45	403	74	1	9	5 carb, 3 1/2 fat
Pineapple Shake	large	820	24	26	24	60	537	99	1	12	6 1/2 carb, 5 fat
Pineapple Sundae	1	399	11	25	11	26	242	53	0	5	3 1/2 carb, 2 fat
Slush Float Drink	large	608	17	25	17	43	365	75	0	9	5 carb, 3 1/2 fat
Slush Float Drink	regular	423	12	26	12	30	253	52	0	6	3 1/2 carb, 2 1/2 fat
Sonic Blast	regular	658	30	41	23	47	478	52	1	13	3 1/2 carb, 6 fat

✔ = Healthiest Bets

(*Continued*)

FROZEN FAVORITES DESSERTS (*Continued*)	Amount	Cal.	Fat (g)	% Cal. Fat	Sat. Fat (g)	Chol. (mg)	Sod. (mg)	Carb. (g)	Fiber (g)	Pro. (g)	Servings/Exchanges
Sonic Blast	large	963	45	42	32	64	689	78	2	19	5 carb, 9 fat
Strawberry Shake	large	680	24	32	24	60	484	61	1	13	4 carb, 5 fat
Strawberry Shake	regular	510	18	32	18	45	363	46	1	9	3 carb, 3 1/2 fat
Strawberry Sundae	1	322	11	31	11	26	213	32	1	6	2 carb, 2 fat
Vanilla Shake	regular	454	18	36	18	45	363	32	0	9	2 carb, 3 1/2 fat
Vanilla Shake	large	605	24	36	24	60	484	42	0	12	3 carb, 5 fat
KID'S MEAL											
✓Chicken Strips	2	184	9	44	1	23	507	15	0	13	1 starch, 1 lean meat, 1 fat
✓Corn Dog	1	262	17	58	5	15	480	23	1	6	1 1/2 starch, 1 high-fat meat, 1 1/2 fat
Grilled Cheese	1	282	12	38	5	15	830	39	2	12	2 1/2 starch, 1 high-fat meat, 1 fat

Hot Dog Plain	1	262	16	55	5	30	657	22	1	8	1 1/2 starch, 1 high-fat meat, 1 1/2 fat
Jr. Burger	1	353	21	54	6	45	1294	27	1	14	1 1/2 carb, 2 high-fat meat, 1 fat
✓Pancake on a Stick (Sausage 'n Pancake)	1	240	14	53	7	30	520	22	0	7	1 1/2 starch, 1 high-fat meat, 1 fat
Regular French Fries	1	195	11	51	2	0	648	22	4	2	1 1/2 starch, 2 fat
Regular Tots	1	259	16	56	3	0	1046	27	3	0	1 1/2 starch, 3 fat
SALADS AND DRESSING											
Fat Free Golden Italian Dressing	4 T	50	0	0	0	0	600	13	0	0	1 carb
Grilled Chicken Salad	4 T	355	17	43	7	95	807	20	3	33	4 veg, 3 lean meat, 2 fat
Honey Mustard Dressing	4 T	240	21	79	3	15	300	14	0	1	1 carb, 4 fat
Jumbo Popcorn Chicken Salad	1	485	26	48	8	60	1397	39	4	26	1 starch, 4 veg, 3 lean meat, 3 1/2 fat

✓ = Healthiest Bets

(Continued)

SALADS AND DRESSING (*Continued*)	Amount	Cal.	Fat (g)	% Cal. Fat	Sat. Fat (g)	Chol. (mg)	Sod. (mg)	Carb. (g)	Fiber (g)	Pro. (g)	Servings/Exchanges
Light Original Ranch Dressing	4 T	120	7	53	1	15	740	14	0	1	1 carb, 1 1/2 fat
Original Ranch Dressing	4 T	260	28	97	5	20	490	0	0	0	6 fat
Santa Fe Chicken Salad	1	426	18	38	7	95	882	33	6	36	1 starch, 4 veg, 5 lean meat
SANDWICHES AND TOASTER SANDWICHES											
Bacon Cheddar Burger	1	675	38	51	11	59	1786	60	4	26	4 starch, 2 high-fat meat, 4 fat
BLT	1	581	41	64	9	47	1307	42	3	19	3 starch, 1 high-fat meat, 5 1/2 fat
Chicken Club	1	675	29	39	8	85	1458	75	3	39	5 starch, 3 lean meat, 4 fat
Country Fried Steak	1	708	45	57	11	60	944	55	3	26	3 1/2 starch, 2 high-fat meat, 5 fat

Country Fried Steak Sandwich	1	748	47	57	12	60	804	56	2	24	3 1/2 starch, 2 high-fat meat, 6 fat
Grilled Cheese	1	282	12	38	5	15	830	39	2	12	2 1/2 starch, 1 high-fat meat, 1/2 fat
WRAPS											
Chicken Strip Wrap	1	574	29	45	5	28	1071	55	2	20	3 1/2 starch, 1 lean meat, 5 fat
Chicken Strip Wrap w/out Ranch	1	428	13	27	2	23	856	53	2	20	3 1/2 starch, 1 lean meat, 1 1/2 fat
Fritos Chili Cheese Wrap	1	743	42	51	14	52	1172	68	5	23	4 1/2 starch, 1 high-fat meat, 6 1/2 fat
Grilled Chicken Wrap	1	539	27	45	5	70	1035	40	2	29	2 1/2 starch, 3 lean meat, 4 fat
Grilled Chicken Wrap w/out Ranch	1	393	12	27	3	65	820	38	2	29	2 1/2 starch, 3 lean meat, 1/2 fat

✓ = Healthiest Bets

Wendy's

❖ Wendy's provides nutrition information for all its menu items on its Web site at www.wendys.com.

Light 'n Lean Choice

Mandarin Chicken Salad
Roasted Almonds ***(1 pkt)***
Low-Fat Honey Mustard ***(2 T, 1/2 pkt)***
Jr. Frosty

Calories	535	Sodium (mg)	1,055
Fat (g)	20	Carbohydrate (g)	59
% calories from fat	34	Fiber (g)	5
Saturated fat (g)	4.5	Protein (g)	31
Cholesterol (mg)	65		

Exchanges: 2 veg, 2 carb, 3 lean meat, 2 fat

Healthy 'n Hearty Choice

Plain Baked Potato
Chili ***(large)***
Side Salad
Reduced-Fat Creamy Ranch Salad Dressing ***(2 T)***

Calories	655	Sodium (mg)	1,630
Fat (g)	11	Carbohydrate (g)	102
% calories from fat	15	Fiber (g)	18
Saturated fat (g)	4	Protein (g)	35
Cholesterol (mg)	58		

Exchanges: 6 starch, 1 veg, 2 medium-fat meat

Wendy's

	Amount	Cal.	Fat (g)	% Cal. Fat	Sat. Fat (g)	Chol. (mg)	Sod. (mg)	Carb. (g)	Fiber (g)	Pro. (g)	Servings/Exchanges
BAKED POTATOES											
Bacon and Cheese	1	560	25	40	7	35	910	67	7	16	4 1/2 starch, 4 1/2 fat
✔Broccoli and Cheese	1	440	15	31	3	10	540	70	9	10	4 1/2 starch, 3 fat
✔Plain	1	270	0	0	0	0	25	61	7	7	4 starch
✔Sour Cream and Chives	1	340	6	16	3.5	15	40	62	7	8	4 starch, 1 fat
CHICKEN STRIPS AND NUGGETS											
✔Chicken Nuggets	5 pc.	220	14	57	3	35	490	13	0	10	1 starch, 1 lean meat, 2 fat
✔Chicken Nuggets Kids' Meal	4 pc.	180	11	55	2.5	25	390	10	0	8	1/2 starch, 1 lean meat, 1 1/2 fat
Home style Chicken Strips	3 ea.	410	18	40	3.5	60	1470	33	0	28	2 starch, 3 lean meat, 2 fat

✔ = Healthiest Bets

(*Continued*)

	Amount	Cal.	Fat (g)	% Cal. Fat	Sat. Fat (g)	Chol. (mg)	Sod. (mg)	Carb. (g)	Fiber (g)	Pro. (g)	Servings/Exchanges
CHILI AND FIXINGS											
Cheddar Cheese, shredded	2 T	70	6	77	3.5	15	110	1	0	4	1 medium-fat meat
Large Chili	1	300	7	21	3	50	1310	31	7	25	2 starch, 3 lean meat
✔Saltine Crackers	2 ea.	25	1	36	0	0	70	5	0	1	1/2 starch
Small Chili	1	200	5	23	2	35	870	21	5	17	1 1/2 starch, 2 lean meat
FRIES											
Biggie	5.6 oz	440	19	39	3.5	0	380	63	7	5	4 starch, 2 fat
Great Biggie	6.7 oz	530	23	39	4.5	0	450	75	8	6	5 starch, 4 1/2 fat
Kids' Meal	3.2 oz	250	11	40	2	0	220	36	4	3	2 starch, 2 fat
Medium	5.0 oz	390	17	39	3	0	340	56	6	4	3 1/2 starch, 3 1/2 fat

FROSTY											
✓Frosty Junior	6 oz	160	4	23	2.5	15	75	28	0	4	2 carb, 1 fat
Frosty Medium	16 oz	430	11	23	7	45	200	74	0	10	5 carb, 2 fat
Frosty Small	12 oz	330	8	22	5	35	150	56	0	8	3 1/2 carb, 1 1/2 fat
SALADS											
✓Caesar Side	1	70	5	64	2	10	190	2	1	6	1 veg, 1 fat
Chicken BLT	1	360	19	48	9	95	1140	10	4	34	2 veg, 4 medium-fat meat
Home style Chicken Strips	1	450	22	44	9	70	1190	34	5	29	1 1/2 starch, 2 veg, 3 lean meat, 2 1/2 fat
✓Mandarin Chicken	1	190	3	14	1	50	740	17	3	22	1/2 starch, 2 veg, 3 lean meat
✓Side	1	35	0	0	0	0	20	7	3	2	1 veg
✓Spring Mix	1	180	11	55	6	30	230	12	5	11	2 veg, 1 lean meat, 1 1/2 fat
Taco Supremo	1	360	16	40	8	65	1090	29	8	27	1 starch, 2 veg, 3 lean meat, 1 1/2 fat

✓ = Healthiest Bets

(*Continued*)

	Amount	Cal.	Fat (g)	% Cal. Fat	Sat. Fat (g)	Chol. (mg)	Sod. (mg)	Carb. (g)	Fiber (g)	Pro. (g)	Servings/Exchanges
SANDWICHES											
Big Bacon Classic	1	580	29	45	12	95	1430	45	3	33	3 starch, 3 high-fat meat, 1 fat
Cheeseburger Kids' Meal	1	310	12	35	6	45	820	33	1	17	2 starch, 2 medium-fat meat
Classic Single w/ Everything	1	410	19	42	7	70	910	37	2	25	2 1/2 starch, 2 high-fat meat
✓Hamburger Kids' Meal	1	270	9	30	3.5	30	610	33	1	15	2 starch, 1 high-fat meat, 1 fat
Home style Chicken Fillet	1	540	22	37	4	55	1320	57	2	29	3 1/2 starch, 2 lean meat, 3 fat
Jr. Bacon Cheeseburger	1	380	19	45	7	55	830	34	2	20	2 starch, 2 high-fat meat
✓Jr. Cheeseburger	1	310	12	35	6	45	820	34	2	17	2 starch, 1 high-fat meat, 1 fat

Jr. Cheeseburger Deluxe	1	350	15	39	6	45	880	36	2	18	2 starch, 2 high-fat meat
✓Jr. Hamburger	1	270	9	30	3.5	30	610	34	2	15	2 starch, 1 high-fat meat
Spicy Chicken Fillet Sandwich	1	510	19	34	3.5	55	1480	57	2	29	4 starch, 2 lean meat, 2 1/2 fat
Ultimate Grilled Chicken Sandwich	1	360	7	18	1.5	75	1100	44	2	31	3 starch, 2 lean meat, 1/2 fat
TOPPINGS AND DRESSINGS											
✓Barbeque Sauce	1 pkt/4 T	40	0	0	0	0	160	10	0	1	1/2 carb
Caesar Dressing	1 pkt/4 T	150	16	96	2.5	20	240	1	0	1	3 fat
Creamy Ranch Dressing	1 pkt/4 T	230	23	90	4	15	580	5	0	1	5 fat
Crispy Noodles	1 pkt.	60	2	30	0	0	170	10	0	1	1/2 starch
Deli Honey Mustard Sauce	1 pkt.	170	16	85	2.5	15	190	6	0	0	1/2 carb, 3 fat

✓ = Healthiest Bets

(*Continued*)

TOPPINGS AND DRESSINGS (*Continued*)	Amount	Cal.	Fat (g)	% Cal. Fat	Sat. Fat (g)	Chol. (mg)	Sod. (mg)	Carb. (g)	Fiber (g)	Pro. (g)	Servings/Exchanges
Fat Free French Style Dressing	1 pkt/4 T	80	0	0	0	0	210	19	0	0	1 carb
Heartland Ranch Sauce	1 pkt/4 T	200	21	95	3.5	20	280	1	0	0	4 fat
Home style Garlic Croutons	1 pkt	70	3	39	0	0	120	9	0	1	1/2 starch, 1/2 fat
Honey Mustard Dressing	1 pkt/4 T	280	26	84	4	25	350	11	0	1	1 carb, 5 fat
Honey Mustard Sauce	1 pkt/4 T	130	12	83	2	10	220	6	0	0	1/2 carb, 2 fat
Honey Roasted Pecans	1 pkt	130	13	90	12	0	65	5	2	2	2 1/2 fat
House Vinaigrette Dressing	1 pkt/4 T	190	18	85	2.5	0	750	8	0	0	1/2 carb, 3 fat
Low Fat Honey Mustard Dressing	1 pkt/4 T	110	3	25	0	0	340	21	0	0	1 1/2 carb
Oriental Sesame Dressing	1 pkt/4 T	250	19	68	2.5	0	560	19	0	1	1 carb, 3 fat

Reduced Fat Creamy Ranch Dressing	1 pkt/4 T	100	8	72	1.5	15	550	6	1	1	2 fat
Roasted Almonds	1 pkt	130	11	76	1	0	70	4	2	5	2 1/2 fat
Salsa	1 pkt	30	0	0	0	0	440	6	0	1	1 veg
Sour Cream	2 T	60	5	75	3.5	20	20	2	0	1	1 fat
Spicy Southwest Chipotle Sauce	2 T	140	13	84	2	20	170	5	0	0	3 fat
✓Sweet and Sour Sauce	2 T	45	0	0	0	0	120	12	0	0	1 carb
Taco Chips	1 pkt	220	11	45	2	0	200	27	0	3	2 starch, 2 fat

✓ = Healthiest Bets

Chicken—Fried, Roasted, or Grilled

RESTAURANTS

Chick-fil-A
Church's Chicken
El Pollo Loco
KFC

NUTRITION PROS

- No foods greet you at the table. What you order is what you eat. This puts you in the driver's seat.
- There's no waiting for food. You order and then eat.
- You can be in the know. Most large chicken chains provide full disclosure of nutrition information.
- You know the menu well, so you can plan what to order before you walk in the door.
- Order à la carte. That makes it easier for you to order and eat smaller quantities.
- Fried is not the only option in some chicken chains. They've mastered roasting or grilling.
- Healthier side items can fill your plate—corn, green beans, baked beans, rice, potatoes—but make sure they're not swimming in butter or gravy.
- You can sometimes get a salad. But take control: You pour the dressing.

NUTRITION CONS

- Portions are often enough for two people or two meals.

Healthy Tips

- ★ You are better off skinless. If the chicken is served with skin, take the skin off and save some fat grams. You'll also lighten up on cholesterol and saturated fat.
- ★ If there's enough for two meals, ask for a take-out container and split the meal into two before you dig in.
- ★ To keep fat grams and calories down, go with the quarter white meat. Wings and thighs have the most fat.
- ★ If you are going to eat the meal at home, a better buy (price and healthwise) is a whole chicken and several sides. That way you—rather than the server—can decide on your portions.
- ★ Split a quarter of a chicken meal and add an extra side or two. This keeps the protein portion where it should be, about 2–3 ounces.

- Some chicken chains stick to the tried and true, high-fat battered and fried chicken.
- Some side items are sure candidates for the high-fat column: french fries, fried okra, potato salad, coleslaw, and biscuits.
- Some side items hide their fat grams: baked beans, mashed potatoes, and pasta salad.
- Unadulterated cooked vegetables don't appear often.
- Fruit is usually not available unless it's part of a high-fat, high-sugar dessert.

Get It Your Way

- ★ Ask to have the skin removed if you can't trust yourself to do it.
- ★ Ask the server to take the wing off the breast.
- ★ Ask for the gravy, butter, or salad dressing on the side.

Chick-fil-A

❖ Chick-fil-A provides nutrition information for all its menu items on its Web site at www.chickfila.com.

Light 'n Lean Choice

Spicy Chicken Cool Wrap
Waffle Potato Fries *(small, 1/2)*
Fresh Fruit Cup

Calories....................580
Fat (g)........................13
% calories from fat..20
Saturated fat (g)........6
Cholesterol (mg).........68
Sodium (mg)..........1,145
Carbohydrate (g).........85
Fiber (g)......................8
Protein (g)...................33

Exchanges: 2 starch, 1 fruit, 4 lean meat

Healthy 'n Hearty Choice

Chargrilled Chicken Club Sandwich
Carrot and Raisin Salad
Icedream *(small cone)*

Calories....................710
Fat (g)........................21
% calories from fat..27
Saturated fat (g)...........8
Cholesterol (mg).......115
Sodium (mg)..........1,610
Carbohydrate (g).........89
Fiber (g)......................5
Protein (g)...................40

Exchanges: 3 1/2 starch, 1 veg, 2 carb, 4 lean meat, 1/2 fat

Chick-fil-A

	Amount	Cal.	Fat (g)	% Cal. Fat	Sat. Fat (g)	Chol. (mg)	Sod. (mg)	Carb. (g)	Fiber (g)	Pro. (g)	Servings/Exchanges
BEVERAGES											
✓Diet Lemonade	9 oz	25	0	0	0	0	5	5	0	0	free
✓Iced Tea (sweetened)	9 oz	80	0	0	0	0	0	19	0	0	1 carb
Lemonade	9 oz	170	1	5	0	0	10	41	0	0	2 1/2 carb
BREAKFAST BISCUITS											
Chicken	1	400	18	41	4.5	30	1200	43	2	16	3 starch, 2 medium-fat meat, 1/2 fat
Chicken w/ Cheese	1	450	23	46	7	45	1430	43	2	19	3 starch, 2 high-fat meat, 1 1/2 fat
Hot Buttered	1	270	12	40	3	0	680	38	1	4	1 1/2 starch, 2 1/2 fat

✓ = Healthiest Bets

(Continued)

BREAKFAST BISCUITS (*Continued*)	**Amount**	**Cal.**	**Fat (g)**	**% Cal. Fat**	**Sat. Fat (g)**	**Chol. (mg)**	**Sod. (mg)**	**Carb. (g)**	**Fiber (g)**	**Pro. (g)**	**Servings/Exchanges**
Plain	1	260	11	38	2.5	0	670	38	1	4	1 1/2 starch, 2 fat
✓w/ Bacon	1	300	14	42	4	5	780	38	1	6	2 1/2 starch, 1 high-fat meat
w/ Bacon & Egg	1	390	20	46	6	250	860	38	1	13	2 1/2 starch, 1 medium-fat meat, 1 high-fat meat, 1/2 fat
w/ Bacon, Egg & Cheese	1	430	24	50	9	265	1070	38	1	16	2 1/2 starch, 2 medium-fat meat, 1 high-fat meat
✓w/ Egg	1	340	16	42	4.5	245	740	38	1	11	2 1/2 starch, 1 high-fat meat, 1 fat
w/ Egg & Cheese	1	390	21	48	7	260	960	38	1	13	2 1/2 starch, 1 medium-fat meat,1 high-fat meat
w/ Gravy	1	310	13	38	0.5	5	930	44	1	5	3 starch, 1 lean meat, 1/2 fat

w/ Sausage	1	410	23	50	9	20	740	42	1	9	3 starch, 1 high-fat meat, 1 1/2 fat
w/ Sausage & Egg	1	500	29	52	11	265	810	43	1	15	3 starch, 2 high-fat meat, 1 1/2 fat
w/ Sausage, Egg, & Cheese	1	540	33	55	13	280	1030	43	1	18	3 starch, 1 medium-fat meat, 2 high-fat meat, 1/2 fat
BREAKFAST ITEMS											
Danish	1	430	17	36	4.5	25	160	63	2	6	4 starch, 3 1/2 fat
Hash browns	1	170	9	48	4.5	10	350	20	2	2	1 starch, 2 fat
CHARGRILLED CHICKEN SANDWICHES											
Chargrilled Chicken	1	270	3.5	12	1	65	940	33	3	28	2 starch, 3 lean meat
✓Chargrilled Chicken (no bun or pickle)	1	100	2	18	0	65	610	1	0	21	3 lean meat

✓ = Healthiest Bets

(Continued)

CHARGRILLED CHICKEN SANDWICHES (*Continued*)	Amount	Cal.	Fat (g)	% Cal. Fat	Sat. Fat (g)	Chol. (mg)	Sod. (mg)	Carb. (g)	Fiber (g)	Pro. (g)	Servings/Exchanges
Chargrilled Chicken Club (no sauce)	1	380	11	26	5	90	1420	33	3	35	2 starch, 3 lean meat, 1 fat
CHICKEN SANDWICHES											
Chicken	1	410	16	35	3.5	60	1300	38	1	28	2 1/2 starch, 3 lean meat, 1 fat
Chicken w/out butter	1	380	13	31	3	60	1290	37	1	28	2 1/2 starch, 3 lean meat, 1 fat
Chicken (no bun or pickle)	1	230	11	43	2.5	60	990	10	0	23	1/2 starch, 3 lean meat, 1/2 fat
Chicken Deluxe	1	420	16	34	3.5	60	1300	39	2	28	2 1/2 starch, 3 lean meat, 1 1/2 fat
COOL WRAPS											
Chargrilled Chicken	1	390	7	16	3	65	1020	54	3	29	3 1/2 starch, 2 lean meat

Chicken Caesar	1	460	10	20	6	82	1350	52	3	36	3 1/2 starch, 4 lean meat
Spicy Chicken	1	380	6	14	3	60	1090	52	3	30	3 1/2 starch, 2 lean meat
CROUTONS/KERNELS											
✓Garlic & Butter Croutons	1 pkt	50	3	54	0	0	90	6	0	0	1/2 starch, 1/2 fat
Honey Roasted Sunflower Kernels	1 pkt	80	7	79	1	0	38	3	1	2	1 1/2 fat
✓Tortilla Strips	1 pkt	70	4	51	0.5	0	53	9	1	2	1/2 starch, 1 fat
DESSERTS											
Cheesecake	1 slice	340	21	56	12	90	270	30	2	6	2 carb, 4 fat
Cheesecake w/ Blueberry Topping	1 slice	370	21	51	12	90	280	39	2	6	2 1/2 carb, 4 fat
Cheesecake w/ Strawberry Topping	1 slice	360	21	53	12	90	290	38	2	6	2 1/2 carb, 4 fat

✓ = Healthiest Bets

(*Continued*)

DESSERTS (*Continued*)	Amount	Cal.	Fat (g)	% Cal. Fat	Sat. Fat (g)	Chol. (mg)	Sod. (mg)	Carb. (g)	Fiber (g)	Pro. (g)	Servings/Exchanges
Fudge Nut Brownie	1	330	15	41	3.5	20	210	45	2	4	3 carb, 3 fat
Icedream	small cup	230	6	23	3.5	25	100	38	0	5	2 1/2 carb, 1 fat
✓Icedream	small cone	160	4	23	2	15	80	28	0	4	2 carb, 1 fat
Lemon Pie	1 slice	320	10	28	3.5	110	220	51	3	7	3 1/2 carb, 2 fat
DIPPING SAUCES											
✓Barbecue Sauce	2 T	45	0	0	0	0	180	11	0	0	1/2 carb
Buffalo Sauce	2 T	15	2	100	0	0	410	1	0	0	free
Honey Mustard Sauce	2 T	110	12	98	2	5	200	1	0	0	2 1/2 fat
Honey Roasted BBQ Sauce	2 T	60	6	90	1	5	90	2	0	0	1 fat
Polynesian Sauce	2 T	110	6	49	1	0	210	13	0	0	1/2 carb, 1 fat

DRESSINGS											
Blue Cheese Dressing	2 T	150	16	96	3	20	300	1	0	1	3 fat
Buttermilk Ranch Dressing	2 T	160	16	90	2.5	5	270	1	0	0	3 1/2 fat
Caesar Dressing	2 T	160	17	96	2.5	30	240	1	0	1	3 1/2 fat
Fat Free Honey Mustard Dressing	2 T	60	0	0	0	0	200	14	0	0	1 carb
Light Italian Dressing	2 T	15	1	60	0	0	570	2	0	0	free
✔Reduced Fat Raspberry Vinaigrette	2 T	80	2	23	0	0	190	15	0	0	1 carb
Spicy Dressing	2 T	140	14	90	2	5	130	2	0	0	3 fat
Thousand Island	2 T	150	14	84	2	10	250	5	0	0	3 fat

✔ = Healthiest Bets

(Continued)

	Amount	Cal.	Fat (g)	% Cal. Fat	Sat. Fat (g)	Chol. (mg)	Sod. (mg)	Carb. (g)	Fiber (g)	Pro. (g)	Servings/Exchanges
SALADS											
✓Chargrilled Chicken Garden	1	180	6	30	3	65	620	9	3	22	2 veg, 2 lean meat, 1/2 fat
Chick - n - Strips	1	390	18	42	5	80	860	22	4	34	1/2 starch, 2 veg, 4 lean meat, 2 fat
✓Side	1	60	3	45	1.5	10	75	4	2	3	1 veg, 1/2 fat
✓Southwest Chargrilled	1	240	8	30	3.5	60	770	17	5	25	3 veg, 3 lean meat
SIDES											
Carrot & Raisin	1 small	170	6	32	1	10	110	28	2	1	2 veg, 1 fruit, 1 fat
Cole Slaw	1 small	260	21	73	3.5	25	220	17	2	2	1/2 starch, 2 veg, 4 fat
✓Fresh Fruit Cup	medium order	60	0	0	0	0	0	16	2	1	1 fruit

Waffle Potato Fries (salted)	small order	280	14	45	5	15	105	37	5	3	2 1/2 starch, 3 fat
SPECIALTIES											
✓Chick - n - Strips	4	290	13	40	2.5	65	730	14	1	29	1 starch, 4 lean meat
Chicken Nuggets	8	260	12	42	2.5	70	1090	12	0	26	1 starch, 3 lean meat, 1/2 fat
Chicken Salad	1	350	15	39	3	65	880	32	5	20	2 starch, 1 lean meat, 2 1/2 fat
Hearty Breast of Chicken Soup	8 oz	140	4	26	1	25	900	18	1	8	1 starch, 1 1/2 fat

✓ = Healthiest Bets

Church's Chicken

❖ Church's Chicken provides nutrition information for all its menu items on its Web site at www.churchs.com.

Light 'n Lean Choice

Crunchy Tenders *(2)*
Corn on the Cob
Mashed Potatoes and Gravy
Collard Greens

Calories....................528
Fat (g) 16
% calories from fat..27
Saturated fat (g).....n/a
Cholesterol (mg) 50
Sodium (mg) 1,567
Carbohydrate (g).........65
Fiber (g)....................12
Protein (g) 18

Exchanges: 3 1/2 starch, 2 veg, 2 lean meat, 2 fat

Healthy 'n Hearty Choice

Chicken Breast *(fried)*
Corn on the Cob
Cajun Rice
Cole Slaw
Apple Pie *(1/2 slice)*

Calories....................701
Fat (g) 34
% calories from fat..43
Saturated fat (g).....n/a
Cholesterol (mg) 72
Sodium (mg) 1,185
Carbohydrate (g).........72
Fiber (g)....................13
Protein (g) 33

Exchanges: 3 starch, 1 veg, 1 1/2 carb, 3 lean meat, 3 fat

Church's Chicken

	Amount	Cal.	Fat (g)	% Cal. Fat	Sat. Fat (g)	Chol. (mg)	Sod. (mg)	Carb. (g)	Fiber (g)	Pro. (g)	Servings/Exchanges
DESSERTS											
Apple Pie	1 serving	280	12	39	n/a	4	340	41	1	2	3 carb, 2 fat
Edward's Double Lemon Pie	1 serving	300	14	42	n/a	25	160	39	0	5	3 1/2 carb, 3 fat
Edward's Strawberry Cream Cheese Pie	1 serving	280	15	48	n/a	15	130	32	2	4	2 carb, 3 fat
FRIED CHICKEN											
Breast	1 piece	200	12	54	n/a	65	510	4	0	19	3 medium-fat meat
Crunchy Tenders	6-8 pieces	411	15	33	n/a	74	1294	32	1	34	2 starch, 4 lean meat, 1 fat

n/a = not available

(*Continued*)

FRIED CHICKEN (*Continued*)	Amount	Cal.	Fat (g)	% Cal. Fat	Sat. Fat (g)	Chol. (mg)	Sod. (mg)	Carb. (g)	Fiber (g)	Pro. (g)	Servings/Exchanges
Crunchy Tenders	1 piece	137	5	33	n/a	25	431	11	0	11	1 starch, 1 lean meat
Leg	1 piece	140	9	58	n/a	45	160	2	0	13	2 lean meat, 1 fat
Thigh	1 piece	230	16	63	n/a	80	520	5	0	16	2 lean meat, 2 fat
Wing	1 piece	250	16	58	n/a	60	540	8	0	19	1/2 starch, 2 lean meat, 2 fat
FRIED CHICKEN W/OUT BATTER AND SKIN											
Breast	1 piece	145	6	37	n/a	60	480	1	0	21	3 lean meat
Leg	1 piece	118	6	46	n/a	40	145	1	0	14	2 lean meat
Thigh	1 piece	180	11	55	n/a	70	470	3	0	17	2 medium-fat meat, 1/2 fat
Wing	1 piece	160	8	45	n/a	56	475	2	0	20	3 lean meat

SAUCES											
✔BBQ	1 T	29	0	0	n/a	0	181	7	0	0	1/2 carb
Creamy Jalapeno	1 T	102	11	97	n/a	10	137	1	0	0	2 fat
Honey Mustard	1 T	111	11	89	n/a	10	130	4	0	0	2 fat
✔Purple Pepper	1 T	46	0	0	n/a	0	26	12	0	0	1 starch
✔Sweet and Sour	1 T	31	0	0	n/a	0	116	8	0	0	1/2 starch
SIDES											
Cajun Rice	1	130	7	48	n/a	5	260	16	0	1	1 starch, 1 1/2 fat
Chicken Fried Steak w/ White Gravy	1	470	28	54	n/a	65	1615	36	1	21	2 starch, 3 medium-fat meat, 2 fat
Cole Slaw	1	92	6	59	n/a	0	230	8	2	8	1/2 starch, 1 veg, 1 fat
✔Collard Greens	1	25	0	0	n/a	0	170	5	2	2	1 veg
✔Corn on the Cob	1	139	3	19	n/a	0	15	24	9	4	1 1/2 starch, 1/2 fat

✔ = Healthiest Bets; n/a = not available

(*Continued*)

SIDES (*Continued*)	Amount	Cal.	Fat (g)	% Cal. Fat	Sat. Fat (g)	Chol. (mg)	Sod. (mg)	Carb. (g)	Fiber (g)	Pro. (g)	Servings/Exchanges
French Fries	1	210	11	47	n/a	0	60	29	2	3	2 starch, 2 fat
Honey Butter Biscuits	1	250	16	58	n/a	4	640	26	1	2	1 1/2 starch, 3 fat
Jalapeno Cheese Bombers	1	240	10	38	n/a	28	968	29	3	8	2 starch, 1 high-fat meat
Macaroni & Cheese	1	210	11	47	n/a	15	690	23	1	8	1 1/2 starch, 1 high-fat meat
Mashed Potatoes and Gravy	1	90	3	30	n/a	0	520	14	1	1	1 starch, 1/2 fat
Okra	1	210	16	69	n/a	0	520	19	4	3	1 starch, 1 veg, 3 fat
Sweet Corn Nuggets	1	250	12	43	n/a	0	530	30	2	3	2 starch, 2 1/2 fat
✓Whole Jalapeno Peppers	1	10	0	0	n/a	0	390	2	1	0	free

✓ = Healthiest Bets; n/a = not available

El Pollo Loco

❖ El Pollo Loco provides nutrition information for all its menu items on its Web site at www.elpolloloco.com.

Light 'n Lean Choice

Grilled Chicken Breast *(no skin)*
Corn Cobbette
Spanish Rice
Fresh Vegetables
Avocado Salsa *(2 T)*

Calories	447	Sodium (mg)	1,072
Fat (g)	10	Carbohydrate (g)	50
% calories from fat	20	Fiber (g)	5
Saturated fat (g)	2	Protein (g)	36
Cholesterol (mg)	95		

Exchanges: 2 starch, 1 veg, 4 lean meat, 1 fat

Healthy 'n Hearty Choice

Tostada Salad *(without shell)*
Pico de Gallo *(2 T)*
Corn Tortilla *(2 of 3 in order)*
Fresh Vegetables

Calories	632	Sodium (mg)	1,759
Fat (g)	22	Carbohydrate (g)	79
% calories from fat	31	Fiber (g)	14
Saturated fat (g)	7	Protein (g)	41
Cholesterol (mg)	65		

Exchanges: 5 starch, 2 veg, 3 lean meat

(*Continued*)

El Pollo Loco

	Amount	Cal.	Fat (g)	% Cal. Fat	Sat. Fat (g)	Chol. (mg)	Sod. (mg)	Carb. (g)	Fiber (g)	Pro. (g)	Servings/Exchanges
BOWLS											
Chicken Caesar Bowl	1	535	29	49	6	51	1451	47	5	25	2 starch, 2 veg, 3 lean meat, 2 fat
Pollo Bowl	1	543	10	17	1	42	2159	84	12	31	4 starch, 3 veg, 3 lean meat
BURRITOS											
BRC Burrito	1	528	15	26	5	15	1394	79	6	17	5 starch, 1 lean meat, 1 1/2 fat
Chicken Lover's Burrito	1	526	18	31	6	101	1808	55	2	34	3 1/2 starch, 3 lean meat, 2 fat
Classic Chicken Burrito	1	636	19	27	6	63	1749	81	6	32	5 starch, 2 lean meat, 3 fat
Grilled Fiesta Burrito	1	1068	54	46	13	124	3006	91	5	55	6 starch, 5 high-fat meat, 2 fat

Spicy Chicken Burrito	1	555	19	31	6	72	1962	64	6	29	4 starch, 2 lean meat, 2 1/2 fat
Twice Grilled Burrito	1	853	41	43	17	151	2936	62	2	59	4 starch, 7 lean meat, 4 fat
Ultimate Chicken Burrito	1	701	24	31	8	65	2281	84	6	35	5 1/2 starch, 2 lean meat, 3 1/2 fat
DESSERTS											
Caramel Flan	1	303	12	36	11	54	160	43	0	4	3 carb, 1 1/2 fat
✔Churro	1	181	11	55	3	5	221	24	1	3	1 1/2 carb, 1 1/2 fat
✔Foster's Freeze Soft Serve (in cup)	1 order	180	5	25	3	20	100	30	0	4	2 carb, 1/2 fat
DRESSINGS											
Buttermilk Ranch Dressing	3 T	220	24	98	4	10	420	2	0	1	5 fat
Creamy Chipotle Dressing	4 T	269	28	94	4	13	354	3	1	1	5 1/2 fat
Creamy Cilantro Dressing	4 T	275	29	95	4	13	292	1	0	1	6 fat

✔ = Healthiest Bets

(*Continued*)

DRESSINGS (*Continued*)	Amount	Cal.	Fat (g)	% Cal. Fat	Sat. Fat (g)	Chol. (mg)	Sod. (mg)	Carb. (g)	Fiber (g)	Pro. (g)	Servings/Exchanges
Light Italian Dressing	3 T	20	1	45	0	0	780	2	0	0	free
Lite Creamy Cilantro Dressing	4 T	83	7	76	2	8	430	5	0	0	2 fat
Thousand Island Dressing	3 T	220	21	86	3	30	360	7	0	0	4 1/2 fat
FLAME-GRILLED CHICKEN											
✓Breast w/ skin	1 piece	187	7	34	2	128	540	0	0	30	4 lean meat
✓Breast w/out skin	1 piece	153	4	24	1	95	540	0	0	29	4 lean meat
✓Leg	1 piece	86	3	31	0	80	206	0	0	14	2 lean meat
✓Thigh	1 piece	120	7	53	2	82	225	0	0	14	2 lean meat
✓Wing	1 piece	83	3	33	1	58	334	0	0	13	2 lean meat
INDIVIDUAL SIDE DISHES											
Black Beans	1	306	16	47	6	13	731	35	5	7	2 starch, 3 fat

Cole Slaw	1	206	16	70	3	11	358	12	2	2	2 veg, 3 fat
✓Corn Cobbette	1	42	0	0	0	0	7	10	0	1	1/2 starch
French Fries	1	444	19	39	5	0	605	61	0	6	4 starch, 3 fat
✓Fresh Vegetables	1	68	4	53	1	0	78	6	4	3	1 veg, 1/2 fat
✓Garden Salad	1	111	7	57	3	15	271	8	2	5	2 veg, 1 1/2 fat
Macaroni and Cheese	1	381	26	61	16	65	891	25	2	11	1 1/2 starch, 1 high-fat meat, 3 1/2 fat
✓Mashed Potatoes w/ Gravy	1	110	1	8	0	0	406	23	2	2	1 1/2 starch
Pinto Beans	1	154	4	23	0	0	674	24	9	7	1 1/2 starch, 1 fat
✓Spanish Rice	1	161	1	6	0	0	421	33	1	3	2 starch
KIDS' MEALS											
BBQ Sauce	2 T	44	0	0	0	0	226	11	1	0	1/2 carb

✓ = Healthiest Bets

(*Continued*)

KIDS' MEALS (*Continued*)	Amount	Cal.	Fat (g)	% Cal. Fat	Sat. Fat (g)	Chol. (mg)	Sod. (mg)	Carb. (g)	Fiber (g)	Pro. (g)	Servings/Exchanges
Drumstick Chicken	1	86	3	31	0	80	206	0	0	14	2 lean meat
✓French Fries	1	242	10	37	3	0	330	33	0	3	2 starch, 2 fat
✓Popcorn Chicken	1	226	12	48	2	53	787	15	0	17	1 starch, 2 lean meat, 1 fat
LOCO FAVORITES											
Cheese Quesadilla	1	543	26	43	14	60	1177	51	2	22	3 1/2 starch, 2 high-fat meat, 1 1/2 fat
Chicken Nachos	1	1299	77	53	31	202	2340	90	12	65	6 starch, 6 medium-fat meat, 8 fat
Chicken Quesadilla	1	654	30	41	15	108	1530	53	3	38	3 1/2 starch, 4 lean meat, 3 1/2 fat
✓Chicken Soft Taco	1	237	11	42	5	45	526	18	1	17	1 starch, 2 lean meat, 1 fat
✓Chicken Taquitos (2)	1	370	17	41	4	25	690	43	3	15	3 starch, 1 medium-fat meat, 3 fat

✓Taco al Carbon	1	134	3	20	1	29	224	28	1	9	2 starch
POLLO SALADS											
Caesar Pollo	1	535	42	71	7	59	1242	17	4	23	1/2 starch, 2 veg, 3 medium-fat meat, 5 fat
Caesar Pollo w/out dressing	1	221	9	37	2	44	908	15	4	22	3 veg, 3 lean meat
Fiesta Pollo	1	747	57	69	15	97	1654	29	5	31	1 starch, 3 veg, 4 medium-fat meat, 6 1/2 fat
Fiesta Pollo w/out dressing	1	439	26	53	11	82	1249	26	4	30	1/2 starch, 3 veg, 4 lean meat
Monterrey Pollo	1	258	13	45	3	52	1266	17	3	22	1/2 starch, 2 veg, 3 lean meat, 1/2 fat
Monterrey Pollo w/out dressing	1	176	6	31	1	44	836	12	3	22	2 veg, 3 lean meat

✓ = Healthiest Bets

(*Continued*)

POLLO SALADS (*Continued*)	Amount	Cal.	Fat (g)	% Cal. Fat	Sat. Fat (g)	Chol. (mg)	Sod. (mg)	Carb. (g)	Fiber (g)	Pro. (g)	Servings/Exchanges
Tostada	1	740	33	40	9	65	1823	83	11	34	4 1/2 starch, 3 veg, 3 lean meat, 3 fat
Tostada w/out shell	1	414	16	35	6	65	1479	42	7	29	1 1/2 starch, 3 veg, 3 lean meat, 1 1/2 fat
SALSAS AND MORE											
✓Avocado Salsa	2 T	18	1	50	0	0	26	1	0	0	free
✓Fried Serrano Pepper	1 T	23	1	39	0	0	2	3	0	0	1/2 starch
Guacamole	3 T	51	3	53	0	0	272	5	0	0	1 fat
✓House Salsa	2 T	6	0	0	0	0	87	1	0	0	free
✓Jalapeno Hot Sauce	1 pkt.	3	0	0	0	0	112	0	0	0	free
✓Ketchup	1 pkt.	10	0	0	0	0	100	2	0	0	free
Pico de Gallo Salsa	2 T	10	0	0	0	0	136	1	0	0	free

Sour Cream	3 T	104	10	87	7	22	26	2	0	2	2 fat
✔Spicy Chipotle Salsa	2 T	7	0	0	0	0	180	1	0	0	free
Tortilla Chips	2 oz	304	17	50	4	0	430	34	3	4	2 starch, 3 fat
TORTILLAS FOR CHICKEN MEALS											
✔6.0″ Corn Tortilla (3)	3 oz	210	3	13	0	0	105	42	3	3	3 starch
✔6.5″ Flour Tortilla (3)	3 oz	330	12	33	3	0	630	48	3	9	3 starch, 2 fat

✔ = Healthiest Bets

KFC

❖ KFC provides nutrition information for all its menu items on its Web site at www.kfc.com.

Light 'n Lean Choice

Original Drumsticks *(2)*
Corn on the Cob *(large)*
Green Beans

Calories	480	Sodium (mg)	1,350
Fat (g)	21	Carbohydrate (g)	35
% calories from fat	40	Fiber (g)	9
Saturated fat (g)	6	Protein (g)	40
Cholesterol (mg)	155		

Exchanges: 2 1/2 starch, 1 veg, 4 lean meat, 1 1/2 fat

Healthy 'n Hearty Choice

Original Chicken Breast
BBQ Beans
Macaroni and Cheese

Calories	740	Sodium (mg)	2,480
Fat (g)	26	Carbohydrate (g)	72
% calories from fat	32	Fiber (g)	8
Saturated fat (g)	9	Protein (g)	53
Cholesterol (mg)	150		

Exchanges: 4 starch, 5 lean meat, 3 fat

KFC

	Amount	Cal.	Fat (g)	% Cal. Fat	Sat. Fat (g)	Chol. (mg)	Sod. (mg)	Carb. (g)	Fiber (g)	Pro. (g)	Servings/Exchanges
CHICKEN											
Boneless Wings in HBBQ Sauce (7)	1 order	600	26	39	5	75	1950	49	2	35	3 starch, 4 lean meat, 3 fat
Chicken Pot Pie	1	770	40	47	15	115	1680	70	5	33	4 1/2 starch, 2 lean meat, 6 1/2 fat
Crispy Strips (3)	1 order	400	24	54	5	75	1250	17	0	29	1 starch, 4 lean meat, 2 1/2 fat
Extra Crispy Breast	1	460	28	55	8	135	1230	19	0	34	1 starch, 4 lean meat, 1 1/2 fat
✓Extra Crispy Drumstick	1	160	10	56	2.5	70	420	5	0	12	2 lean meat, 1 fat
Extra Crispy Thigh	1	370	26	63	7	120	710	12	0	21	1 starch, 2 lean meat, 4 fat

✓ = Healthiest Bets

(*Continued*)

CHICKEN (*Continued*)	Amount	Cal.	Fat (g)	% Cal. Fat	Sat. Fat (g)	Chol. (mg)	Sod. (mg)	Carb. (g)	Fiber (g)	Pro. (g)	Servings/Exchanges
✓Extra Crispy Whole Wing	1	190	12	57	4	55	390	10	0	10	1/2 starch, 1 lean meat, 2 1/2 fat
Hot and Spicy Breast	1	460	27	53	8	130	1450	20	0	33	1 starch, 4 lean meat, 3 1/2 fat
✓Hot and Spicy Drumstick	1	160	9	51	2.5	65	380	4	0	13	2 lean meat, 1 fat
Hot and Spicy Thigh	1	400	28	63	8	125	1240	14	0	22	1 starch, 3 lean meat, 3 1/2 fat
Hot and Spicy Wing	1	180	11	55	3	60	420	9	0	11	1/2 starch, 1 lean meat, 2 fat
Hot Wings (6)	1	450	29	58	6	145	1120	23	1	24	1 1/2 starch, 3 lean meat, 3 1/2 fat
Individual Popcorn	1	450	30	60	7	50	1030	25	0	19	1 1/2 starch, 2 lean meat, 5 fat
✓Kids Popcorn	1	270	18	60	4	30	640	16	0	12	1 starch, 1 lean meat, 3 fat
Large Popcorn	1	660	44	60	10	75	1530	37	0	29	2 1/2 starch, 3 lean meat, 6 1/2 fat

Original Breast	1	380	19	45	6	145	1150	11	0	40	1 starch, 5 lean meat, 1 1/2 fat
✓Original Breast w/out skin or breading	1	140	3	19	1	95	410	0	0	29	4 lean meat
✓Original Drumstick	1	140	8	51	2	75	440	4	0	14	2 lean meat, 1 fat
Original Thigh	1	360	25	63	7	165	1060	12	0	22	1 starch, 3 lean meat, 3 fat
✓Original Whole Wing	1	150	9	54	2.5	60	370	5	0	11	1 lean meat, 2 fat
Wings in HBBQ Sauce (6)	1 order	540	33	55	7	150	1130	36	1	25	2 starch, 3 lean meat, 5 fat
DESSERTS											
Apple Pie Slice	1	270	9	30	2	0	200	45	4	3	2 carb, 1 fruit, 1 fat
Cherry Cheesecake Parfait	1	300	11	33	5	4	130	46	2	3	3 carb, 1 1/2 fat
Double Chocolate Chip Cake	1	400	29	65	5	45	230	31	2	4	2 carb, 5 1/2 fat

✓ = Healthiest Bets

(*Continued*)

DESSERTS (*Continued*)	Amount	Cal.	Fat (g)	% Cal. Fat	Sat. Fat (g)	Chol. (mg)	Sod. (mg)	Carb. (g)	Fiber (g)	Pro. (g)	Servings/Exchanges
Lemon Meringue Pie	1	310	11	32	5	40	160	47	3	5	3 carb, 1 1/2 fat
Lil' Bucket Chocolate Cream	1	270	13	43	8	0	180	37	2	2	2 1/2 starch, 2 fat
Lil' Bucket Fudge Brownie	1	270	9	30	4	30	170	44	1	2	3 carb, 2 fat
Lil' Bucket Lemon Crème	1	400	14	32	7	5	210	65	2	4	4 carb, 3 fat
Lil' Bucket Strawberry Short Cake	1	200	6	27	4	20	110	34	0	2	2 carb, 1 fat
Pecan Pie Slice	1	370	15	36	2.5	40	190	55	2	4	3 1/2 carb, 2 1/2 fat
Strawberry Crème Pie Slice	1	270	12	40	7	10	200	37	0	3	2 1/2 carb, 2 fat

SANDWICHES											
✔HBBQ	1	300	6	18	1.5	50	640	41	4	21	3 starch, 2 lean meat
Original w/ sauce	1	450	27	54	6	65	1010	22	0	29	1 1/2 starch, 3 lean meat, 3 1/2 fat
Original w/out sauce	1	320	13	37	4	60	890	21	0	29	1 1/2 starch, 3 lean meat, 1 fat
TC w/out sauce	1	540	26	43	6	75	1510	41	1	35	3 starch, 4 lean meat, 2 1/2 fat
TC w/ sauce	1	670	40	54	8	80	1640	42	1	36	3 starch, 4 lean meat, 5 fat
TR w/ sauce	1	390	19	44	4	70	810	24	1	31	1 1/2 starch, 4 lean meat, 1 1/2 fat
✔TR w/out sauce	1	260	5	17	1.5	65	690	23	1	31	1 1/2 starch, 4 lean meat, 1/2 fat
Twister	1	670	38	51	7	60	1650	55	3	21	3 1/2 starch, 2 lean meat, 6 fat
Zinger w/ sauce	1	680	41	54	8	90	1650	42	1	35	3 starch, 4 lean meat, 5 fat
Zinger w/out sauce	1	540	26	43	6	75	1510	41	1	35	3 starch, 4 lean meat, 2 fat
SIDE DISHES											
BBQ Beans	1	230	1	4	1	0	720	46	7	8	3 starch

✔ = Healthiest Bets

(Continued)

SIDE DISHES (*Continued*)	Amount	Cal.	Fat (g)	% Cal. Fat	Sat. Fat (g)	Chol. (mg)	Sod. (mg)	Carb. (g)	Fiber (g)	Pro. (g)	Servings/Exchanges
Biscuit	1	190	10	47	2	2	580	23	0	2	1 1/2 starch, 2 fat
Cole Slaw	1	190	11	52	2	5	300	22	3	1	1 starch, 2 veg, 2 fat
✓Corn on the Cob 3″	1	70	2	26	0.5	0	5	13	3	2	1 starch
✓Corn on the Cob 5.5″	1	150	3	18	1	0	10	26	7	5	2 starch
✓Green Beans	1	50	2	36	0.5	5	460	5	2	5	1 veg, 1/2 fat
Mac and Cheese	1	130	6	42	2	5	610	15	1	5	1 starch, 1 medium-fat meat
✓Mashed Potatoes w/ Gravy	1	120	5	38	1	0	380	18	1	2	1 starch, 1 fat
✓Mashed Potatoes w/out Gravy	1	110	4	33	1	0	260	16	1	2	1 starch, 1/2 fat
Potato Salad	1	180	9	45	1.5	5	470	22	1	2	1 1/2 starch, 2 fat
Potato Wedges (small)	1	240	12	45	3	0	830	30	3	1	2 starch, 2 fat

✓ = Healthiest Bets

Seafood Catches

RESTAURANTS

Captain D's
Long John Silver's
Red Lobster

NUTRITION PROS

- Fish and seafood are naturally low in total and saturated fat and low in calories.
- During the years of nutrition and health consciousness, some fast-food restaurants began to bake, broil, or grill seafood. Today, Red Lobster is offering some healthier items under its LightHouse fare.
- Some healthy sides are available: baked potatoes, rice, salad, and cooked vegetables.

NUTRITION CONS

- The nutritional virtues of fish and seafood are lost in most chain seafood restaurants because their favorite preparation method is frying.
- After fish and seafood have been battered and fried, you wonder what happened to the fish. When you read the nutrition numbers, there's not much fish to speak of.
- Fried fish is often surrounded by high-fat plate fillers—hush puppies, french fries, or creamy coleslaw. Thus, the once-healthy seafood is now part of a fat- and calorie-dense meal.

- Seafood restaurants load their starches—hush puppies, biscuits, cornbread, french fries, etc.—with fat.
- Fruit is nowhere to be found.

Healthy Tips

★ If you order a baked potato, have butter and sour cream held or served on the side.
★ Lemon is plentiful. Use it to add flavor without calories.
★ Use low-fat, low-calorie cocktail sauce to add flavor without extra calories. Substitute this for higher calorie tartar sauce.
★ Not all coleslaw is created equal. Some is high in fat, and some is relatively low. Check the nutrition numbers to know the score in the restaurant you choose.

Get It Your Way

★ Hold the tartar sauce and opt for lemon or vinegar.
★ Substitute a baked potato or rice for french fries or hush puppies.
★ Substitute a cooked vegetable, such as green beans or corn, for french fries.
★ Substitute breadsticks or a yeast roll for biscuits or corn bread if you have the option.

Captain D's

❖ Captain D's provides nutrition information only for its Lighter Fare menu items on its Web site, www.captainds.com.

Light 'n Lean Choice

Baked Fish Dinner *(with rice, broccoli, and vegetables)*
Breadstick

Calories	540	Sodium (mg)	900
Fat (g)	11	Carbohydrate (g)	71
% calories from fat	18	Fiber (g)	6
Saturated fat (g)	3	Protein (g)	39
Cholesterol (mg)	15		

Exchanges: 4 starch, 2 veg, 5 very lean meat

Healthy 'n Hearty Choice

Baked Salmon Dinner *(with rice, broccoli, and vegetables)*
Corn on the Cob

Calories	620	Sodium (mg)	960
Fat (g)	11	Carbohydrate (g)	92
% calories from fat	16	Fiber (g)	7
Saturated fat (g)	0	Protein (g)	46
Cholesterol (mg)	30		

Exchanges: 5 starch, 2 veg, 4 very lean meat, 1 fat

(*Continued*)

Captain D's

	Amount	Cal.	Fat (g)	% Cal. Fat	Sat. Fat (g)	Chol. (mg)	Sod. (mg)	Carb. (g)	Fiber (g)	Pro. (g)	Servings/Exchanges
CARB COUNTERS											
Baked Chicken Dinner (1 piece)	1	320	15	42	2.5	70	1010	19	6	27	1 starch, 4 lean meat
✓Baked Fish Dinner (3 pieces)	1	350	17	44	2	20	880	19	6	33	1 starch, 4 lean meat, 1 fat
LOW-CAL FARE											
✓Baked Chicken Dinner (1 piece)	1	350	4	10	0.6	60	880	49	5	30	3 starch, 3 lean meat
✓Baked Fish Dinner (3 pieces)	1	390	5	12	0	10	750	49	5	36	2 1/2 starch, 4 lean meat
✓Baked Salmon Dinner (1 piece)	1	470	8	15	0	30	940	58	5	40	4 starch, 4 lean meat

✓Baked Scampi Dinner (10 pieces)	1	370	5	12	0.6	170	340	50	5	29	3 1/2 starch, 3 lean meat
SIDE DISHES											
✓Baked Potato	1	190	0	0	0	0	15	44	4	4	3 starch
Breadstick	1	150	6	36	2	5	150	22	1	3	1 1/2 starch, 1 fat
Cole Slaw	1	170	12	64	1.5	10	305	13	2	1	1/2 starch, 1 1/2 veg, 2 fat
✓Corn on the Cob	1	150	3	18	0	0	20	34	2	5	2 starch, 1/2 fat
✓Fresh Steamed Broccoli	1	25	1	36	0	0	25	5	3	3	1 veg
✓Green Beans	1	90	3	30	1	5	505	15	4	2	1/2 starch, 1 veg, 1/2 fat
Rice Pilaf	1	160	1	6	0	0	625	35	1	4	2 starch
✓Side Salad w/out dressing	1	30	1	30	0	0	20	6	2	2	1 veg
✓Tuscan-Style Vegetables	1	30	0	0	0	0	10	7	2	1	1 veg

✓ = Healthiest Bets

Long John Silver's

❖ Long John Silver's provides nutrition information for its menu items on its Web site at www.longjohnsilvers.com.

Light 'n Lean Choice

Baked Cod *(1 piece)*
Corn Cobbette
Rice
Cole Slaw *(1/2 serving)*

Calories	490	Sodium (mg)	950
Fat (g)	19	Carbohydrate (g)	56
% calories from fat	35	Fiber (g)	10
Saturated fat (g)	4	Protein (g)	19
Cholesterol (mg)	10		

Exchanges: 3 starch, 1 veg, 3 very lean meat, 3 fat

Healthy 'n Hearty Choice

Clam Chowder
Baked Cod
Corn Cobbette
Hush Puppies *(3)*

Calories	610	Sodium (mg)	1,650
Fat (g)	24	Carbohydrate (g)	64
% calories from fat	36	Fiber (g)	7
Saturated fat (g)	7	Protein (g)	24
Cholesterol (mg)	115		

Exchanges: 4 starch, 4 very lean meat, 3 fat

Long John Silver's

	Amount	Cal.	Fat (g)	% Cal. Fat	Sat. Fat (g)	Chol. (mg)	Sod. (mg)	Carb. (g)	Fiber (g)	Pro. (g)	Servings/Exchanges
CHICKEN											
✓Battered Chicken	1 piece	140	8	51	2.5	20	400	9	0	8	1/2 starch, 1 high-fat meat
DESSERTS											
Chocolate Cream Pie	1	310	22	64	14	15	170	24	1	5	1 1/2 carb, 4 fat
Pecan Pie	1	370	15	36	2.5	40	190	55	2	4	3 1/2 carb, 3 fat
Pineapple Cream Pie	1	290	13	40	7	15	210	39	1	4	2 1/2 starch, 2 fat
FISH AND SEAFOOD											
✓Baked Cod	1 piece	120	5	38	1	90	240	0	1	22	3 lean meat

✓ = Healthiest Bets

(*Continued*)

FISH AND SEAFOOD (*Continued*)	Amount	Cal.	Fat (g)	% Cal. Fat	Sat. Fat (g)	Chol. (mg)	Sod. (mg)	Carb. (g)	Fiber (g)	Pro. (g)	Servings/Exchanges
Battered Fish	1 piece	230	13	51	4	30	700	16	0	11	1 starch, 1 lean meat, 2 fat
Battered Shrimp	1 piece	45	3	60	1	15	125	3	0	2	1 fat
Breaded Clams	1 order	240	13	49	2	10	1110	22	1	8	1 1/2 starch, 1 lean meat, 1 1/2 fat
Crunchy Shrimp Basket	22 pieces	330	18	49	5	105	700	31	2	12	2 starch, 2 lean meat, 2 fat
SANDWICHES											
Chicken	1	360	15	38	3.5	25	810	41	3	13	3 starch, 1 lean meat, 1 1/2 fat
Fish	1	440	20	41	5	35	1120	48	3	17	3 starch, 2 lean meat, 3 fat
Ultimate Fish	1	500	25	45	8	50	1310	48	3	20	3 starch, 2 lean meat, 3 1/2 fat

SIDES AND STARTERS											
Cheese sticks	3	140	8	51	2	10	320	12	1	4	1 starch, 1 1/2 fat
✓Clam Chowder	1	220	10	41	4	25	810	23	0	9	1/2 starch, 1 milk, 2 fat
Corn Cobbette	1	90	3	30	0.5	0	0	14	3	3	1 starch
Crumblies	1	170	12	64	2.5	0	420	14	1	1	1 starch, 2 fat
✓Hushpuppies	1	60	3	45	0.5	0	200	9	1	1	1/2 starch, 1 fat
Large Fries	1	390	17	39	4	0	580	56	5	4	3 1/2 starch, 3 fat
Regular Fries	1	230	10	39	2.5	0	350	34	3	3	2 starch, 2 fat
✓Rice	1	180	4	20	1	0	540	34	3	3	2 starch, 1/2 fat
Slaw	1	200	15	68	2.5	20	340	15	3	1	1/2 starch, 2 veg, 3 fat

✓ = Healthiest Bets

Red Lobster

❖ Red Lobster provides some nutrition information for its LightHouse Selections (healthier offerings) on its Web site, www.redlobster.com. Red Lobster does not provide nutrition information for its regular menu. Insufficient information is available to determine healthiest bets.

Light 'n Lean Choice

(from LightHouse Selections Menu)
Jumbo Shrimp Cocktail Appetizer *(ask for as main course)*
Garden Salad with Red Wine Vinaigrette
Wild Rice Pilaf
Buttered Fresh Vegetables

Calories........................598
Fat (g) 21
% calories from fat..32
Saturated fat (g).....n/a
Cholesterol (mg).........n/a
Sodium (mg)..............n/a
Carbohydrate (g).........64
Fiber (g)......................5
Protein (g)..................n/a

Exchanges: Insufficient information provided to calculate.

Healthy 'n Hearty Choice

(from LightHouse Selections Menu)
King Crab Legs with Melted Butter *(1 serving)*
Baked Potato with Pico de Gallo
Seasoned Broccoli
Garden Salad with Red Wine Vinaigrette

Calories	692	Sodium (mg)	n/a
Fat (g)	31	Carbohydrate (g)	63
% calories from fat	40	Fiber (g)	10
Saturated fat (g)	n/a	Protein (g)	n/a
Cholesterol (mg)	n/a		

Exchanges: Insufficient information provided to calculate.

(Continued)

Red Lobster

	Amount	Cal.	Fat (g)	% Cal. Fat	Sat. Fat (g)	Chol. (mg)	Sod. (mg)	Carb. (g)	Fiber (g)	Pro. (g)	Servings/Exchanges
ACCOMPANIMENTS											
Baked Potato	1	179	2	10	n/a	n/a	n/a	36	4	n/a	2 starch
Baked Potato with Pico de Gallo	1	185	2	10	n/a	n/a	n/a	37	4	n/a	2 starch
Fresh Buttered Vegetables	1	143	12	76	n/a	n/a	n/a	9	3	n/a	2 veg, 2 fat
Seasoned Broccoli	1	60	0	0	n/a	n/a	n/a	12	5	n/a	2 veg
Wild Rice Pilaf	1	208	5	22	n/a	n/a	n/a	36	2	n/a	2 starch, 1 fat
DIPPING SAUCES											
Large Cocktail Sauce	1 serving	68	0	0	n/a	n/a	n/a	17	0	n/a	1 carb
Lemon Wedge	1	8	0	0	n/a	n/a	n/a	2	0	n/a	free

ENTREES

Broiled Founder	1	240	5	19	n/a	n/a	n/a	0	0	n/a	insufficient info. to calculate
Grilled Chicken	1	528	14	24	n/a	n/a	n/a	38	2	n/a	insufficient info. to calculate
Jumbo Shrimp Cocktail Dinner	1	243	3	11	n/a	n/a	n/a	2	0	n/a	insufficient info. to calculate
King Crab Legs	1	490	9	17	n/a	n/a	n/a	0	0	n/a	insufficient info. to calculate
Live Maine Lobster	1	145	1	6	n/a	n/a	n/a	2	0	n/a	insufficient info. to calculate
Rainbow Trout (dinner portion)	1	512	25	44	n/a	n/a	n/a	6	0	n/a	insufficient info. to calculate
Rainbow Trout (lunch portion)	1	273	14	46	n/a	n/a	n/a	2	0	n/a	insufficient info. to calculate

✔ = Healthiest Bets; n/a = not available

(*Continued*)

ENTREES (*Continued*)	Amount	Cal.	Fat (g)	% Cal. Fat	Sat. Fat (g)	Chol. (mg)	Sod. (mg)	Carb. (g)	Fiber (g)	Pro. (g)	Servings/Exchanges
Rock Lobster Tail	1	258	3	10	n/a	n/a	n/a	2	0	n/a	insufficient info. to calculate
Salmon (dinner portion)	1	578	31	48	n/a	n/a	n/a	0	0	n/a	insufficient info. to calculate
Salmon (lunch portion)	1	258	12	42	n/a	n/a	n/a	0	0	n/a	insufficient info. to calculate
Snow Crab Legs	1	262	4.5	15	n/a	n/a	n/a	0	0	n/a	insufficient info. to calculate
Tilapia (dinner portion)	1	186	6	29	n/a	n/a	n/a	0	0	n/a	insufficient info. to calculate
Tilapia (lunch portion)	1	346	10	26	n/a	n/a	n/a	0	0	n/a	insufficient info. to calculate
GREAT SHELLFISH ADDITIONS											
King Crab Legs	1	163	3	17	n/a	n/a	n/a	0	0	n/a	insufficient info. to calculate

Maine Lobster Tail	1	104	5	43	n/a	n/a	n/a	2	0	n/a	insufficient info. to calculate
Snow Crab Legs	1	129	2	14	n/a	n/a	n/a	0	0	n/a	insufficient info. to calculate
STARTERS AND SALAD											
Cheddar Bay Biscuits	1 order	160	9	51	n/a	n/a	n/a	17	0	n/a	insufficient info. to calculate
Garden Salad	1	52	2	35	n/a	n/a	n/a	9	0	n/a	insufficient info. to calculate
Jumbo Shrimp Cocktail	1	146	2	12	n/a	n/a	n/a	2	0	n/a	insufficient info. to calculate
Petite Shrimp Topping	1	30	1	30	n/a	n/a	n/a	1	0	n/a	insufficient info. to calculate
Red Wine Vinaigrette Dressing	1 serving	49	3	55	n/a	n/a	n/a	5	0	n/a	insufficient info. to calculate

✓ = Healthiest Bets; n/a = not available

Sit-Down Family Fare

RESTAURANTS

Bob Evans Restaurants

Boston Market

Chili's Grill & Bar

Denny's

Ruby Tuesday

Note: Nutrition information provided by most restaurants in this category is far from complete. You might not find a few large chains you expect to see in this chapter because they don't provide nutrition information for their complete menu.

NUTRITION PROS

- Many sit-down American restaurants have added healthier options to their menus.
- You can pick and choose among the appetizers, salads, soups, and side dishes to put together healthy, portion-controlled meals.
- Healthier preparation methods are available—stir-frying, grilling, and blackening.
- Time and a desire to please is on your side. This makes special requests easier for you and possible for the kitchen.
- Portions are large, but take-home containers are at the ready.
- Some of these restaurants serve their breakfast-to-dinner menu 24 hours a day. This puts variety on your side.

- These restaurants hardly limit their menu to American specialties. They globe trot to bring you Mexican fajitas or salads, Italian pastas or pizzas, and Chinese pot stickers or stir-fry dishes. This helps to widen the variety of healthier choices.
- Raw and cooked vegetables are easier to find here than in fast-food restaurants. Just be careful they aren't drenched in fat or fried.
- Condiments to help you add taste without fat might be found in the kitchen—teriyaki or soy sauce, lemons, limes, a variety of vinegars, ketchup, barbecue sauce, and low-calorie salad dressings. Ask, and maybe you'll receive.

NUTRITION CONS

- Bread, rolls, crackers, or breadsticks and butter might greet you at the table.
- These restaurants love to fry—from fried mozzarella sticks to fried shrimp, chicken fingers, french fries, and onion rings.
- Sandwiches and other entrees may be accompanied by french fries, onion rings, potato chips, or creamy coleslaw.
- Some foods get a healthy start—vegetables, potatoes, or pasta. But then they are drenched in salad dressing or cheese sauce, or dropped a foot deep in oil and fried.
- Salads can start off healthy but end up with high-fat toppers—avocado, cheese, bacon, or croutons.
- Portions are frequently too big . . . many are way too big.
- Plain fruit is often not available. The apples buried between a double crust are not the healthiest way to count your fruits.

- Cheese is in, on, and around a startling number of menu items—melted cheese on a sandwich or cheese sauce on vegetables or pasta. This makes the calories, saturated fat, and cholesterol rise.

Healthy Tips

★ Combine a soup, salad, and side dish or combine one or two appetizers and a salad for a healthy, portion-controlled meal.

★ Share two complementary entrees—pasta topped with a tomato-based sauce or vegetables and a Mexican salad, for example.

★ Split everything with your dining partner, from appetizer to dessert.

★ Request a take-home container when you order your meal. Pack up the portion to take home when your food arrives.

Get It Your Way

★ Ask for your salad dressing on the side—all of the time.

★ Ask that high-fat salad toppers be used lightly or left in the kitchen.

★ Request to substitute high-fat, high-calorie sides with lower-fat, lower-calorie items. Substitute a baked potato for french fries or onion rings, request a sandwich on whole-

(*Continued*)

wheat bread rather than on a croissant, opt for mustard rather than mayonnaise.

★ Ask the kitchen to hold the butter or cheese sauce on vegetables.

★ Forgo the fried tortilla shell in which big salads are served.

★ Request some lemon or lime slices, vinegar, or soy or teriyaki sauce on the side to flavor menu items with few calories.

Bob Evans Restaurants

❖ Bob Evans Restaurants provides nutrition information for all its menu items on its Web site at www.bobevans.com.

Light 'n Lean Choice

Fruit Cup *(1/2 serving)*
Egg Beaters Omelette
Lite Sausage Link *(2)*
Grits *(1 serving)*

Calories	618	Sodium (mg)	1,171
Fat (g)	34	Carbohydrate (g)	52
% calories from fat	48	Fiber (g)	8
Saturated fat (g)	11	Protein (g)	39
Cholesterol (mg)	41		

Exchanges: 2 starch, 1 fruit, 4 medium-fat meat, 2 fat

Healthy 'n Hearty Choice

Salmon with Wildfire Barbecue Sauce
Buttered Corn
Glazed Carrots
Applesauce

Calories	837	Sodium (mg)	786
Fat (g)	39	Carbohydrate (g)	96
% calories from fat	42	Fiber (g)	11
Saturated fat (g)	9	Protein (g)	31
Cholesterol (mg)	93		

Exchanges: 2 starch, 2 veg, 2 fruit, 2 carb, 3 lean meat, 4 fat

(Continued)

Bob Evans Restaurants

	Amount	Cal.	Fat (g)	% Cal. Fat	Sat. Fat (g)	Chol. (mg)	Sod. (mg)	Carb. (g)	Fiber (g)	Pro. (g)	Servings/Exchanges
BEEF & PORK											
Country Fried Steak w/ gravy	1	535	37	62	13	60	1763	31	0	20	2 starch, 2 medium-fat meat, 5 1/2 fat
Country Fried Steak w/out gravy	1	481	33	62	12	60	1217	26	0	20	1 1/2 starch, 2 medium-fat meat, 4 1/2 fat
Meatloaf	1	627	44	63	19	157	1043	14	1	42	1 starch, 6 medium-fat meat, 3 fat
Open-faced Roast Beef Dinner	1	416	22	48	7	103	1004	20	1	35	1 starch, 4 medium-fat meat, 2 fat
Pork Chop (plain)	1	477	28	53	9	129	829	2	0	48	7 lean meat, 1 1/2 fat
Pork Chop w/ garlic herb butter	1	635	39	55	11	120	1234	16	2	50	1 starch, 7 lean meat, 5 1/2 fat

Pork Chop w/ Wildfire Barbecue Sauce	1	654	35	48	10	129	1099	29	2	49	2 starch, 6 lean meat, 3 1/2 fat
Steak Monterey	1	600	41	62	17	126	1671	7	1	44	1/2 starch, 6 lean meat, 4 1/2 fat
Steak Tips & Noodles	1	1051	39	33	11	266	3464	98	9	78	6 1/2 starch, 8 lean meat, 3 fat
Strip Steak (plain)	1	677	50	66	17	128	1140	12	1	50	1 starch, 7 lean meat, 6 fat
Strip Steak w/ garlic herb butter	1	771	59	69	19	129	1375	15	2	50	1 starch, 7 lean meat, 8 fat
BEVERAGES											
✓Hot Chocolate	1	142	3	19	2	5	168	28	1	2	2 carb, 1/2 fat
✓Ice Blue Raspberry Lemonade Kool Aid - kids cup	1	70	0	0	0	0	41	18	0	0	1 carb
✓Iced Raspberry Tea	1	81	0	0	0	0	8	20	0	0	1 carb

✓ = Healthiest Bets

(Continued)

BEVERAGES (*Continued*)	Amount	Cal.	Fat (g)	% Cal. Fat	Sat. Fat (g)	Chol. (mg)	Sod. (mg)	Carb. (g)	Fiber (g)	Pro. (g)	Servings/Exchanges
✓Iced Strawberry Tea	1	80	0	0	0	0	8	20	0	0	1 carb
✓Iced Tea	1	5	0	0	0	0	9	5	0	0	free
Lemonade	1	136	0	0	0	0	10	36	0	0	2 carb
Raspberry Lemonade	1	201	0	0	0	0	9	51	0	0	3 1/2 carb
Strawberry Lemonade	1	201	0	0	0	0	9	51	0	0	3 1/2 carb
BREAKFAST A LA CARTE											
✓Fruit Cup	9 oz	164	1	5	0	0	11	42	4	2	3 fruit
✓Grits	7 oz	187	7	34	3	0	186	29	2	3	1 1/2 starch, 1 fat
✓Oatmeal (plain)	12 oz	185	3	15	0	0	301	34	5	7	2 starch
Sausage Gravy	7 oz	217	15	62	9	18	901	14	0	7	1 starch, 1 medium-fat meat, 2 fat
Sausage Gravy	13 oz	403	27	60	17	34	1673	26	0	14	1 1/2 starch, 1 1/2 medium-fat meat, 4 fat

✓Strawberry Yogurt	5 oz	145	1	6	1	5	85	28	1	6	1 carb, 1 milk
BREAKFAST COMBINATIONS											
Country Biscuit Breakfast	1	852	49	52	16	261	2455	71	4	30	4 1/2 starch, 3 medium-fat meat, 7 fat
Fruit & Yogurt Plate	1	414	2	4	1	5	106	96	8	9	1 1/2 carb, 4 fruit, 1 milk
Home Fries	1	193	7	33	1	0	577	28	3	4	2 starch, 1 1/2 fat
Lite Sausage	1	404	20	45	5	22	844	48	3	32	3 starch, 3 medium-fat meat, 1 fat
Pot Roast Hash	1	752	46	55	17	529	1261	37	4	45	2 1/2 starch, 5 1/2 medium-fat meat, 5 fat
Sirloin Steak	1	423	29	62	9	82	3	0	0	35	5 medium-fat meat, 1 fat
BREAKFAST MEATS											
✓Bacon	1 slice	36	4	100	2	5	54	0	0	1	1 high-fat meat
✓Canadian Bacon	1 slice	21	1	43	0	9	261	0	0	4	1 lean meat

✓ = Healthiest Bets

(*Continued*)

BREAKFAST MEATS (*Continued*)	Amount	Cal.	Fat (g)	% Cal. Fat	Sat. Fat (g)	Chol. (mg)	Sod. (mg)	Carb. (g)	Fiber (g)	Pro. (g)	Servings/Exchanges
Ham	1 slice	66	2	27	1	40	857	2	0	11	1 lean meat
Lite Sausage Link	1	100	7	63	3	19	278	0	0	10	1 high-fat meat
Sausage Link	1	125	11	79	3	14	184	0	0	5	1 high-fat meat, 1/2 fat
Sausage Patty	1	117	9	69	4	22	279	0	0	8	1 high-fat meat
BURGERS FROM THE GRILL											
Bacon Cheeseburger (plain)	1	1006	76	68	34	153	1374	31	1	45	2 starch, 5 1/2 high-fat meat, 7 fat
Cheeseburger (plain)	1	692	46	60	19	104	979	31	1	38	2 starch, 4 high-fat meat, 1 fat
Hamburger (plain)	1	605	38	57	15	82	429	30	1	34	2 starch, 4 medium-fat meat, 3 1/2 fat
Hamburger Patty	1	388	30	70	13	82	64	0	0	28	4 medium-fat meat, 2 fat

CHEESE											
✓American Cheese	1 slice	51	5	88	3	15	238	1	0	3	1 medium-fat meat
Bleu Cheese (crumbled)	2 T	97	8	74	5	22	381	0	0	6	1 high-fat meat
Monterey Jack Cheese	1 slice	76	6	71	5	23	365	0	0	4	1 medium-fat meat
CHICKEN & TURKEY											
Chicken - n - Noodles	1	407	22	49	5	115	659	32	2	20	2 starch, 2 medium-fat meat, 2 1/2 fat
Chicken Pot Pie	1 order	758	49	58	22	209	1754	46	2	32	3 starch, 3 medium-fat meat, 6 1/2 fat
Fried Chicken	1 piece	291	15	46	3	77	666	9	1	31	1/2 starch, 4 lean meat, 1/2 fat
Fried Chicken Strips	1 order	127	7	50	1	14	321	9	0	7	1/2 starch, 1 lean meat, 1 fat
Grilled Chicken (plain)	1 piece	214	9	38	2	84	544	0	0	33	5 lean meat
Grilled Chicken Tenders	1 piece	101	7	62	1	28	191	0	0	10	1 lean meat, 1 fat

✓ = Healthiest Bets

(*Continued*)

CHICKEN & TURKEY (*Continued*)	Amount	Cal.	Fat (g)	% Cal. Fat	Sat. Fat (g)	Chol. (mg)	Sod. (mg)	Carb. (g)	Fiber (g)	Pro. (g)	Servings/Exchanges
Grilled Chicken w/ garlic herb butter	1 piece	373	20	48	4	85	949	15	2	34	1 starch, 5 lean meat, 2 1/2 fat
Grilled Chicken w/ Wildfire Barbecue Sauce	1 piece	392	16	37	3	84	813	27	2	34	2 starch, 4 medium-fat meat, 1 fat
✓Turkey	1 slice	47	0	0	0	34	30	1	1	10	1 lean meat
Turkey & Dressing	1	542	24	40	7	105	1400	41	4	37	4 starch, 3 medium-fat meat, 1 fat
CONDIMENTS											
✓Butter	1 t	37	4	97	2	11	30	0	0	0	1 fat
✓Honey	1 T	43	0	0	0	0	1	12	0	0	1/2 carb
✓Margarine	1 t	31	3	87	1	0	34	0	0	0	1/2 fat
Mayonnaise	1 T	90	10	100	2	5	65	0	0	0	2 fat

✓Saltines	1 pkt	52	2	35	1	0	109	8	0	1	1/2 starch, 1/2 fat
Sour Cream	2 T	57	17	100	12	69	80	5	0	3	3 fat
CRACKERS											
✓Captains Wafer	1 pkt	60	3	45	1	0	95	9	0	1	1/2 starch, 1/2 fat
DESSERTS											
Apple Dumpling Pie	1	682	30	40	8	7	276	100	5	5	6 1/2 carb, 6 fat
Apple Dumpling Pie a la Mode	1	840	37	40	13	41	327	119	5	8	8 carb, 7 1/2 fat
Coconut Cream Pie	1	461	23	45	16	11	391	57	1	7	4 carb, 4 1/2 fat
Fudge Sundae	1	501	19	34	13	64	193	78	1	7	5 carb, 4 fat
Hershey's Hot Fudge Cake	1	688	25	33	20	34	528	94	4	1	6 carb, 5 fat
Hershey's Hot Fudge Cake a la Mode	1	846	33	35	25	67	580	113	4	4	7 1/2 carb, 6 1/2 fat

✓ = Healthiest Bets

(*Continued*)

DESSERTS (*Continued*)	**Amount**	**Cal.**	**Fat (g)**	**% Cal. Fat**	**Sat. Fat (g)**	**Chol. (mg)**	**Sod. (mg)**	**Carb. (g)**	**Fiber (g)**	**Pro. (g)**	**Servings/Exchanges**
No-Sugar-Added Apple Pie	1	483	27	50	7	0	350	52	2	3	3 1/2 starch, 5 fat
No-Sugar-Added Apple Pie a la Mode	1	642	36	50	12	34	401	71	2	7	4 1/2 starch, 7 fat
Oregon Berry Cobbler	1	631	31	44	7	0	546	85	5	3	5 1/2 starch, 6 fat
Oregon Berry Cobbler a la Mode	1	790	39	44	12	24	597	105	5	7	7 starch, 8 fat
Pumpkin Pie	1	545	27	45	13	53	72	69	3	7	4 1/2 starch, 5 1/2 fat
Reese's Peanut Butter Cup Pie	1	1130	60	48	33	22	763	129	4	18	8 1/2 starch, 12 fat
Reese's Sundae	1	769	35	41	19	67	352	104	3	13	7 starch, 6 fat
✓Vanilla Ice Cream	1	159	8	45	6	34	51	19	0	3	1 carb, 1 1/2 fat

FARM FRESH EGGS											
✓Egg Beaters Omelette	1	149	12	72	2	3	423	2	0	19	3 lean meat, 1/2 fat
✓Egg, hardboiled	1	60	4	60	2	190	55	1	0	6	1 medium-fat meat
✓Egg, over easy	1	95	7	66	2	213	63	1	0	6	1 medium-fat meat
✓Egg, scrambled	1	170	11	58	3	482	142	1	0	14	2 medium-fat meat
✓Egg, scrambled Egg Beaters	1	149	12	72	2	3	423	2	0	19	3 medium-fat meat
Eggs Benedict	1	418	20	43	5	442	1008	35	2	25	2 starch, 2 medium-fat meat, 2 1/2 fat
✓Omelette	1	285	24	76	5	482	142	1	0	14	2 medium-fat meat, 3 fat
FARM FRESH SALADS											
Chicken Salad Plate	1	781	46	53	7	87	1132	77	12	23	4 starch, 3 veg, 2 lean meat, 8 fat

✓ = Healthiest Bets

(*Continued*)

FARM FRESH SALADS (*Continued*)	Amount	Cal.	Fat (g)	% Cal. Fat	Sat. Fat (g)	Chol. (mg)	Sod. (mg)	Carb. (g)	Fiber (g)	Pro. (g)	Servings/Exchanges
Cobb w/ Grilled Chicken	1	753	50	60	20	360	1708	15	6	64	1/2 starch, 2 veg, 9 medium-fat meat, 2 fat
Country Spinach Salad w/ Grilled Chicken	1	624	40	58	10	314	1350	13	5	55	3 veg, 8 medium-fat meat
Frisco Salad w/ Fried Chicken	1	648	38	53	12	91	1577	40	6	38	1 1/2 starch, 3 veg, 5 medium-fat meat, 2 1/2 fat
Frisco Salad w/ Grilled Chicken	1	595	38	57	13	148	1272	14	6	52	3 veg, 7 medium-fat meat
✓Salad Base	1	40	1	23	0	0	27	8	4	3	2 veg
Specialty Side	1	174	9	47	4	22	119	16	2	9	1/2 starch, 2 veg, 1 lean meat, 1 fat
Specialty Side w/out croutons	1	113	7	56	4	22	267	5	2	7	1 veg, 1 lean meat, 1/2 fat

Wildfire Chicken w/ Fried Chicken	1	798	36	41	10	66	1518	88	11	35	5 starch, 3 veg, 3 lean meat, 3 1/2 fat
Wildfire Chicken w/ Grilled Chicken	1	745	36	43	10	122	1213	68	10	49	3 1/2 starch, 3 veg, 5 lean meat, 2 1/2 fat
GARNISH											
Cranberry Relish	2 T	54	0	0	0	0	6	13	1	0	1 starch
✓Dill Pickle	.6 oz	2	0	0	0	0	146	0	0	0	free
✓Lettuce & Tomato	.7 oz	4	0	0	0	0	2	1	0	0	free
✓Lettuce, Tomato & Pickle	1.3 oz	6	0	0	0	0	148	1	1	0	free
✓Onion Rings	1.5 oz	115	7	55	1	0	170	12	1	1	1/2 starch, 1 veg, 1 1/2 fat
✓Tomato Slices	.7 oz	4	0	0	0	0	2	1	0	1	free
GRAVY											
✓Beef Gravy	6 T	29	1	31	1	1	502	4	0	1	1/2 fat
Chicken Gravy	6 T	60	4	60	1	4	448	4	0	1	1 1/2 fat

✓ = Healthiest Bets

(*Continued*)

GRAVY (*Continued*)	Amount	Cal.	Fat (g)	% Cal. Fat	Sat. Fat (g)	Chol. (mg)	Sod. (mg)	Carb. (g)	Fiber (g)	Pro. (g)	Servings/Exchanges
Country Gravy	6 T	54	4	67	1	0	546	6	0	0	1 1/2 fat
GRIDDLE ITEMS											
✓Belgian Waffle	1	342	10	26	4	18	735	57	2	7	4 starch, 2 fat
✓Blueberry Hotcake	1	187	5	24	2	9	369	32	2	4	2 starch, 1 fat
✓Buttermilk Hotcake	1	171	5	26	2	9	367	28	1	3	2 starch, 1 fat
✓Mush	1 slice	65	0	0	0	0	196	14	0	1	1 starch
Stuffed French Toast	1 order	566	15	24	9	84	659	55	3	11	3 1/2 starch, 2 fat
✓Stuffed French Toast (breakfast savors)	1 order	397	12	27	8	54	419	38	2	7	2 1/2 starch, 1 1/2 fat
HEARTY SOUPS											
✓Bean Soup	1 cup	125	3	22	1	10	902	16	5	8	1 starch, 1 lean meat
Bean Soup	1 bowl	176	5	26	1	14	1268	23	7	11	1 1/2 starch, 1 lean meat, 1/2 fat

Cheddar Baked Potato Soup	1 cup	307	18	53	11	49	1200	25	1	14	1 1/2 starch, 1 medium-fat meat, 2 1/2 fat
Cheddar Baked Potato Soup	1 bowl	387	22	51	13	62	1515	31	2	17	1 starch, 2 medium-fat meat, 2 fat
Sausage Chili	1 cup	268	17	57	6	42	687	19	8	16	1 starch, 2 medium-fat meat, 1 1/2 fat
Sausage Chili	1 bowl	376	24	57	9	59	962	26	10	22	1 1/2 starch, 3 medium-fat meat, 1 fat
✓Vegetable Beef Soup	1 cup	127	5	35	2	7	556	13	2	7	1/2 starch, 1 lean meat, 1/2 fat
✓Vegetable Beef Soup	1 bowl	219	9	37	4	29	962	23	4	11	1 1/2 starch, 1 lean meat, 1 fat
JELLIES & JAMS											
✓Apple Butter	1 pkt/1 T	33	0	0	0	0	2	8	0	0	1/2 carb
✓Apple Jelly	1 pkt/1 T	35	0	0	0	0	0	9	0	0	1/2 carb

✓ = Healthiest Bets

(Continued)

JELLIES & JAMS (*Continued*)	Amount	Cal.	Fat (g)	% Cal. Fat	Sat. Fat (g)	Chol. (mg)	Sod. (mg)	Carb. (g)	Fiber (g)	Pro. (g)	Servings/Exchanges
✓Blackberry Lemonade	1 pkt/1 T	5	0	0	0	0	5	2	0	0	free
✓Grape Jelly	1 pkt/1 T	36	0	0	0	0	2	9	0	0	1/2 carb
✓Orange Marmalade	1 pkt/1 T	35	0	0	0	0	0	9	0	0	1/2 carb
✓Strawberry Jam	1 pkt/1 T	36	0	0	0	0	1	9	0	0	1/2 carb
KIDS' DESSERTS											
Fudge Blast Sundae	1	254	10	35	7	30	92	37	1	3	2 1/2 carb, 2 fat
Oreo Cookies 'n' Cream Sundae	1	376	13	31	7	21	200	64	2	3	4 carb, 2 1/2 fat
Rainbow Sundae	1	320	14	39	9	30	92	46	2	4	3 carb, 3 fat
Reese's I'm Smiling Sundae	1	325	15	42	9	31	130	42	1	5	3 carb, 3 fat

KIDS' ITEMS

Chicken Quesadilla	1	542	31	51	12	73	1238	39	2	28	2 1/2 starch, 3 lean meat, 4 1/2 fat
Colorful Cool Cakes	1	530	17	29	8	25	980	85	3	10	5 1/2 carb, 3 1/2 fat
Hot Diggety Dog	1	361	26	65	10	39	843	23	1	10	1 1/2 starch, 1 high-fat meat, 3 1/2 fat
✓Kids Garden Salad	1	41	2	44	1	7	54	3	2	3	1 veg, 1/2 fat
L'il Homesteader	1	446	26	52	8	261	774	33	2	16	2 starch, 1 lean meat, 1 fat
✓Mac & Cheese	1	330	12	33	4	20	610	56	2	11	3 1/2 starch, 1 high-fat meat
✓Mini Cheeseburgers	1	252	14	50	4	25	288	20	1	9	1 starch, 1 medium-fat meat, 2 fat
Pizza Pizzazz	1	505	23	41	8	18	796	57	2	18	3 1/2 starch, 1 medium-fat meat, 4 fat
Plenty-O-Pancakes	1	503	17	30	9	24	982	79	2	9	5 starch, 3 1/2 fat

✓ = Healthiest Bets

(*Continued*)

KIDS' ITEMS (*Continued*)	Amount	Cal.	Fat (g)	% Cal. Fat	Sat. Fat (g)	Chol. (mg)	Sod. (mg)	Carb. (g)	Fiber (g)	Pro. (g)	Servings/Exchanges
Smiley Face Potatoes	1	340	13	34	1	0	780	48	4	4	3 starch, 2 1/2 fat
Spaghetti & Meatballs	1	523	21	36	9	51	999	57	6	27	3 1/2 starch, 2 lean meat, 3 fat
LUNCH SAVORS PASTA & STIR-FRY											
Grilled Chicken Stir-Fry	1	497	18	33	4	66	1295	55	5	31	3 1/2 starch, 3 lean meat, 2 fat
Steak Tips & Noodles	1	567	25	40	6	134	1654	46	3	38	3 starch, 4 lean meat, 2 1/2 fat
Vegetable Stir-Fry	1	278	4	13	1	0	855	55	4	7	1 1/2 starch, 2 veg, 1 fat
LUNCH SAVORS SALADS											
Country Spinach	1	545	38	63	1	282	1106	11	4	42	2 veg, 6 medium-fat meat, 1 fat
Frisco w/ Fried Chicken	1	496	31	56	12	77	1243	26	4	29	1/2 starch, 2 veg, 4 lean meat, 4 fat

Frisco w/ Grilled Chicken	1	461	31	61	12	115	1040	9	3	39	2 veg, 6 medium-fat meat
Grilled Chicken Cobb	1	574	39	61	16	319	1321	9	3	48	2 veg, 7 medium-fat meat
Wild Fire Chicken w/ Grilled Chicken	1	610	29	43	9	89	981	57	8	35	3 starch, 2 veg, 3 medium-fat meat, 2 fat
Wild Fire Chicken w/ Fried Chicken	1	646	29	40	9	52	1184	74	8	26	4 starch, 3 veg, 2 medium-fat meat, 4 fat
LUNCH SAVORS SANDWICHES											
Pulled Pork Sandwich	1	464	48	93	2	59	579	54	3	24	3 starch, 2 veg, 2 medium-fat meat, 1 fat
OMELETTES											
Cheese	1	477	40	75	15	530	428	3	1	25	3 high-fat meat, 4 fat
Egg Beaters Cheese	1	328	26	71	11	51	709	4	1	30	4 lean meat, 3 fat
Egg Beaters Farmer's Market	1	493	36	66	16	78	2273	12	1	37	1/2 starch, 5 lean meat, 4 fat

✔ = Healthiest Bets

(Continued)

OMELETTES (*Continued*)	Amount	Cal.	Fat (g)	% Cal. Fat	Sat. Fat (g)	Chol. (mg)	Sod. (mg)	Carb. (g)	Fiber (g)	Pro. (g)	Servings/Exchanges
Egg Beaters Ham & Cheese	1	356	25	63	9	67	1560	3	1	39	4 medium-fat meat, 2 fat
Egg Beaters Sausage & Cheese	1	530	43	73	16	76	1312	3	1	42	6 medium-fat meat, 2 fat
Egg Beaters Southwest Chicken	1	551	40	65	14	111	1839	5	2	50	7 lean meat, 3 fat
Egg Beaters Western	1	399	28	63	9	67	1449	7	2	40	1/2 starch, 6 lean meat, 1 fat
Farmer's Market	1	642	50	70	20	556	1991	11	1	32	1/2 starch, 5 medium-fat meat, 3 fat
Ham & Cheese	1	505	39	70	13	546	1278	2	0	34	5 medium-fat meat, 5 fat
Sausage & Cheese	1	679	57	76	20	554	1030	2	0	37	5 high-fat meat, 4 fat
Southwest Chicken	1	674	51	68	17	590	1669	5	1	45	6 medium-fat meat, 5 fat
Western	1	522	39	67	13	546	1279	6	1	35	7 medium-fat meat

PASTA & STIR-FRY											
Buttered Pasta Noodles	1	287	13	41	2	47	120	35	2	7	2 starch, 2 1/2 fat
Spaghetti & Marinara Sauce	1	619	7	10	3	15	1128	104	10	34	7 starch, 2 lean meat
Spaghetti & Meatballs	1	1087	45	37	17	107	1965	116	13	54	7 1/2 starch, 6 medium-fat meat, 1 fat
Vegetable Stir-Fry	1	502	7	13	1	5	1416	99	12	15	5 starch, 4 veg, 5 fat
SALAD DRESSING - SIDE PORTION											
Bleu Cheese Dressing	3 T	440	47	96	9	44	675	6	0	3	9 1/2 fat
Colonial Dressing	3 T	464	41	80	6	0	387	23	0	0	1 1/2 starch, 8 fat
French Dressing	3 T	219	21	86	3	14	247	10	0	0	1/2 starch, 4 fat
Honey Mustard Dressing	3 T	192	18	84	3	21	247	8	0	0	3 1/2 fat
Hot Bacon Dressing	3 T	106	3	25	1	4	189	18	0	0	1 starch, 1/2 fat
Lite Italian Dressing	3 T	82	7	77	1	0	590	4	0	0	1 1/2 fat

✓ = Healthiest Bets

(*Continued*)

SALAD DRESSING - SIDE PORTION (*Continued*)	Amount	Cal.	Fat (g)	% Cal. Fat	Sat. Fat (g)	Chol. (mg)	Sod. (mg)	Carb. (g)	Fiber (g)	Pro. (g)	Servings/Exchanges
Lite Ranch Dressing	3 T	103	10	87	2	11	377	0	0	1	2 fat
Thousand Island Dressing	3 T	213	20	85	3	14	354	7	0	0	1/2 starch, 4 fat
✓Vinegar & Oil Dressing	3 T	26	3	104	0	0	0	0	0	0	1/2 fat
Wildfire Ranch Dressing	3 T	121	9	67	1	8	307	9	0	1	1/2 starch, 2 fat
SAUCES											
Cocktail Sauce	2 T	25	0	0	0	0	334	6	0	0	1/2 starch
Garlic Herb Butter	2 T	43	4	84	1	1	235	2	1	0	1 fat
Hollandaise Sauce	4 T	52	3	52	1	2	219	6	0	1	1 fat
✓Ranchero Picante Sauce	2 T	28	0	0	0	0	71	0	0	7	1/2 starch
Spaghetti Sauce	6 oz	94	2	19	0	0	889	17	4	3	1 starch, 1/2 fat
Stir-Fry Sauce	3 oz	73	2	25	0	0	340	15	0	1	1 starch, 1/2 fat
Tartar Sauce	1 oz	166	18	98	3	20	176	1	0	0	3 fat

Wildfire Barbecue Sauce	3 T	94	0	0	0	0	149	22	2	0	1 1/2 starch
SEAFOOD											
Fried Shrimp (plain)	1	330	20	55	2	284	1499	8	0	32	1/2 starch, 5 lean meat, 1/2 fat
Grilled New Orleans Style Catfish	1 piece	270	19	63	3	58	896	4	2	22	3 medium-fat meat, 1 fat
✓Grilled Shrimp (combo portion)	1	229	17	67	3	142	749	4	0	16	2 lean meat, 2 fat
Salmon (plain)	1	376	23	55	4	74	232	12	1	27	4 medium-fat meat, 1/2 fat
Salmon w/ garlic herb butter	1	424	28	59	5	75	467	15	2	28	4 medium-fat meat, 2 1/2 fat
Salmon w/ Wildfire Barbecue Sauce	1	443	24	49	4	74	331	27	2	27	1 1/2 starch, 3 medium-fat meat, 2 fat

✓ = Healthiest Bets

(Continued)

	Amount	Cal.	Fat (g)	% Cal. Fat	Sat. Fat (g)	Chol. (mg)	Sod. (mg)	Carb. (g)	Fiber (g)	Pro. (g)	Servings/Exchanges
SENIOR ITEMS											
Grilled Chicken Stir-Fry	1	480	18	34	4	57	1236	55	5	28	3 1/2 starch, 3 lean meat, 1 1/2 fat
Spaghetti & Meatballs	1	617	29	42	11	69	1166	59	7	31	4 starch, 3 medium-fat meat, 3 fat
Steak Tips & Noodles	1	567	25	40	6	134	1654	46	3	38	3 starch, 4 medium-fat meat, 1 fat
SIDE ITEMS											
✓Applesauce	1	101	0	0	0	0	17	26	2	0	1 1/2 starch, 1 1/2 fruit
✓Baked Potato - plain	1	207	0	0	0	0	16	54	6	8	3 1/2 starch
Baked Potato - seasoned	1	433	18	37	10	54	612	57	7	22	3 1/2 starch, 1 medium-fat meat, 2 fat
Bread & Celery Dressing	1	362	20	50	5	0	1013	36	0	6	2 starch, 4 fat

✓Broccoli Florets	1	44	1	20	0	0	41	8	5	5	2 veg
Cheddar Broccoli Florets	1	162	9	50	4	20	367	14	5	10	2 veg, 1 medium-fat meat
Coleslaw	1	198	13	59	2	12	229	17	2	1	1/2 starch, 2 veg, 2 fat
Corn - buttered sweet	1	156	9	52	3	12	313	18	2	3	1 starch, 2 fat
✓Cottage Cheese	1	122	5	37	3	37	436	4	0	15	2 lean meat
✓French Fries	1	217	7	29	2	0	300	35	3	3	2 starch, 1 1/2 fat
✓Fruit Dish	1	91	1	10	0	0	10	23	2	1	1 1/2 fruit
✓Garden Side Salad w/out dressing	1	152	4	24	0	0	396	26	2	6	1 starch, 2 veg, 1/2 fat
✓Garden Side Salad w/out dressing & croutons	1	23	0	0	0	0	10	5	2	1	1 veg
Glazed Carrots	1	137	6	39	2	7	125	21	5	1	1 starch, 1 veg, 1 fat
Green Beans & Ham	1	53	2	34	1	7	641	5	2	2	1 veg, 1/2 fat

✓ = Healthiest Bets

(Continued)

SIDE ITEMS (*Continued*)	Amount	Cal.	Fat (g)	% Cal. Fat	Sat. Fat (g)	Chol. (mg)	Sod. (mg)	Carb. (g)	Fiber (g)	Pro. (g)	Servings/Exchanges
✓Grilled Garden Vegetables	1	260	20	69	4	0	203	16	5	5	1/2 starch, 1 veg, 4 fat
Grilled Mushrooms	1	152	12	71	2	0	1003	10	5	4	1/2 starch, 1 veg, 2 1/2 fat
Home Fries	1	193	7	33	1	0	577	28	3	4	2 starch, 1 1/2 fat
Mashed Potatoes	1	171	6	32	4	18	382	15	1	2	1 starch, 1 fat
Onion Rings	1	461	27	53	5	1	680	49	3	5	3 starch, 1 veg, 5 1/2 fat
Rice Pilaf	1	163	3	17	1	0	606	32	1	3	2 starch, 1/2 fat
Specialty Side Salad w/out dressing	1	174	9	47	4	22	449	16	2	9	1/2 starch, 2 veg, 1 lean meat, 2 fat
Specialty Side Salad w/out dressing & croutons	1	113	7	56	4	22	267	5	2	7	1 veg, 1 lean meat, 1 fat
SKILLETS											
Sunshine Skillet	1	780	56	65	17	530	1781	35	4	33	2 starch, 4 high-fat meat, 5 fat

SPECIALTY BREADS											
✔Banana Nut Bread	1 slice	186	7	34	1	7	275	30	3	1	2 starch, 1 1/2 fat
Cinnamon Swirl Roll - frosted	1	557	24	39	6	9	550	76	0	9	5 starch, 5 fat
Cinnamon Swirl Roll - unfrosted	1	460	21	41	5	5	514	59	0	9	4 starch, 4 fat
✔English Muffin	1	139	1	6	0	0	229	28	2	5	2 starch
✔French Toast Bread	1 slice	137	2	13	0	25	175	14	1	3	1 1/2 starch, 1/2 fat
Garlic Bread	1 slice	218	16	66	3	0	386	16	1	3	1 starch, 3 fat
✔Kaiser Bun	1	167	2	11	0	0	310	30	1	6	2 starch, 1/2 fat
✔Mini Bun	1	105	1	9	0	0	211	20	1	3	1 1/2 starch
Plain Biscuit	1	277	12	39	3	0	764	26	0	5	1 1/2 starch, 3 1/2 fat
✔Plain Dinner Roll	1	201	5	22	1	9	268	34	1	5	2 starch, 1 fat

✔ = Healthiest Bets

(Continued)

SPECIALTY BREADS (*Continued*)	Amount	Cal.	Fat (g)	% Cal. Fat	Sat. Fat (g)	Chol. (mg)	Sod. (mg)	Carb. (g)	Fiber (g)	Pro. (g)	Servings/Exchanges
✓Pumpkin Bread	1 slice	161	5	28	1	3	244	27	1	3	1 1/2 starch, 1 fat
✓Sourdough Bread	1 slice	130	1	7	0	0	253	26	0	4	1 1/2 starch
✓Texas Toast	1 slice	120	1	8	0	0	126	12	1	2	1 starch, 1 fat
✓Wheat Bread	1 slice	69	1	13	0	0	148	13	2	3	1 starch
✓Wheat Bread - toasted	1 slice	65	1	14	0	0	132	12	1	2	1 starch
Wheat Bread - toasted w/ margarine	1 slice	115	7	55	1	0	188	12	1	2	1 starch, 1 1/2 fat
✓White Bread	1 slice	67	1	13	0	0	134	12	1	2	1 starch
✓White Bread - toasted	1 slice	65	1	14	0	0	131	12	1	2	1 starch
White Bread - toasted w/ margarine	1 slice	115	6	47	1	0	187	12	1	2	1 starch, 1 1/2 fat

SPECIALTY SANDWICHES

Bacon Turkey Melt	1	825	47	51	20	152	1567	56	3	45	3 1/2 starch, 5 medium-fat meat, 4 1/2 fat
✓Bacon Turkey Melt (1/2 Combo)	1	343	17	45	8	70	743	29	1	21	2 starch, 2 medium-fat meat, 2 1/2 fat
Big BLT	1	418	29	62	11	30	686	29	2	10	2 starch, 2 high-fat meat, 1 1/2 fat
✓Big BLT (1/2 Combo)	1	211	15	64	5	15	344	15	1	5	1 starch, 1 high-fat meat, 1 fat
Bob's BLT & E	1	798	57	64	20	269	1319	48	0	23	3 starch, 3 high-fat meat, 5 1/2 fat
Chicken Salad (plain)	1	694	43	56	7	60	1329	55	3	21	3 1/2 starch, 2 high-fat meat, 5 fat
Fish Market Haddock	1	570	25	39	4	32	944	65	0	21	4 starch, 2 lean meat, 3 fat

✓ = Healthiest Bets

(Continued)

SPECIALTY SANDWICHES (*Continued*)	Amount	Cal.	Fat (g)	% Cal. Fat	Sat. Fat (g)	Chol. (mg)	Sod. (mg)	Carb. (g)	Fiber (g)	Pro. (g)	Servings/Exchanges
Fried Chicken (plain)	1	508	23	41	4	77	1032	39	2	36	2 1/2 starch, 4 lean meat, 2 1/2 fat
Fried Chicken Club	1	888	59	60	22	141	1856	40	2	47	2 1/2 starch, 6 medium-fat meat, 5 fat
Grilled Cheese	1	392	17	39	7	30	782	25	2	9	1 1/2 starch, 1 medium-fat meat, 3 fat
Grilled Chicken Club	1	822	54	59	21	154	1772	32	2	51	2 starch, 6 medium-fat meat, 4 1/2 fat
Grilled Chicken Club (plain)	1	442	17	35	3	90	947	30	2	41	2 starch, 5 lean meat, 1/2 fat
Pot Roast	1	655	31	43	12	98	1455	62	1	34	4 starch, 3 medium-fat meat, 3 fat
Pot Roast (1/2 Combo)	1	435	23	48	10	81	1051	33	0	25	2 starch, 2 medium-fat meat, 3 fat

SYRUP											
Syrup	6 T	213	0	0	0	0	101	55	0	0	3 1/2 carb
✔Syrup - sugar free	6 T	47	0	0	0	0	149	11	0	0	1/2 carb
TOPPINGS											
Raspberry Topping	6 T	108	0	0	0	0	8	27	4	1	1 1/2 carb
Roasted Apple Topping	6 T	94	1	10	0	0	34	20	2	0	1/2 carb, 1 fruit
Whipped Topping	2 T	93	7	68	6	0	5	7	0	0	1/2 starch, 1 1/2 fat

✔ = Healthiest Bets

Boston Market

❖ Boston Market provides nutrition information for all its menu items on its Web site at www.bostonmarket.com.

Light 'n Lean Choice

Macaroni and Cheese
Butternut Squash
Steamed Broccoli with Hollandaise
Fruit Salad

Calories	590	Sodium (mg)	1,635
Fat (g)	23	Carbohydrate (g)	81
% calories from fat	35	Fiber (g)	10
Saturated fat (g)	13.5	Protein (g)	19
Cholesterol (mg)	75		

Exchanges: 3 1/2 starch, 1 veg, 1 fruit, 1 high-fat meat, 3 fat

Healthy 'n Hearty Choice

1/4 White Meat Chicken *(no skin or wing)*
Sweet Corn
Green Bean Casserole
Apple Pie *(1/2 serving)*

Calories	680	Sodium (mg)	1,495
Fat (g)	22	Carbohydrate (g)	73
% calories from fat	29	Fiber (g)	5
Saturated fat (g)	6	Protein (g)	41
Cholesterol (mg)	93		

Exchanges: 2 starch, 1 veg, 1 carb, 4 lean meat, 3 fat

Boston Market

	Amount	Cal.	Fat (g)	% Cal. Fat	Sat. Fat (g)	Chol. (mg)	Sod. (mg)	Carb. (g)	Fiber (g)	Pro. (g)	Servings/Exchanges
COLD SIDES											
Caesar Side Salad	1	300	26	78	4.5	15	690	13	0	5	2 veg, 1 medium-fat meat, 4 fat
✔Cranberry Walnut Relish	1	350	5	13	0	0	0	75	3	3	1 starch, 3 carb, 1 fat
✔Fruit Salad	1	70	0	0	0	0	15	16	1	1	1 veg
Garden Fresh Coleslaw	1	310	22	64	3	20	230	29	10	7	1 starch, 1 veg, 4 fat
DESSERTS											
Apple Pie	1	490	24	44	6	15	350	65	2	3	4 carb, 4 fat
Caramel Pecan Brownie	1	900	47	47	9	120	150	114	6	9	7 1/2 carb, 7 fat

✔ = Healthiest Bets

(*Continued*)

DESSERTS (*Continued*)	Amount	Cal.	Fat (g)	% Cal. Fat	Sat. Fat (g)	Chol. (mg)	Sod. (mg)	Carb. (g)	Fiber (g)	Pro. (g)	Servings/Exchanges
Chocolate Brownie	1	580	23	36	5	95	350	88	6	9	6 carb, 3 fat
Chocolate Cake	1	650	32	44	8	60	320	86	2	4	6 carb, 4 fat
Chocolate Chip Cookie	1	390	19	44	6	15	350	51	2	4	3 1/2 carb, 3 fat
Chocolate Mania	1	490	33	61	17	95	170	36	1	4	2 1/2 carb, 6 fat
✔Cornbread	1	200	6	27	1.5	25	390	33	1	3	2 starch, 1 fat
Family Size Apple Pie	1	350	14	36	3	0	390	54	2	4	3 1/2 carb, 3 fat
✔Family Size Caramel Brownie	1	160	8	45	2	25	85	22	0	2	1 1/2 carb, 1 1/2 fat
✔Family Size Chocolate Brownie	1	160	8	45	2	25	85	22	0	2	1 1/2 carb, 1 1/2 fat
Family Size Pecan Pie	1	560	29	47	7	85	230	70	2	6	4 1/2 carb, 3 fat
Family Size Pumpkin Pie	1	360	18	45	5	35	240	44	2	5	3 carb, 2 1/2 fat

Oatmeal Scotchie Cookie	1	390	20	46	5	30	340	47	2	5	3 carb, 4 fat
Pecan Pie	1	700	36	46	9	105	290	88	3	7	6 carb, 5 fat
Pumpkin Pie	1	450	22	44	6	45	310	55	2	6	3 1/2 carb, 4 fat
ENTREES											
1/2 Chicken w/ skin	1	590	33	50	10	290	1010	4	0	70	10 lean meat, 1/2 fat
1/4 Dark Chicken w/ skin	1	320	21	59	6	155	500	2	0	30	4 lean meat, 1 1/2 fat
✔1/4 Dark Chicken w/out skin	1	190	10	47	3	115	440	1	0	22	3 lean meat
✔1/4 White Chicken w/ skin & wing	1	280	12	39	3.5	135	510	2	0	40	6 lean meat
✔1/4 White Chicken w/out skin or wing	1	170	4	21	1	85	480	2	0	33	5 lean meat
✔Asian Grilled Chicken	1	430	12	25	2	145	690	34	0	48	2 starch, 6 lean meat
Chicken Pot Pie	1	750	46	55	14	110	1530	57	2	26	3 1/2 starch, 2 medium-fat meat, 7 fat

✔ = Healthiest Bets

(*Continued*)

ENTREES (*Continued*)	Amount	Cal.	Fat (g)	% Cal. Fat	Sat. Fat (g)	Chol. (mg)	Sod. (mg)	Carb. (g)	Fiber (g)	Pro. (g)	Servings/Exchanges
Chipotle Meatloaf w/ chipotle gravy	1	860	55	58	23	210	1750	47	3	48	3 starch, 6 lean meat, 6 1/2 fat
Double Sauced Meatloaf	1	510	34	60	15	140	890	22	2	32	1 1/2 starch, 4 lean meat, 5 fat
Double Sauced Meatloaf & Chunky Tomato	1	550	34	56	15	140	1270	30	3	33	2 starch, 4 lean meat, 5 fat
Double Sauced Meatloaf w/ beef gravy	1	580	39	61	16	140	1270	27	2	33	1 1/2 starch, 5 medium-fat 2 fat
Hand Carved Ham	1	210	8	34	3	75	1460	10	0	24	4 lean meat
Hand Carved Turkey	1	170	1	5	0	100	850	3	0	36	4 lean meat
HOT SIDES											
Butternut Squash	1	150	6	36	4	20	560	25	6	2	1 1/2 starch, 1/2 fat
Creamed Spinach	1	260	20	69	13	55	740	11	2	9	1/2 starch, 1 veg, 4 fat
✓Fresh Steamed Broccoli	1	30	0	0	0	0	30	6	2	3	1 veg

✓Garlic Dill New Potatoes	1	130	3	21	0	0	150	25	2	3	1 1/2 starch, 1/2 fat
Green Bean Casserole	1	80	5	56	1.5	5	670	9	2	1	1/2 starch, 1 veg, 1 fat
✓Green Beans	1	70	4	51	0.5	0	250	6	2	1	1 veg, 1 fat
Home style Mashed Potatoes	1	210	9	39	5	25	590	30	2	4	2 starch, 1 1/2 fat
Home style Mashed Potatoes w/ Gravy	1	230	9	35	5	25	780	32	3	4	2 starch, 2 fat
✓Hot Cinnamon Apples	1	250	2	7	0.5	0	45	56	3	0	1 1/2 carb, 2 fruit
Macaroni and Cheese	1	280	11	35	6	30	890	33	1	13	2 starch, 1 medium-fat meat, 1 fat
Potatoes Au Gratin	1	250	18	65	11	60	410	17	2	7	1 starch, 1 medium-fat meat, 2 fat
✓Poultry Gravy	1	15	1	60	0	0	180	2	0	0	free
Savory Stuffing	1	190	8	38	1.5	5	620	27	2	4	2 starch, 1 1/2 fat

✓ = Healthiest Bets

(*Continued*)

HOT SIDES (*Continued*)	Amount	Cal.	Fat (g)	% Cal. Fat	Sat. Fat (g)	Chol. (mg)	Sod. (mg)	Carb. (g)	Fiber (g)	Pro. (g)	Servings/Exchanges
Squash Casserole	1	330	24	65	13	70	1110	20	3	7	1 starch, 1 veg, 5 fat
✓Steam Vegetable Medley	1	30	0	0	0	0	135	2	2	6	1 veg
Steamed Broccoli w/ Hollandaise Sauce	1	90	6	60	3.5	25	170	7	2	3	1/2 starch, 1 veg, 1 fat
✓Sweet Corn	1	180	1	5	0.2	0	170	30	2	5	2 starch
Sweet Potato Casserole	1	280	13	42	4.5	10	190	39	2	3	2 1/2 starch, 2 1/2 fat
Vegetable Rice Pilaf	1	140	4	26	0.5	0	520	34	1	2	2 starch, 1 fat
SALADS & SOUPS											
Asian Grilled Chicken Salad w/ dressing & noodles	1	570	19	30	3.5	95	1810	56	8	39	3 1/2 starch, 3 lean meat, 2 fat
✓Asian Grilled Chicken Salad w/out dressing & noodles	1	300	9	27	1.5	95	440	21	7	36	1 1/2 starch, 4 lean meat

Caesar Salad Entrée	1	470	40	77	9	35	1070	17	3	14	3 veg, 1 medium-fat meat, 7 fat
Chicken Caesar Salad	1	800	62	70	13	140	1770	18	3	47	3 veg, 5 medium-fat meat, 7 1/2 fat
✓Hearty Chicken Noodle Soup	1	100	5	45	1.5	30	500	8	0	6	1/2 starch, 1 lean meat, 1/2 fat
Tortilla Soup w/ toppings	1	170	8	42	2.5	25	1060	18	2	8	1 starch, 1 lean meat, 1 fat
✓Tortilla Soup w/out toppings	1	80	5	56	1	15	930	7	1	5	1/2 starch, 1 lean meat
SANDWICHES											
Chicken Carver w/ cheese & sauce	1	640	29	41	7	90	980	61	4	38	4 starch, 4 medium-fat meat
✓Chicken Carver w/out cheese & sauce	1	400	6	14	0.5	55	860	60	4	32	4 starch, 3 lean meat
Chicken Queso	1	550	21	34	7	150	1590	62	3	38	4 starch, 4 lean meat, 2 fat

✓ = Healthiest Bets

(*Continued*)

SANDWICHES (*Continued*)	Amount	Cal.	Fat (g)	% Cal. Fat	Sat. Fat (g)	Chol. (mg)	Sod. (mg)	Carb. (g)	Fiber (g)	Pro. (g)	Servings/Exchanges
Marinated Grilled Chicken w/ mayo	1	670	36	48	6	105	810	45	2	42	3 starch, 5 lean meat, 3 1/2 fat
Meatloaf Carver w/ cheese	1	730	29	36	12	100	1590	85	5	39	5 starch, 4 medium-fat meat, 1 fat
Turkey Carver w/ cheese & sauce	1	630	26	37	7	110	1350	64	4	40	4 starch, 4 medium-fat meat
Turkey Carver w/out cheese & sauce	1	400	2	5	0	60	1080	61	4	34	4 starch, 2 lean meat

✔ = Healthiest Bets

Chili's Grill & Bar

Chili's Grill & Bar gives minimal nutrition information for its "Guiltless Gourmet" items at its Web site, www.chilis.com. No meals or healthiest bets are provided due to the minimal information available.

(*Continued*)

Chili's Grill & Bar

	Amount	Cal.	Fat (g)	% Cal. Fat	Sat. Fat (g)	Chol. (mg)	Sod. (mg)	Carb. (g)	Fiber (g)	Pro. (g)	Servings/Exchanges
GUILTLESS GRILL MENU ITEMS											
Chicken Pita	1	544	9	15	n/a	n/a	n/a	77	15	39	5 starch, 3 lean meat
Chicken Platter	1	563	9	14	n/a	n/a	n/a	83	4	38	5 1/2 starch, 3 lean meat
Chicken Sandwich	1	527	9	15	n/a	n/a	n/a	70	11	44	4 1/2 starch, 5 lean meat
Tomato Basil Pasta	1	671	15	20	n/a	n/a	n/a	106	n/a	28	7 starch, 2 1/2 fat

n/a = not available

Denny's

❖ Denny's provides nutrition information for all its menu items on its Web site at www.dennys.com.

Light 'n Lean Choice

Grapefruit *(1/2)*
Veggie-Cheese Egg Beaters Omelette
English Muffin *(order dry)*
Cream Cheese *(1/2 serving)*

Calories....................581
Fat (g)........................28
% calories from fat..43
Saturated fat (g)......10
Cholesterol (mg).........38
Sodium (mg)..........1,092
Carbohydrate (g).........52
Fiber (g)...................10
Protein (g)...................32

Exchanges: 2 starch, 1 veg, 1 fruit, 3 medium-fat meat, 2 fat

Healthy 'n Hearty Choice

Vegetable Beef Soup *(1 serving)*
Pot Roast with Gravy
Baked Potato *(plain)*
Whipped Margarine *(1 serving)*
Carrots in Butter Sauce

Calories....................728
Fat (g)........................23
% calories from fat..28
Saturated fat (g)........8
Cholesterol (mg).........92
Sodium (mg)..........2,001
Carbohydrate (g).........75
Fiber (g).....................9
Protein (g)...................53

Exchanges: 3 starch, 2 veg, 5 medium-fat meat, 1 1/2 fat

(Continued)

Denny's

	Amount	Cal.	Fat (g)	% Cal. Fat	Sat. Fat (g)	Chol. (mg)	Sod. (mg)	Carb. (g)	Fiber (g)	Pro. (g)	Servings/Exchanges
APPETIZERS											
Buffalo Chicken Strips	5	734	42	51	4	96	1673	43	0	48	3 starch, 6 medium-fat meat, 1 fat
Buffalo Wings	9	974	72	67	18	267	4049	44	5	67	3 starch, 8 medium-fat meat, 3 fat
Chicken Strips	5	720	33	41	4	95	1666	56	0	47	3 1/2 starch, 6 lean meat, 2 1/2 fat
Mozzarella Sticks	8	710	41	52	24	48	5220	49	6	36	3 starch, 4 high-fat meat, 1 1/2 fat
Nachos	1	1278	64	45	31	181	1654	177	11	54	12 starch, 3 high-fat meat
Sampler	1	1405	80	51	24	75	5305	124	4	47	8 starch, 5 high-fat meat, 6 fat

Smothered Cheese Fries	1	767	48	56	17	78	875	69	0	27	4 1/2 starch, 3 high-fat meat, 2 1/2 fat
BEVERAGES											
✓Apple Juice	10 oz	126	0	0	0	0	24	33	0	0	2 fruit
Floats	12 oz	280	10	32	6	39	109	47	0	3	3 fruit, 1 1/2 fat
✓French Vanilla Cappuccino	8 oz	100	2	18	2	0	220	28	1	3	1 1/2 carb
✓Hot Chocolate	8 oz	100	2	18	2	0	219	28	1	3	1 1/2 carb
Lemonade	16 oz	150	0	0	0	0	38	35	0	0	2 carb
Malted Milkshake	12 oz	583	26	40	16	100	278	82	0	12	5 1/2 carb, 3 1/2 fat
Milkshake	12 oz	560	26	42	16	100	272	76	0	11	5 carb, 4 fat
✓Orange Juice	10 oz	126	0	0	0	0	31	31	0	2	2 fruit
Oreo Blender Blaster	15 oz	895	46	46	23	125	280	112	2	16	7 1/2 carb, 6 1/2 fat
✓Original Flavor Cappuccino	8 oz	100	3	27	3	0	100	17	0	2	1 carb, 1/2 fat
✓Raspberry Iced Tea	16 oz	78	0	0	0	0	0	21	0	0	1 1/2 carb

✓ = Healthiest Bets

(Continued)

BEVERAGES (*Continued*)	Amount	Cal.	Fat (g)	% Cal. Fat	Sat. Fat (g)	Chol. (mg)	Sod. (mg)	Carb. (g)	Fiber (g)	Pro. (g)	Servings/Exchanges
✓Ruby Red Grapefruit Juice	10 oz	162	0	0	0	0	43	41	0	0	1/2 carb
✓Tomato Juice	10 oz	56	0	0	0	0	921	11	2	2	2 veg
BREAKFAST											
All American Slam	1	816	67	74	24	828	1826	3	1	46	7 high-fat meat, 2 1/2 fat
Bacon	4 strips	162	18	100	5	36	640	1	0	12	2 high-fat meat
✓Bagel, dry	1	235	1	4	0	0	498	46	0	9	3 starch
Belgian Waffle Platter	1	619	45	65	22	274	1683	28	0	22	2 starch, 2 medium-fat meat, 6 fat
✓Biscuit	1	192	10	47	2	0	519	22	0	3	1 1/2 starch, 1 1/2 fat
Blueberry Topping	1 order	106	0	0	0	0	15	26	0	0	1 1/2 starch
Breakfast Dagwood	1	1446	90	56	35	765	4003	81	1	82	5 starch, 9 high-fat meat, 3 fat

Buttermilk Pancake Platter	1	466	23	44	7	17	2077	17	2	20	1 starch, 3 high-fat meat, 2 fat
✓Buttermilk Pancakes	3	223	4	16	1	0	901	47	2	6	3 starch
Cherry Topping	1 order	86	0	0	0	0	5	21	0	0	1 1/2 carb
Chicken Fajita Skillet	1	855	49	52	15	515	1863	30	11	26	2 starch, 4 medium-fat meat, 9 fat
Corned Beef Hash Slam	1	668	55	74	19	535	816	11	1	32	1/2 starch, 4 high-fat meat, 5 fat
Country Fried Potatoes	1	394	20	46	6	9	938	23	10	3	1 1/2 starch, 6 fat
Country Fried Steak & Eggs	1	464	34	66	9	527	828	13	6	29	1 starch, 4 high-fat meat
Country Scramble	1	1038	62	54	19	481	3935	79	4	42	5 starch, 4 high-fat meat, 5 1/2 fat
Cream Cheese	1 order	100	10	90	6	31	90	1	0	2	2 fat

✓ = Healthiest Bets

(Continued)

BREAKFAST (*Continued*)	Amount	Cal.	Fat (g)	% Cal. Fat	Sat. Fat (g)	Chol. (mg)	Sod. (mg)	Carb. (g)	Fiber (g)	Pro. (g)	Servings/Exchanges
Denver Scramble	1	940	51	49	15	551	3331	75	4	48	5 starch, 5 high-fat meat, 1 fat
✓Egg	1	120	10	75	3	210	120	0	0	6	1 medium-fat meat, 1 fat
✓Egg Beaters Egg Substitute	1 order	56	0	0	0	0	186	2	0	11	1 lean meat
✓English Muffin, dry	1	125	1	7	0	0	198	24	1	5	1 1/2 starch
Farmer's Slam	1	1200	80	60	24	704	3204	82	3	51	5 1/2 starch, 5 high-fat meat, 1 1/2 fat
Fiesta Scramble	1	910	52	51	16	493	2945	74	4	40	5 starch, 4 high-fat meat, 2 1/2 fat
French Slam	1	1119	77	62	25	705	2265	71	3	46	4 1/2 starch, 5 high-fat meat, 6 fat
French Toast Platter	1	1146	71	56	24	298	2441	104	3	26	7 starch, 2 medium-fat meat, 7 1/2 fat

✓Fresh Fruit Bowl w/ Bagel	1	407	4	9	1	0	659	86	5	13	3 starch, 3 fruit
Grand Slam Slugger	1	927	55	53	15	476	2399	84	3	34	5 1/2 starch, 3 high-fat meat, 4 fat
Grilled Ham Slice	1	85	3	32	2	19	1700	6	0	15	2 lean meat
Grits	1	80	0	0	0	0	520	18	0	2	1 starch
Ham & Cheddar Egg Beater Omelette	1	468	32	62	11	58	1351	5	0	37	5 medium-fat meat, 2 1/2 fat
Ham & Cheddar Omelette	1	595	47	71	16	782	7831	5	0	41	6 medium-fat meat, 3 fat
Hashed Browns	1	197	12	55	2	0	446	20	2	2	1 starch, 2 1/2 fat
Lumberjack Slam w/ Hash Browns	1	1035	58	50	17	589	4462	73	3	51	5 starch, 5 high-fat meat, 3 fat
Maple - Flavored Syrup	3 T	143	0	0	0	0	26	36	0	0	2 carb
Meat Lovers Breakfast	1	1027	60	53	18	497	3462	72	3	44	4 1/2 starch, 5 high-fat meat, 4 fat

✓ = Healthiest Bets

(*Continued*)

BREAKFAST (*Continued*)	Amount	Cal.	Fat (g)	% Cal. Fat	Sat. Fat (g)	Chol. (mg)	Sod. (mg)	Carb. (g)	Fiber (g)	Pro. (g)	Servings/Exchanges
Meat Lovers Skillet	1	1031	74	65	24	528	2374	27	10	39	1 1/2 starch, 5 high-fat meat, 9 fat
Moons Over My Hammy	1	841	51	55	22	580	2699	42	2	54	3 starch, 6 medium-fat meat, 3 1/2 fat
✓Oatmeal	1	100	2	18	0	0	175	18	3	5	1 starch
Oatmeal Deluxe	1 order	460	6	12	3	11	87	95	7	13	6 starch
Original Grand Slam	1	665	49	66	15	515	1106	33	2	26	2 starch, 3 high-fat meat, 4 1/2 fat
Sausage	4 links	354	32	81	12	64	944	0	0	16	2 high-fat meat, 3 fat
Sirloin Steak & Eggs	1	675	45	60	16	643	368	1	1	62	9 medium-fat meat
Skinny Moons (fit fare)	1	492	10	18	4	49	2378	59	3	33	3 1/2 starch, 3 lean meat
Slim Slam (fit fare)	1	421	13	28	4	50	2625	69	1	32	4 1/2 starch, 3 lean meat, 1 fat

Strawberry Topping	1	115	1	8	0	0	12	26	1	1	1 1/2 carb
✓Sugar-Free Maple - Flavored Syrup	3 T	23	0	0	0	0	71	9	0	0	1/2 carb
T-bone Steak & Eggs	1	991	77	70	31	657	1003	1	1	73	9 high-fat meat, 2 fat
✓Toast, dry	1 slice	90	1	10	0	0	166	17	1	3	1 starch
Two Egg Breakfast w/ Hash Browns	1	825	67	73	17	538	1765	24	2	31	1 1/2 starch, 4 high-fat meat, 6 1/2 fat
Ultimate Omelette	1	619	50	73	16	770	1214	8	1	36	1/2 starch, 5 medium-fat meat, 2 fat
Veggie-Cheese Egg Beater Omelette	1	346	22	57	7	23	849	11	3	25	1/2 starch, 3 medium-fat meat, 2 fat
Veggie-Cheese Omelette	1	494	39	71	12	747	719	11	2	30	1/2 starch, 4 medium-fat meat, 3 1/2 fat
✓Veggie Egg Beater Omelette (fit fare)	1	332	8	22	3	0	853	38	5	25	2 1/2 starch, 2 lean meat

✓ = Healthiest Bets

(Continued)

BREAKFAST (*Continued*)	Amount	Cal.	Fat (g)	% Cal. Fat	Sat. Fat (g)	Chol. (mg)	Sod. (mg)	Carb. (g)	Fiber (g)	Pro. (g)	Servings/Exchanges
Whipped Cream, dollop	1	23	2	78	0	7	1	2	0	0	1/2 fat
Whipped Margarine	1 order	87	10	100	2	0	117	0	0	0	2 fat
DESSERTS											
Apple Crisp a la mode	1	723	21	26	8	32	394	133	6	6	8 carb, 1 fruit, 1/2 fat
Apple Pie	1	470	24	46	6	0	470	64	1	3	4 carb, 1 fruit, 2 fat
Banana Split	1	894	43	43	19	78	177	121	6	15	7 carb, 1 fruit, 6 fat
Blueberry Topping	1	71	0	0	0	0	10	17	0	0	1 carb
Carrot Cake	1	799	45	51	13	125	630	99	2	9	6 1/2 carb, 8 1/2 fat
Cheesecake	1	580	38	59	24	174	380	51	0	8	3 1/2 carb, 6 1/2 fat
Chocolate Peanut Butter Pie	1	653	39	54	19	27	319	64	3	15	4 carb, 1 high-fat meat, 5 fat
Chocolate Topping	1	133	1	7	0	0	109	34	1	2	2 carb

Coconut Cream Pie	1	582	33	51	15	0	482	63	3	5	4 carb, 6 fat
Double Scoop Sundae	1	375	27	65	12	74	86	29	0	6	2 carb, 4 1/2 fat
French Silk Pie	1	690	49	64	24	80	225	54	4	7	3 1/2 carb, 9 fat
Fudge Topping	4 T	201	10	45	7	3	96	30	1	1	2 carb, 1 fat
Hot Fudge Brownie a la mode	1 serving	997	42	38	6	14	82	147	6	12	10 carb, 4 1/2 fat
Whipped Cream	2 T	23	2	78	0	7	3	2	0	0	1/2 fat
DINNERS & PLATES											
Chicken Strips	1	635	25	35	1	95	1510	55	0	47	3 1/2 starch, 5 lean meat, 2 fat
Country Fried Steak	1	644	46	64	40	89	2149	30	11	28	2 starch, 4 high-fat meat, 2 fat
Fish & Chips	1	958	54	51	30	88	1390	83	6	34	5 1/2 starch, 3 medium-fat meat, 6 1/2 fat

✓ = Healthiest Bets

(*Continued*)

DINNERS & PLATES (*Continued*)	Amount	Cal.	Fat (g)	% Cal. Fat	Sat. Fat (g)	Chol. (mg)	Sod. (mg)	Carb. (g)	Fiber (g)	Pro. (g)	Servings/Exchanges
Fisherman's Platter	1	1027	62	54	32	121	1103	89	10	24	6 starch, 3 medium-fat meat, 7 fat
Fried Shrimp & Shrimp Scampi	1	346	20	52	4	240	1104	15	1	27	1 starch, 3 lean meat, 2 fat
✓Fried Shrimp Dinner	1	219	10	41	2	133	774	18	1	17	1 starch, 2 lean meat, 1 fat
✓Grilled Chicken Dinner	1	200	5	23	1	67	824	15	1	25	1 starch, 3 lean meat
Mini Burgers w/ Onion Rings	1	2044	122	54	38	145	3834	179	10	61	12 starch, 5 high-fat meat, 21 fat
Pot Roast w/ gravy Dinner	1	292	11	34	5	87	927	5	0	42	6 lean meat
Roast Turkey w/ stuffing & gravy	1	435	10	21	0	100	4620	62	2	42	4 starch, 4 lean meat
✓Shrimp Scampi Skillet Dinner	1	289	19	59	4	192	766	3	0	25	4 lean meat, 1 1/2 fat

Sirloin Steak Dinner	1	337	28	75	8	687	344	1	1	18	2 high-fat meat, 3 fat
Steak and Shrimp Dinner	1	645	42	59	14	150	1143	31	2	36	2 starch, 4 medium-fat meat, 4 fat
T-bone Steak Dinner	1	860	65	68	29	196	867	0	0	65	9 medium-fat meat, 4 fat
DRESSINGS											
Blue Cheese Dressing	2 T	163	18	99	3	20	205	1	0	1	3 1/2 fat
Caesar Dressing	2 T	133	14	95	2	2	380	1	0	1	3 fat
Fat Free Ranch Dressing	2 T	25	0	0	0	0	300	6	0	0	1/2 carb
French Dressing	2 T	106	10	85	2	7	274	3	0	0	2 fat
Honey Mustard Dressing	2 T	160	15	84	8	20	123	20	0	0	1 carb, 3 fat
Low Calorie Italian Dressing	2 T	15	1	60	0	0	390	3	0	0	free
Ranch Dressing	2 T	129	14	98	2	8	189	1	0	0	3 fat
Thousand Island Dressing	2 T	118	11	84	2	15	170	5	0	0	2 fat

✔ = Healthiest Bets

(*Continued*)

	Amount	Cal.	Fat (g)	% Cal. Fat	Sat. Fat (g)	Chol. (mg)	Sod. (mg)	Carb. (g)	Fiber (g)	Pro. (g)	Servings/Exchanges
FRUITS											
✓Banana	1	110	0	0	0	0	0	29	4	1	2 fruit
✓Cantaloupe	1/4	32	0	0	0	0	16	8	1	1	1/2 fruit
✓Grapefruit	1/2	60	0	0	0	0	0	16	6	1	1 fruit
✓Grapes	1 serving	55	1	16	0	0	0	15	1	1	1 fruit
✓Honeydew	1/4	31	0	0	0	0	22	8	1	1	1/2 fruit
KIDS' MEALS											
✓Burgerlicious	1	296	17	52	6	28	368	24	1	13	1 1/2 starch, 2 medium-fat meat, 1/2 fat
Charming Cheese Burger	1	735	37	45	11	50	2129	73	7	25	5 starch, 3 high-fat meat, 1 fat
✓Deep Sea Salad w/ Rowdy Ranch	1	240	20	75	3	16	359	13	1	3	1 starch, 1 veg, 3 fat

✔Dennysaur Chicken Nuggets	1	190	13	62	4	30	340	9	0	9	1/2 starch, 2 medium-fat meat
Enchanting Chicken Strips	1	696	31	40	4	56	978	71	4	33	4 1/2 starch, 3 medium-fat meat, 3 1/2 fat
French Toastix	1	627	71	100	13	190	1068	71	1	18	4 1/2 starch, 1 medium-fat meat, 4 fat
Jr. Dippers w/ Marinara & Applesauce	1	566	27	43	12	22	1504	50	5	27	2 starch, 1 fruit, 3 medium-fat meat, 2 1/2 fat
Jr. Dippers w/ Marinara & Fries	1	860	43	45	17	22	1679	80	8	32	5 starch, 4 medium-fat meat, 3 1/2 fat
Junior Grand Slam	1	397	25	57	7	230	1118	33	1	17	2 starch, 2 medium-fat meat, 2 fat
✔Macaroni & Cheese	1	353	13	33	4	19	651	48	2	12	3 starch, 2 medium-fat meat, 1 fat

✔ = Healthiest Bets

(Continued)

KIDS' MEALS (*Continued*)	Amount	Cal.	Fat (g)	% Cal. Fat	Sat. Fat (g)	Chol. (mg)	Sod. (mg)	Carb. (g)	Fiber (g)	Pro. (g)	Servings/Exchanges
Pizza Party	1	400	15	34	3	10	1090	47	7	18	3 starch, 2 medium-fat meat, 1/2 fat
Smiley Face Hotcakes w/ meat	1	463	22	43	7	38	1410	63	2	14	4 starch, 2 medium-fat meat
Smiley Face Hotcakes w/out meat	1	344	9	24	3	13	1014	62	2	7	4 starch, 1 fat
Thanksgiving Jr.	1	290	14	43	4	27	3881	49	2	12	2 1/2 starch, 2 lean meat
✓The Big Cheese	1	334	20	54	20	24	828	28	2	9	2 starch, 1 high-fat meat, 1 1/2 fat
SALADS											
Chef's	1	365	16	39	7	289	1376	14	4	41	3 veg, 5 lean meat
Fried Chicken Strip	1	438	26	53	6	78	1030	26	4	33	1/2 starch, 3 veg, 4 lean meat, 2 fat

✔Grilled Chicken Breast	1	264	11	38	5	89	714	10	4	32	2 veg, 4 lean meat
Side Caesar w/ dressing	1	362	26	65	7	23	913	20	3	11	1/2 starch, 2 veg, 2 medium-fat meat, 2 1/2 fat
✔Side Caesar w/out dressing	1	113	7	56	5	0	144	6	2	7	1 veg, 1 medium-fat meat
✔Turkey Breast w/out dressing	1	248	8	29	4	86	798	12	4	31	2 veg, 4 lean meat
SANDWICHES & BURGERS											
Albacore Tuna Melt	1	640	39	55	13	109	1438	42	3	30	3 starch, 3 lean meat, 6 fat
Bacon Cheddar Burger	1	875	52	53	19	163	1672	58	5	53	3 1/2 starch, 6 high-fat meat
Bacon, Lettuce, & Tomato	1	610	38	56	9	35	862	50	2	15	3 1/2 starch, 2 high-fat meat, 3 fat

✔ = Healthiest Bets

(*Continued*)

SANDWICHES & BURGERS (*Continued*)	Amount	Cal.	Fat (g)	% Cal. Fat	Sat. Fat (g)	Chol. (mg)	Sod. (mg)	Carb. (g)	Fiber (g)	Pro. (g)	Servings/Exchanges
BBQ Chicken Sandwich	1	1089	62	51	14	103	1872	86	5	48	5 1/2 starch, 5 medium-fat meat, 6 fat
Boca Burger	1	601	27	40	6	14	1446	64	9	32	4 starch, 3 lean meat, 2 1/2 fat
Boca Burger w/ small fruit bowl (fit fare)	1	508	11	19	3	15	1308	78	10	33	3 starch, 2 fruit, 3 lean meat
Buffalo Chicken Sandwich	1	708	28	36	6	74	1733	80	5	37	5 starch, 3 lean meat, 3 fat
Chicken Ranch Melt	1	758	45	53	14	405	2195	44	3	44	3 starch, 4 lean meat, 6 1/2 fat
Classic Burger	1	694	35	45	12	100	785	56	4	40	3 1/2 starch, 5 medium-fat meat, 1 fat
Classic Burger w/ Cheese	1	852	48	51	20	140	1385	57	4	49	4 starch, 5 medium-fat meat, 3 1/2 fat

Club Sandwich	1	602	38	57	6	41	2450	45	2	31	3 starch, 3 medium-fat meat, 3 fat
Fish Sandwich	1	589	30	46	5	30	1557	30	3	22	3 starch, 2 lean meat, 5 fat
Grilled Chicken Sandwich w/out dressing	1	476	14	26	3	77	1494	56	4	36	3 1/2 starch, 3 lean meat, 1 fat
Ham & Swiss on Rye w/out mayo	1	417	16	35	8	57	1763	39	5	32	2 1/2 starch, 3 medium-fat meat
Hickory Cheeseburger	1	1221	71	52	40	114	1133	84	5	49	5 1/2 starch, 5 high-fat meat, 6 fat
Hoagie Chicken Melt	1	751	44	53	12	93	1834	43	2	46	3 starch, 6 medium-fat meat, 1 1/2 fat
Hoagie Philly Melt	1	874	50	51	16	114	2444	58	5	47	3 1/2 starch, 5 high-fat meat, 2 fat
Italian Chicken Melt	1	1134	62	49	20	115	3735	68	7	51	4 1/2 starch, 6 medium-fat meat, 7 fat

✔ = Healthiest Bets

(Continued)

SANDWICHES & BURGERS (*Continued*)	Amount	Cal.	Fat (g)	% Cal. Fat	Sat. Fat (g)	Chol. (mg)	Sod. (mg)	Carb. (g)	Fiber (g)	Pro. (g)	Servings/Exchanges
Mushroom Swiss Burger	1	880	49	50	17	137	1617	63	5	51	4 starch, 6 medium-fat meat, 2 1/2 fat
Patty Melt	1	798	51	58	21	127	1285	37	4	45	2 1/2 starch, 5 high-fat meat, 2 fat
The Superbird Sandwich	1	479	29	54	11	47	1764	32	2	24	2 starch, 3 medium-fat meat, 2 fat
Turkey Breast on Multigrain w/out mayo	1	277	4	13	0	15	1607	41	5	23	3 starch, 2 lean meat
SIDES											
✓Applesauce	1	60	0	0	0	0	13	15	1	0	1 fruit
✓Baked Potato, plain w/ skin	1	220	0	0	0	0	16	51	5	5	3 1/2 starch
BBQ Sauce	3 T	47	1	19	0	0	595	11	0	0	1/2 carb
✓Bread Stuffing, plain	1	100	1	9	0	0	409	19	1	3	1 starch, 1/2 fat

✔Brown Gravy	2 T	13	0	0	0	0	184	2	0	0	free
✔Carrots in butter sauce	1	50	1	18	0	0	121	8	2	0	2 veg
Coleslaw	1	274	24	79	30	37	588	14	2	2	3 veg, 4 1/2 fat
✔Corn in butter sauce	1	93	2	19	1	2	113	18	1	2	1 starch
✔Cottage Cheese	1	72	3	38	2	10	281	2	0	9	1 medium-fat meat
✔Country Gravy	2 T	17	1	53	0	0	93	2	0	0	free
French Fries, unsalted	1	423	20	43	5	0	221	57	5	6	3 1/2 starch, 3 fat
Garlic Dinner Bread	2 pc.	170	11	58	2	0	325	15	15	2	1 starch, 2 fat
✔Green Beans in sauce	1	40	1	23	0	2	115	5	2	1	1 veg
✔Marinara Sauce	1 serving	48	2	38	1	0	206	7	1	1	1 veg
Mashed Potatoes, plain	1	68	7	93	3	8	498	23	2	3	1 1/2 starch
Onion Rings	1	381	23	54	6	6	1003	38	1	5	2 starch, 1 veg, 4 1/2 fat
✔Pico de Gallo	1 serving	21	0	0	0	0	125	5	1	1	free

✔ = Healthiest Bets

(Continued)

SIDES (*Continued*)	Amount	Cal.	Fat (g)	% Cal. Fat	Sat. Fat (g)	Chol. (mg)	Sod. (mg)	Carb. (g)	Fiber (g)	Pro. (g)	Servings/Exchanges
Salad Croutons	1 serving	112	6	48	1	0	195	12	1	2	1 starch, 1 fat
Seasoned Fries	1 order	261	12	41	3	0	556	35	0	5	2 starch, 2 1/2 fat
✔Slice Tomatoes	3 slices	13	0	0	0	0	6	3	1	1	1 veg
Sour Cream	3 T	91	9	89	6	19	23	2	0	1	2 fat
Tartar Sauce	3 T	225	23	92	4	15	157	3	0	0	4 1/2 fat
Turkey Gravy	4 T	125	9	65	2	69	3323	29	0	4	2 starch, 1 1/2 fat
SOUPS											
Chicken Noodle	8 oz	118	5	38	2	30	1130	14	1	1	1 starch, 1 fat
Clam Chowder	8 oz	624	42	61	34	5	1474	55	4	7	2 starch, 1 milk, 8 fat
Cream of Broccoli	8 oz	574	46	72	67	0	1174	41	2	6	2 starch, 1 milk, 7 1/2 fat
✔Vegetable Beef	8 oz	79	1	11	1	5	820	11	2	6	1 veg, 1 lean meat

✔ = Healthiest Bets

Ruby Tuesday

Ruby Tuesday has made an effort to be open and provide some nutrition information for its menu offerings on its Web site at www.rubytuesday.com. They provide only calories, fat grams, fiber grams, and "net carb grams." The Ruby Tuesday menu provides this information for the "Smart Eating" items.

The following chart with Ruby Tuesday's menu items provides only calories, fat grams, and fiber grams. It doesn't provide "net carb" grams because this information isn't helpful. No meals were developed or healthiest bets provided due to the minimal information available.

(*Continued*)

Ruby Tuesday

	Amount	Cal.	Fat (g)	% Cal. Fat	Sat. Fat (g)	Chol. (mg)	Sod. (mg)	Carb. (g)	Fiber (g)	Pro. (g)	Servings/Exchanges
BURGERS											
Alpine	1	1081	73	61	n/a	n/a	n/a	n/a	5	n/a	insufficient info. to calculate
American	1	942	62	59	n/a	n/a	n/a	n/a	3	n/a	insufficient info. to calculate
Bacon Cheeseburger	1	1009	67	60	n/a	n/a	n/a	n/a	3	n/a	insufficient info. to calculate
Black & Bleu	1	995	64	58	n/a	n/a	n/a	n/a	3	n/a	insufficient info. to calculate
Classic	1	830	53	57	n/a	n/a	n/a	n/a	3	n/a	insufficient info. to calculate
Colossal B	1	1677	114	61	n/a	n/a	n/a	n/a	5	n/a	insufficient info. to calculate
Old English Bacon Cheeseburger	1	1076	73	61	n/a	n/a	n/a	n/a	3	n/a	insufficient info. to calculate
Pepper Jack Bacon	1	1134	75	60	n/a	n/a	n/a	n/a	3	n/a	insufficient info. to calculate
Smokehouse	1	1144	73	57	n/a	n/a	n/a	n/a	4	n/a	insufficient info. to calculate

Turkey Club	1	776	41	48	n/a	n/a	n/a	n/a	3	n/a	insufficient info. to calculate
Veggie	1	805	41	46	n/a	n/a	n/a	n/a	11	n/a	insufficient info. to calculate
DESSERTS											
Blondie	1	705	37	47	n/a	n/a	n/a	n/a	2	n/a	insufficient info. to calculate
Blueberry D'Lite	1	213	5	21	n/a	n/a	n/a	n/a	4	n/a	insufficient info. to calculate
Brownie	1	999	46	41	n/a	n/a	n/a	n/a	8	n/a	insufficient info. to calculate
Candy Bar Ice Cream Pie	1	827	42	46	n/a	n/a	n/a	n/a	1	n/a	insufficient info. to calculate
Low Carb Cheese Cake	1	400	32	72	n/a	n/a	n/a	n/a	5	n/a	insufficient info. to calculate
Low Carb Chocolate Lava Cake	1	632	40	57	n/a	n/a	n/a	n/a	10	n/a	insufficient info. to calculate
Tallcake	1	632	40	57	n/a	n/a	n/a	n/a	10	n/a	insufficient info. to calculate
ENTRÉE SALADS											
Carolina Chicken w/out dressing	1	880	62	63	n/a	n/a	n/a	n/a	6	n/a	insufficient info. to calculate

n/a = not available

(*Continued*)

ENTRÉE SALADS (*Continued*)	Amount	Cal.	Fat (g)	% Cal. Fat	Sat. Fat (g)	Chol. (mg)	Sod. (mg)	Carb. (g)	Fiber (g)	Pro. (g)	Servings/Exchanges
Low Carb Chicken Caesar	1	501	35	63	n/a	n/a	n/a	n/a	4	n/a	insufficient info. to calculate
Low Carb Chicken Cobb w/out dressing	1	618	41	60	n/a	n/a	n/a	n/a	3	n/a	insufficient info. to calculate
Low Carb Peppercorn Salmon Caesar	1	656	46	63	n/a	n/a	n/a	n/a	4	n/a	insufficient info. to calculate
Low Carb Spring Chicken w/out dressing	1	399	24	54	n/a	n/a	n/a	n/a	4	n/a	insufficient info. to calculate
GOURMET SANDWICHES											
Beale Street BBQ	1	870	33	34	n/a	n/a	n/a	n/a	7	n/a	insufficient info. to calculate
Buffalo & Bleu	1	894	54	54	n/a	n/a	n/a	n/a	3	n/a	insufficient info. to calculate
Crispy Chicken Club	1	830	46	50	n/a	n/a	n/a	n/a	3	n/a	insufficient info. to calculate
Cuban Panini	1	1164	82	63	n/a	n/a	n/a	n/a	2	n/a	insufficient info. to calculate
Ham Panini	1	1172	82	63	n/a	n/a	n/a	n/a	2	n/a	insufficient info. to calculate

Hickory Chicken	1	891	44	44	n/a	n/a	n/a	n/a	3	n/a	insufficient info. to calculate
Low Carb Chicken Caesar Wrap	1	390	18	42	n/a	n/a	n/a	n/a	11	n/a	insufficient info. to calculate
Low Carb Grilled Chicken Wrap	1	395	18	41	n/a	n/a	n/a	n/a	10	n/a	insufficient info. to calculate
Low Carb Roasted Turkey Wrap	1	276	7	23	n/a	n/a	n/a	n/a	11	n/a	insufficient info. to calculate
Ruby's Chicken	1	638	25	35	n/a	n/a	n/a	n/a	3	n/a	insufficient info. to calculate
Signature Fish	1	920	56	55	n/a	n/a	n/a	n/a	3	n/a	insufficient info. to calculate
Turkey & Bacon Panini	1	1315	87	60	n/a	n/a	n/a	n/a	2	n/a	insufficient info. to calculate
Ultimate Roasted Turkey BLT	1	1119	66	53	n/a	n/a	n/a	n/a	5	n/a	insufficient info. to calculate
PASTAS											
Chicken Marinara	1	846	15	16	n/a	n/a	n/a	n/a	12	n/a	insufficient info. to calculate

n/a = not available

(*Continued*)

PASTAS (*Continued*)	Amount	Cal.	Fat (g)	% Cal. Fat	Sat. Fat (g)	Chol. (mg)	Sod. (mg)	Carb. (g)	Fiber (g)	Pro. (g)	Servings/Exchanges
Chicken Parmesan	1	1466	94	58	n/a	n/a	n/a	n/a	7	n/a	insufficient info. to calculate
Pasta Marinara	1	659	10	14	n/a	n/a	n/a	n/a	12	n/a	insufficient info. to calculate
Roma Chicken	1	1183	51	39	n/a	n/a	n/a	n/a	10	n/a	insufficient info. to calculate
Shrimp Alfredo	1	1074	19	16	n/a	n/a	n/a	n/a	10	n/a	insufficient info. to calculate
Sonora Chicken	1 order	1169	41	32	n/a	n/a	n/a	n/a	13	n/a	insufficient info. to calculate
PLATTERS W/OUT GARLIC TOAST											
Classic Baby Back Ribs	full rack	1430	84	53	n/a	n/a	n/a	n/a	9	n/a	insufficient info. to calculate
Classic Baby Back Ribs	half rack	937	51	49	n/a	n/a	n/a	n/a	9	n/a	insufficient info. to calculate
Louisiana Fried Shrimp	1	999	52	47	n/a	n/a	n/a	n/a	10	n/a	insufficient info. to calculate
Original Chicken Tenders	1	963	47	44	n/a	n/a	n/a	n/a	9	n/a	insufficient info. to calculate
Smokehouse Platter	1	954	43	41	n/a	n/a	n/a	n/a	10	n/a	insufficient info. to calculate
Smoky Mountain Chicken	1	942	45	43	n/a	n/a	n/a	n/a	9	n/a	insufficient info. to calculate

Spicy Buffalo Chicken Tenders	1	1188	70	53	n/a	n/a	n/a	n/a	10	n/a	insufficient info. to calculate
Triple Play	1	1474	82	50	n/a	n/a	n/a	n/a	10	n/a	insufficient info. to calculate
SHAREABLE APPETIZERS W/OUT SAUCES											
Asian Pot Stickers	1 serving	121	5	37	n/a	n/a	n/a	n/a	1	n/a	insufficient info. to calculate
Chicken Quesadilla	1 serving	187	11	53	n/a	n/a	n/a	n/a	1	n/a	insufficient info. to calculate
Fried Cheese	1 serving	172	11	58	n/a	n/a	n/a	n/a	2	n/a	insufficient info. to calculate
Loaded Cheese Fries	1 serving	290	18	56	n/a	n/a	n/a	n/a	4	n/a	insufficient info. to calculate
Low Carb Chicken Quesadilla	1 serving	153	10	59	n/a	n/a	n/a	n/a	2	n/a	insufficient info. to calculate
Low Carb Spicy Buffalo Wings	1 serving	228	16	63	n/a	n/a	n/a	n/a	0	n/a	insufficient info. to calculate
Original Chicken Tenders	1 serving	130	7	48	n/a	n/a	n/a	n/a	0	n/a	insufficient info. to calculate
Queso Dip	1 serving	318	22	62	n/a	n/a	n/a	n/a	2	n/a	insufficient info. to calculate

n/a = not available

(*Continued*)

SHAREABLE APPETIZERS W/OUT SAUCES (*Continued*)	Amount	Cal.	Fat (g)	% Cal. Fat	Sat. Fat (g)	Chol. (mg)	Sod. (mg)	Carb. (g)	Fiber (g)	Pro. (g)	Servings/Exchanges
Signature Sampler	1 serving	278	17	55	n/a	n/a	n/a	n/a	3	n/a	insufficient info. to calculate
Southwest Spring Rolls	1 serving	173	10	52	n/a	n/a	n/a	n/a	1	n/a	insufficient info. to calculate
Spicy Buffalo Chicken Tenders	1 serving	187	13	63	n/a	n/a	n/a	n/a	0	n/a	insufficient info. to calculate
Spicy Honey BBQ Chicken Tenders	1 serving	160	7	39	n/a	n/a	n/a	n/a	0	n/a	insufficient info. to calculate
Spinach Dip	1 serving	287	20	63	n/a	n/a	n/a	n/a	2	n/a	insufficient info. to calculate
Tuesday Sampler	1 serving	199	12	54	n/a	n/a	n/a	n/a	1	n/a	insufficient info. to calculate
SIDE ITEMS											
Baked Beans	1	130	3	21	n/a	n/a	n/a	n/a	4	n/a	insufficient info. to calculate
Baked Potato w/ butter & sour cream	1	459	19	37	n/a	n/a	n/a	n/a	11	n/a	insufficient info. to calculate

Brown Rice & Black Beans	1	274	6	20	n/a	n/a	n/a	n/a	5	n/a	insufficient info. to calculate
Brown Rice Pilaf	1	222	6	24	n/a	n/a	n/a	n/a	2	n/a	insufficient info. to calculate
Cole Slaw	1	129	8	56	n/a	n/a	n/a	n/a	0	n/a	insufficient info. to calculate
Creamed Spinach	1	204	17	75	n/a	n/a	n/a	n/a	2	n/a	insufficient info. to calculate
Creamy Mashed Cauliflower	1	166	11	60	n/a	n/a	n/a	n/a	6	n/a	insufficient info. to calculate
Fresh Sautéed Zucchini	1	54	3	50	n/a	n/a	n/a	n/a	2	n/a	insufficient info. to calculate
Fresh Steamed Broccoli	1	129	8	56	n/a	n/a	n/a	n/a	3	n/a	insufficient info. to calculate
Garlic Toast	1	220	12	49	n/a	n/a	n/a	n/a	1	n/a	insufficient info. to calculate
Mashed Potatoes	1	328	15	41	n/a	n/a	n/a	n/a	0	n/a	insufficient info. to calculate
Onion Straws	1	320	23	65	n/a	n/a	n/a	n/a	2	n/a	insufficient info. to calculate
Ruby's Fries	1	185	9	44	n/a	n/a	n/a	n/a	5	n/a	insufficient info. to calculate
Sugar Snap Peas	1	132	6	41	n/a	n/a	n/a	n/a	4	n/a	insufficient info. to calculate

n/a = not available

(*Continued*)

	Amount	Cal.	Fat (g)	% Cal. Fat	Sat. Fat (g)	Chol. (mg)	Sod. (mg)	Carb. (g)	Fiber (g)	Pro. (g)	Servings/Exchanges
SIGNATURE SALAD DRESSINGS											
Bleu Cheese	2 T	177	19	97	n/a	n/a	n/a	n/a	0	n/a	insufficient info. to calculate
Caesar	2 T	97	10	93	n/a	n/a	n/a	n/a	0	n/a	insufficient info. to calculate
Honey Mustard	2 T	92	8	78	n/a	n/a	n/a	n/a	0	n/a	insufficient info. to calculate
Light Balsamic Vinaigrette	2 T	35	2	51	n/a	n/a	n/a	n/a	0	n/a	insufficient info. to calculate
Light Ranch	2 T	55	5	82	n/a	n/a	n/a	n/a	0	n/a	insufficient info. to calculate
Ranch	2 T	101	11	98	n/a	n/a	n/a	n/a	0	n/a	insufficient info. to calculate
Smoky Honey Dijon	2 T	100	8	72	n/a	n/a	n/a	n/a	0	n/a	insufficient info. to calculate
SIGNATURE SAUCES & DRESSING											
Barbecue Sauce	2 T	50	0	0	n/a	n/a	n/a	n/a	0	n/a	insufficient info. to calculate
Bleu Cheese Dressing	2 T	177	19	97	n/a	n/a	n/a	n/a	0	n/a	insufficient info. to calculate

Cocktail Sauce	2 T	23	0	0	n/a	n/a	n/a	n/a	0	n/a	free
Low Carb Chocolate Sauce	2 T	74	2	24	n/a	n/a	n/a	n/a	1	n/a	insufficient info. to calculate
Marinara Sauce	2 T	15	1	60	n/a	n/a	n/a	n/a	0	n/a	free
Ranch Dressing	2 T	101	11	98	n/a	n/a	n/a	n/a	0	n/a	insufficient info. to calculate
Remoulade Sauce	2 T	160	17	96	n/a	n/a	n/a	n/a	0	n/a	insufficient info. to calculate
Salsa	2 T	11	0	0	n/a	n/a	n/a	n/a	0	n/a	free
Side of Turkey Gravy	2 T	30	2	60	n/a	n/a	n/a	n/a	0	n/a	insufficient info. to calculate
Smoky Honey Dijon	2 T	100	8	72	n/a	n/a	n/a	n/a	0	n/a	insufficient info. to calculate
Sour Cream	2 T	30	2	60	n/a	n/a	n/a	n/a	0	n/a	insufficient info. to calculate
Steak Butter	2 T	92	10	98	n/a	n/a	n/a	n/a	0	n/a	insufficient info. to calculate
Thai Peanut Sauce	2 T	66	3	41	n/a	n/a	n/a	n/a	0	n/a	insufficient info. to calculate

n/a = not available

(Continued)

	Amount	Cal.	Fat (g)	% Cal. Fat	Sat. Fat (g)	Chol. (mg)	Sod. (mg)	Carb. (g)	Fiber (g)	Pro. (g)	Servings/Exchanges
SIGNATURE SOUPS											
Baked French Onion Soup	1 serving	547	39	64	n/a	n/a	n/a	n/a	1	n/a	insufficient info. to calculate
Low Carb Broccoli & Cheese Soup	1 serving	332	27	73	n/a	n/a	n/a	n/a	3	n/a	insufficient info. to calculate
Onion Soup	1 serving	198	12	55	n/a	n/a	n/a	n/a	0	n/a	insufficient info. to calculate
White Chicken Chili	1 serving	218	8	33	n/a	n/a	n/a	n/a	6	n/a	insufficient info. to calculate
SPECIALTIES											
Church Street Chicken	1	844	47	50	n/a	n/a	n/a	n/a	8	n/a	insufficient info. to calculate
Creole Catch	1	663	31	42	n/a	n/a	n/a	n/a	5	n/a	insufficient info. to calculate
Eat Your Veggies Platter	1	643	31	43	n/a	n/a	n/a	n/a	10	n/a	insufficient info. to calculate
Glazed Popcorn Salmon	1	774	35	41	n/a	n/a	n/a	n/a	4	n/a	insufficient info. to calculate
New Orleans Seafood	1	858	13	14	n/a	n/a	n/a	n/a	5	n/a	insufficient info. to calculate

Old - Fashion Pot Roast	1	1062	63	53	n/a	n/a	n/a	n/a	3	n/a	insufficient info. to calculate
Oven Roasted Turkey Dinner	1	729	30	37	n/a	n/a	n/a	n/a	3	n/a	insufficient info. to calculate
SPECIALTIES - LOW CARB											
Church Street Chicken	1	788	51	58	n/a	n/a	n/a	n/a	11	n/a	insufficient info. to calculate
Creole Catch	1	607	35	52	n/a	n/a	n/a	n/a	9	n/a	insufficient info. to calculate
Glazed Popcorn Salmon	1	585	32	49	n/a	n/a	n/a	n/a	10	n/a	insufficient info. to calculate
New Orleans Seafood	1	802	50	56	n/a	n/a	n/a	n/a	9	n/a	insufficient info. to calculate
Oven Roasted Turkey Dinner	1	628	24	34	n/a	n/a	n/a	n/a	9	n/a	insufficient info. to calculate
STEAKS & MORE											
Blacken Ribeye	1	645	45	63	n/a	n/a	n/a	n/a	0	n/a	insufficient info. to calculate
Grilled BBQ Chicken - double breast	1	418	10	22	n/a	n/a	n/a	n/a	0	n/a	insufficient info. to calculate

n/a = not available

(*Continued*)

STEAKS & MORE (*Continued*)	Amount	Cal.	Fat (g)	% Cal. Fat	Sat. Fat (g)	Chol. (mg)	Sod. (mg)	Carb. (g)	Fiber (g)	Pro. (g)	Servings/Exchanges
Grilled BBQ Chicken - single breast	1	209	5	22	n/a	n/a	n/a	n/a	0	n/a	insufficient info. to calculate
Honey Dijon Chicken - double breast	1	418	10	22	n/a	n/a	n/a	n/a	0	n/a	insufficient info. to calculate
Honey Dijon Chicken - single breast	1	209	5	22	n/a	n/a	n/a	n/a	0	n/a	insufficient info. to calculate
Peppercorn Mushroom Sirloin	1	613	40	59	n/a	n/a	n/a	n/a	2	n/a	insufficient info. to calculate
Petite Sirloin	1	222	8	32	n/a	n/a	n/a	n/a	0	n/a	insufficient info. to calculate
Ruby's Rib Eye	1	635	44	62	n/a	n/a	n/a	n/a	0	n/a	insufficient info. to calculate
Smothered Sirloin Tips w/out mushrooms	1	990	52	47	n/a	n/a	n/a	n/a	0	n/a	insufficient info. to calculate
Top Sirloin	1	285	11	35	n/a	n/a	n/a	n/a	0	n/a	insufficient info. to calculate

n/a = not available

Soups, Sandwiches, Salads, and Subs

RESTAURANTS

Arby's
Au Bon Pain
Blimpie Subs and Salads
Panera Bread
Quiznos Subs
Schlotzsky's Deli
Subway
Wienerschnitzel

NUTRITION PROS

- Healthier condiments, such as mustard and vinegar, are available. They keep your sub or sandwich moist without adding a lot of calories and fat.
- Subs and sandwiches are often made to order. That's good because you can specify what you want and don't want.
- Healthy breads, even whole wheat with extra fiber, are usually available.
- Healthy sub and sandwich fillers are available—turkey, smoked turkey, ham, chicken breast, or roast beef.
- Healthy broth-based vegetable and grain soups are warm and ready in some sandwich shops.
- Sub shops offer smaller-sized sandwiches. No need to order the foot-long size.

Healthy Tips

- ★ To keep your sodium meter on low, go light on or hold the pickles and olives.
- ★ Complement a sub or sandwich with a healthier side than a fried snack food (potato chips, tortilla chips, and the like). For some crunch, try a side salad, popcorn, baked chips, or pretzels.
- ★ Ask to have large subs cut into two. Pack up half for another day.
- ★ In sandwich shops, order a cup of broth-based vegetable or bean soup. They'll fill you up and not out.
- ★ A Greek salad and piece of pita bread make a moderate-carbohydrate and light-on-protein meal. Ask for dressing on the side.
- ★ Pack a piece of fruit from home to bring to the sub or sandwich shop.

- Salads with light or fat-free salad dressings are an option in most sub and sandwich shops.

NUTRITION CONS

- Large sandwiches and long subs can be stuffed with enough protein for the whole day.
- Common sub and sandwich condiments, such as mayonnaise and oil, are high in fat.
- Tuna fish, chicken, and seafood salads sound healthy, but they are chock full of fat and calories.

- Cheese is a frequent sub or sandwich addition. Some restaurants give their nutrition information minus the cheese. Make sure you read the numbers for the way you eat yours.
- Fruit and cooked vegetables are rarely available.

Get It Your Way

- ★ Hold the mayonnaise and oil. Substitute mustard or vinegar.
- ★ Ask the sub maker to go light on the meat and heavy on the lettuce, onions, tomatoes, and peppers.
- ★ Hold the cheese.
- ★ Ask for the salad dressing on the side.

Arby's

❖ Arby's provides nutrition information for all its menu items on its Web site at www.arbys.com.

Light 'n Lean Choice

Jr. Roast Beef Sandwich
1/2 Curly Fries

Calories	440	Sodium (mg)	1,130
Fat (g)	18	Carbohydrate (g)	54
% calories from fat	37	Fiber (g)	4
Saturated fat (g)	5	Protein (g)	18
Cholesterol (mg)	30		

Exchanges: 3 1/2 starch, 2 medium-fat meat, 1 fat

Healthy 'n Hearty Choice

Martha's Vineyard Salad with Honey Mustard Dipping Sauce *(2 T)*
Baked Potato with Horsey Sauce *(1 T)*

Calories	640	Sodium (mg)	845
Fat (g)	25	Carbohydrate (g)	77
% calories from fat	35	Fiber (g)	8
Saturated fat (g)	7	Protein (g)	30
Cholesterol (mg)	75		

Exchanges: 3 starch, 2 veg, 1 fruit, 3 lean meat, 3 fat

Arby's

	Amount	Cal.	Fat (g)	% Cal. Fat	Sat. Fat (g)	Chol. (mg)	Sod. (mg)	Carb. (g)	Fiber (g)	Pro. (g)	Servings/Exchanges
BREAKFAST BISCUIT											
Bacon	1	300	17	51	5	15	950	27	0	9	2 starch, 1 medium-fat meat, 2 fat
Ham	1	270	13	43	3.5	20	1170	27	0	12	2 starch, 1 lean meat, 1 fat
Plain	1	230	12	47	3	0	710	26	0	5	2 starch, 2 fat
Sausage	1	390	27	62	9	30	1080	26	0	10	2 starch, 1 high-fat meat, 3 fat
Scrambled Egg	1	310	18	52	4.5	145	930	28	0	10	2 starch, 1 medium-fat meat, 2 fat

✓ = Healthiest Bets

(*Continued*)

BREAKFAST BISCUIT (*Continued*)	Amount	Cal.	Fat (g)	% Cal. Fat	Sat. Fat (g)	Chol. (mg)	Sod. (mg)	Carb. (g)	Fiber (g)	Pro. (g)	Servings/Exchanges
Swiss Cheese	1	270	15	50	5	10	910	26	0	8	2 starch, 1 medium-fat meat, 1 fat
w/ butter	1	330	23	63	10	30	825	26	0	5	2 starch, 3 1/2 fat
BREAKFAST CROISSANT											
Bacon 'n Egg	1	410	26	57	12	190	670	31	0	13	2 starch, 2 medium-fat meat, 2 1/2 fat
Ham 'n Cheese	1	350	19	49	11	65	870	30	0	15	2 starch, 2 medium-fat meat, 1 fat
Sausage 'n Egg	1	510	36	64	15	210	800	31	0	14	2 starch, 2 high-fat meat, 3 1/2 fat
BREAKFAST SOURDOUGH											
Bacon, Egg & Swiss	1	500	29	52	10	325	1600	33	1	25	2 starch, 3 high-fat meat, 1 fat

Egg 'n Cheese	1	330	16	44	6	165	1060	31	15	15	2 starch, 2 medium-fat meat, 1 fat
Ham 'n Swiss	1	450	23	46	8	330	1750	33	1	27	2 starch, 3 medium-fat meat, 1 1/2 fat
DESSERTS											
✓Gourmet Chocolate Cookie	1	200	10	45	6	15	210	26	0	2	1 1/2 starch, 2 fat
DESSERTS - TURNOVERS											
Apple w/ icing	1	380	12	28	3.5	0	200	64	2	4	4 starch, 1 fruit
Apple w/out icing	1	250	10	36	3	0	200	35	2	4	2 starch, 1 fruit, 1/2 fat
Cherry w/ icing	1	380	12	28	3.5	0	200	64	2	4	4 starch, 1 fruit
Cherry w/out icing	1	250	10	36	3	0	200	35	2	4	2 starch, 1 fruit, 1/2 fat

✓ = Healthiest Bets

(Continued)

	Amount	Cal.	Fat (g)	% Cal. Fat	Sat. Fat (g)	Chol. (mg)	Sod. (mg)	Carb. (g)	Fiber (g)	Pro. (g)	Servings/Exchanges
MARKET-FRESH SALADS											
Chicken Club	1	530	33	56	10	210	1120	32	5	30	2 starch, 2 veg, 3 lean meat, 3 1/2 fat
✓Martha's Vineyard w/out dressing	1	250	8	29	4.5	60	490	23	4	26	1 starch, 3 veg, 2 lean meat
Santa Fe w/out dressing	1	520	29	50	9	60	1120	40	5	27	2 1/2 starch, 3 veg, 2 medium-fat meat, 3 fat
MARKET-FRESH SANDWICHES											
Chicken Club Wrap	1	680	38	50	14	100	1800	52	31	43	3 1/2 starch, 5 medium-fat meat, 3 fat
Chicken Salad	1	860	44	46	6	60	1270	92	6	26	6 starch, 2 medium-fat meat, 5 fat

Roast Beef and Swiss	1	780	39	45	12	90	1740	74	6	37	5 starch, 3 lean meat, 4 1/2 fat
Roast Ham and Swiss	1	700	31	40	7	85	2140	74	5	36	5 starch, 3 lean meat, 3 fat
Roast Turkey and Swiss	1	720	27	34	6	90	1790	74	5	45	5 starch, 4 lean meat, 2 1/2 fat
Roast Turkey, Ranch, & Bacon	1	830	38	41	10	110	2260	75	5	49	5 starch, 5 lean meat, 3 1/2 fat
Ultimate BLT	1	780	46	53	9	50	1570	75	6	23	5 starch, 2 medium-fat meat, 5 fat
MARKET-FRESH WRAPS											
Chicken Caesar	1	520	27	47	7	65	1530	46	30	33	3 starch, 3 medium-fat meat, 3 fat
Fresh Ultimate BLT	1	650	47	65	11	50	1730	48	31	25	3 starch, 3 medium-fat meat, 5 1/2 fat

✓ = Healthiest Bets

(*Continued*)

MARKET-FRESH WRAPS (*Continued*)	Amount	Cal.	Fat (g)	% Cal. Fat	Sat. Fat (g)	Chol. (mg)	Sod. (mg)	Carb. (g)	Fiber (g)	Pro. (g)	Servings/Exchanges
Roast Turkey Ranch & Bacon	1	710	39	49	11	110	2420	48	30	51	3 starch, 6 lean meat, 3 fat
Southwest Chicken	1	550	30	49	9	75	1690	45	30	35	3 starch, 3 1/2 lean meat, 3 fat
OTHER SANDWICHES											
Chicken Bacon 'n Swiss	1	550	27	44	7	70	1640	49	2	31	3 starch, 3 medium-fat meat, 2 fat
Chicken Breast Fillet	1	490	24	44	4	55	1220	46	2	25	3 starch, 2 lean meat, 3 fat
Chicken Cordon Bleu	1	570	29	46	6	85	1880	46	2	34	3 starch, 4 lean meat, 2 1/2 fat
Chicken Fingers (4 pack)	1 order	640	38	53	8	70	1590	42	3	31	3 starch, 2 medium-fat meat, 5 1/2 fat
Chicken Fingers Combo	1 order	1050	60	51	11	70	2540	89	5	37	6 starch, 3 medium-fat meat, 8 fat

Chicken Fingers Snack	1 order	590	34	52	6	35	1430	53	3	19	3 1/2 starch, 1 medium-fat meat, 5 fat
✓Grilled Chicken Deluxe	1	380	12	28	2	50	920	40	2	29	2 1/2 starch, 3 lean meat, 1/2 fat
Hot Ham 'n Cheese	1	300	9	27	3.5	50	1450	35	1	23	2 1/2 starch, 2 lean meat
Hot Ham 'n Swiss Melt	1	270	8	27	3.5	35	1140	35	1	18	2 starch, 2 lean meat
Roast Chicken Club	1	470	25	48	7	65	1320	39	2	27	2 1/2 starch, 3 lean meat, 2 1/2 fat

PREMIUM POTATOES

✓Baked Potato (plain)	1	200	0	0	0	0	15	46	4	4	3 starch
Baked Potato w/ butter	1	300	11	33	7	30	130	46	4	4	3 starch, 1 1/2 fat
Baked Potato w/ Sour Cream	1	320	12	34	7	25	45	48	4	6	3 starch, 2 fat
Broccoli 'n Cheese Potato	1	460	23	45	15	50	780	56	6	11	3 1/2 starch, 1 veg, 3 fat

✓ = Healthiest Bets

(Continued)

PREMIUM POTATOES (*Continued*)	Amount	Cal.	Fat (g)	% Cal. Fat	Sat. Fat (g)	Chol. (mg)	Sod. (mg)	Carb. (g)	Fiber (g)	Pro. (g)	Servings/Exchanges
Curley Fries - large	1	630	34	49	5	0	1480	73	7	8	5 starch, 5 fat
Curley Fries - medium	1	410	22	48	3	0	950	47	5	5	3 starch, 4 fat
Curley Fries - small	1	340	18	48	3	0	790	39	4	4	2 1/2 starch, 3 fat
Deluxe Potato	1	570	34	54	20	90	750	50	5	18	3 starch, 1 lean meat, 6 fat
Home-style Fries - large	1	570	24	38	3.5	0	1030	82	6	6	5 1/2 starch, 3 fat
Home-style Fries - medium	1	380	16	38	2.5	0	690	55	4	4	3 1/2 starch, 2 1/2 fat
Home-style Fries - small	1	300	13	39	2	0	550	44	3	3	3 starch, 1 1/2 fat
Potato Cakes (2)	1	250	15	54	2	0	390	26	2	2	2 starch, 1 1/2 fat
ROAST BEEF SANDWICHES											
Arby-Q	1	360	11	28	4.5	35	1210	51	2	18	3 1/2 starch, 1 lean meat, 1/2 fat
Beef 'n Cheddar	1	440	21	43	7	50	1270	44	2	22	3 starch, 2 medium-fat meat, 1 fat

Big Montana	1	590	29	44	14	115	2080	41	3	47	3 starch, 5 lean meat, 2 fat
French Dip 'n Swiss	1	320	25	70	11	75	2040	56	3	35	4 starch, 3 medium-fat meat
Giant	1	450	19	38	9	75	1440	41	2	32	3 starch, 3 lean meat, 1 fat
✓Junior	1	270	9	30	4	30	740	34	2	16	2 starch, 1 lean meat, 1 1/2 fat
Philly Beef Supreme	1	450	37	74	13	95	1660	59	3	36	4 starch, 3 lean meat
Regular	1	320	13	37	6	45	950	34	2	21	2 1/2 starch, 3 lean meat
Super	1	440	19	39	7	45	1130	48	3	22	3 starch, 3 lean meat, 1 fat
SAUCES AND CONDIMENTS											
✓Arby's Sauce Packet	1	15	0	0	0	0	180	4	0	0	free
BBQ Dipping Sauce	2 T	40	0	0	0	0	350	10	0	0	1/2 carb
Bronco Berry Sauce	4 T	120	0	0	0	0	35	30	0	0	2 carb

✓ = Healthiest Bets

(Continued)

SAUCES AND CONDIMENTS (*Continued*)	Amount	Cal.	Fat (g)	% Cal. Fat	Sat. Fat (g)	Chol. (mg)	Sod. (mg)	Carb. (g)	Fiber (g)	Pro. (g)	Servings/Exchanges
Buffalo Dipping Sauce	4 T	20	1	45	0	0	1600	3	0	0	free
Buttermilk Ranch Dressing	4 T	290	30	93	5	25	580	3	0	1	6 fat
Cheddar Cheese Sauce (for Fries)	3 T	60	5	75	1	0	360	4	0	1	1 fat
Honey Mustard Dipping Sauce	2 T	130	12	83	2	10	170	5	0	0	2 1/2 fat
Horsey Sauce Packet	1 T	60	5	75	1	5	170	3	0	0	1 fat
✓Marinara Sauce	3 T	15	0	0	0	0	220	4	0	0	free
Raspberry Vinaigrette	2.5 oz	170	12	64	1.5	0	340	16	0	0	1 carb, 2 fat
Red Ranch Sauce	1 T	70	6	77	1	0	105	5	0	0	1 1/2 fat
Santa Fe Ranch Dressing	3 T	300	31	93	5	20	690	4	0	1	6 fat
Seasoned Tortilla Strips	1 T	61	3	44	0.5	0	25	10	0	1	1/2 carb, 1/2 fat

Sliced Almonds	1 T	81	7	78	0	0	0	2	1	4	1 1/2 fat
Tangy Southwest Sauce	4 T	330	35	95	5	30	370	5	0	1	7 fat
✓Three Pepper Sauce Packet	1	20	1	45	0	0	140	3	0	0	free
SHAKES											
Chocolate - Large	1	660	17	23	10	45	450	110	0	17	7 carb, 3 1/2 fat
Chocolate - Regular	1	510	13	23	8	35	360	83	0	13	5 1/2 carb, 2 1/2 fat
Jamocha - Large	1	650	17	24	10	45	510	107	0	17	7 carb, 3 1/2 fat
Jamocha - Regular	1	500	13	23	8	35	390	81	0	13	5 carb, 2 1/2 fat
Strawberry - Large	1	650	17	24	10	45	460	107	0	16	7 carb, 3 1/2 fat
Strawberry - Regular	1	500	13	23	8	35	360	81	0	13	5 carb, 2 1/2 fat
Vanilla - Large	1	650	17	24	10	45	470	107	0	16	7 carb, 3 1/2 fat
Vanilla - Regular	1	500	13	23	8	35	370	82	0	13	5 1/2 carb, 2 1/2 fat

✓ = Healthiest Bets

(*Continued*)

	Amount	Cal.	Fat (g)	% Cal. Fat	Sat. Fat (g)	Chol. (mg)	Sod. (mg)	Carb. (g)	Fiber (g)	Pro. (g)	Servings/Exchanges
SIDE KICKERS											
Jalapeno Bites - Large	1 order	610	37	55	14	55	1050	58	4	11	4 starch, 1 medium-fat meat, 6 fat
Jalapeno Bites - Regular	1 order	310	19	55	7	30	530	29	2	5	2 starch, 1 medium-fat meat, 3 fat
Mozzarella Sticks - Large	1 order	850	45	48	19	90	2740	76	4	36	5 starch, 3 medium-fat meat, 6 fat
Mozzarella Sticks - Regular	1 order	430	23	48	10	45	1370	38	2	18	2 1/2 starch, 1 medium-fat meat, 3 fat
Onion Petals - Large	1 order	830	48	52	7	0	830	88	5	10	5 starch, 2 veg, 9 1/2 fat
Onion Petals - Regular	1 order	330	19	52	3	0	330	35	2	4	2 starch, 1 veg, 4 fat

✓ = Healthiest Bets

Au Bon Pain

❖ Au Bon Pain provides nutrition information for its menu items on its Web site at www.aubonpain.com.

Light 'n Lean Choice

Holiday Turkey Stew Soup *(12 oz)*
Multigrain Bread *(1 slice)*
Garden Salad with Lite Ranch Dressing *(2 T)*

Calories	615	Sodium (mg)	1,642
Fat (g)	22	Carbohydrate (g)	75
% calories from fat	32	Fiber (g)	9
Saturated fat (g)	7	Protein (g)	27
Cholesterol (mg)	75		

Exchanges: 4 starch, 2 veg, 2 lean meat, 3 fat

Healthy 'n Hearty Choice

Wild Mushroom Bisque *(12 oz)*
Honey Dijon Cordon Bleu Wrap

Calories	700	Sodium (mg)	2,480
Fat (g)	17	Carbohydrate (g)	83
% calories from fat	22	Fiber (g)	5
Saturated fat (g)	7.5	Protein (g)	49
Cholesterol (mg)	125		

Exchanges: 5 starch, 2 veg, 4 lean meat, 1 fat

(*Continued*)

Au Bon Pain

	Amount	Cal.	Fat (g)	% Cal. Fat	Sat. Fat (g)	Chol. (mg)	Sod. (mg)	Carb. (g)	Fiber (g)	Pro. (g)	Servings/Exchanges
BAGELS											
✓Asiago Cheese	1	380	8	19	4.5	20	740	59	3	18	4 starch, 1 medium-fat meat
Cinnamon Crisp	1	430	6	13	1	0	430	96	3	11	6 starch
✓Cinnamon Raisin	1	330	1	3	0	0	480	71	3	12	4 1/2 starch
Dutch Apple	1	470	4	8	1	0	540	98	5	13	6 1/2 starch
✓Everything	1	330	3	8	0	0	750	63	3	13	4 starch
French Toast	1	420	7	15	2	0	440	76	3	11	5 starch
✓Honey 9 Grain	1	360	2	5	0	0	550	75	6	14	5 starch
✓Jalapeno Cheddar	1	350	6	15	3.5	15	690	56	2	18	3 1/2 starch, 1 medium-fat meat

✓Plain	1	300	1	3	0	0	470	61	3	12	4 starch
✓Sesame Seed	1	340	4	11	0.5	0	470	62	3	13	4 starch
BEVERAGES											
✓Apple Cider	16 oz	250	0	0	0	0	125	62	0	0	4 starch
✓Café Au Lait (small)	12 oz	80	3	34	2	15	85	9	0	5	1 milk, 1/2 fat
✓Cafe Latte (small)	12 oz	130	5	35	3	20	130	13	0	8	1 milk, 1 fat
✓Fresh Orange Juice	8 oz	110	0	0	0	0	0	27	1	2	2 fruit
✓Home style Lemonade	22 oz	50	0	0	0	0	15	14	2	1	1 carb
✓Hot Cappuccino (small)	12 oz	100	4	36	2.5	15	100	10	0	6	1 milk, 1/2 fat
Hot Chocolate (small)	12 oz	370	11	27	7	30	170	60	2	12	2 carb, 1 1/2 milk, 1 fat
✓Iced Cappuccino (regular)	16 oz	220	8	33	5	35	220	22	2	14	1 1/2 milk, 1 fat
✓Peach Iced Tea	22 oz	120	0	0	0	0	35	30	0	0	2 carb

✓ = Healthiest Bets

(Continued)

	Amount	Cal.	Fat (g)	% Cal. Fat	Sat. Fat (g)	Chol. (mg)	Sod. (mg)	Carb. (g)	Fiber (g)	Pro. (g)	Servings/Exchanges
BLASTS											
Frozen Mocha Blast (regular)	16 oz	410	27	59	17	95	50	41	0	3	3 carb, 4 fat
✓Hot Mocha Blast (small)	12 oz	280	9	29	6	30	160	40	1	11	3 carb, 1 fat
Ice Cream Cookie Blast (regular)	16 oz	720	56	70	30	155	400	88	1	13	6 carb, 5 1/2 fat
Mango Blast (regular)	16 oz	360	10	25	6	35	30	66	2	1	4 1/2 carb, 1 fat
Strawberry Banana Blast (regular)	16 oz	400	10	23	6	35	30	78	5	1	5 carb
Wildberry Blast (regular)	16 oz	360	10	25	6	35	30	66	5	1	4 1/2 carb
BREADS											
✓Artisan Baguette	1 slice	140	0	0	0	0	360	30	1	5	2 starch
✓Artisan Bavarian Rye	1 slice	236	1	4	0	0	542	49	4	8	3 starch

✔Artisan Chocolate Cherry	1 slice	170	3	16	1	0	260	33	2	5	2 starch
✔Artisan French Country White	1 slice	130	0	0	0	0	340	27	1	4	1 1/2 starch
✔Artisan Honey Multigrain Baguette	1 slice	140	0	0	0	0	360	30	2	5	2 starch
✔Artisan Multigrain	1 slice	165	2	11	0	0	342	31	2	5	2 starch
✔Artisan Sundried Tomato Loaf	1 slice	130	0	0	0	0	370	27	2	5	1 1/2 starch
Braided Roll	1	420	14	30	3	40	730	63	3	13	4 starch, 2 fat
Bread Bowl	1	640	3	4	0	0	1830	127	6	28	8 starch
✔Cinnamon w/ Golden Raisins	1 slice	160	2	11	0.5	5	210	30	1	4	2 starch
✔Cranberry Raisin Nut Loaf	1 slice	150	3	18	0	0	330	28	2	4	2 starch

✔ = Healthiest Bets

(Continued)

BREADS (*Continued*)	Amount	Cal.	Fat (g)	% Cal. Fat	Sat. Fat (g)	Chol. (mg)	Sod. (mg)	Carb. (g)	Fiber (g)	Pro. (g)	Servings/Exchanges
Focaccia	1 slice	740	9	11	1.5	0	1700	137	7	26	9 starch, 1/2 fat
✓Garlic	1 slice	190	8	38	5	20	440	25	1	5	1 1/2 starch, 1 1/2 fat
✓Lahvash	1 slice	250	0	0	0	0	280	55	4	9	3 1/2 starch
Rosemary Garlic Stick	1	200	5	23	0.5	0	1430	33	2	6	2 starch, 1 fat
Soft White Roll	1	400	11	25	2.5	30	700	65	2	11	4 starch, 2 fat
BREAKFAST BAGELS											
Egg w/ Bacon	1	480	12	23	3.5	130	960	63	3	30	4 starch, 1 medium-fat meat, 1 high-fat meat
Egg w/ Cheese	1	480	11	21	5	140	980	63	3	31	4 starch, 1 medium-fat meat, 1 high-fat meat
Egg w/ Cheese & Bacon	1	560	18	29	7	155	1100	63	3	35	4 starch, 2 medium-fat meat, 1 high-fat meat
✓w/ Egg	1	400	4	9	1	120	730	63	3	25	4 starch, 1 medium-fat meat

CAKES & BROWNIES											
Apple Crumb Cake	1	540	30	50	12	155	510	62	1	7	4 carb, 5 fat
Blonde w/ Nuts	1	570	36	57	14	65	460	57	2	6	3 1/2 carb, 6 1/2 fat
Butter Crumb Cake	1	790	42	48	17	50	560	96	2	9	6 1/2 carb, 6 fat
Cheesecake Brownie	1	470	26	50	9	95	260	55	1	5	3 1/2 carb, 4 1/2 fat
Chocolate Chip Brownie	1	480	25	47	7	85	220	61	2	5	4 carb, 3 1/2 fat
Pecan Brownie	1	510	31	55	7	80	200	55	3	5	3 1/2 carb, 5 fat
Raspberry Crumb Cake	1	770	41	48	16	50	550	94	2	9	6 carb, 5 1/2 fat
Rocky Road Brownie	1	550	33	54	7	115	410	49	2	13	3 carb, 4 1/2 fat
COOKIES											
Butterscotch Chip w/ Pecans	1	270	11	37	6	15	190	42	1	3	3 carb, 1 fat
Chocolate Chip	1	260	11	38	5	20	240	40	1	3	2 1/2 carb, 1 1/2 fat

✓ = Healthiest Bets

(*Continued*)

COOKIES (*Continued*)	Amount	Cal.	Fat (g)	% Cal. Fat	Sat. Fat (g)	Chol. (mg)	Sod. (mg)	Carb. (g)	Fiber (g)	Pro. (g)	Servings/Exchanges
Chocolate Dipped Cranberry Almond Macaroon	1	320	16	45	8	0	190	42	3	4	3 carb, 2 fat
Chocolate Dipped Shortbread	1	300	10	30	4.5	20	190	52	1	6	3 1/2 carb, 0.2 fat
Chocolate Orange White Chocolate Chip w/ Walnuts	1	270	10	33	5	15	200	42	1	4	3 carb, 1 fat
Christmas Tree	1	170	2	11	1	10	75	35	0	2	2 carb
Coconut Orange Chocolate Macaroon w/ Snowflake	1	370	19	46	10	80	115	49	2	4	3 carb, 3 fat
Confetti w/ M&M's	1	280	13	42	7	35	200	37	1	5	2 1/2 carb, 2 fat
Double Chocolate Shortbread	1	340	19	50	10	40	120	42	2	3	3 carb, 2 fat

English Toffee	1	240	14	53	5	20	180	26	1	2	1 1/2 carb, 2 1/2 fat
Gingerbread Man	1	290	10	31	3.5	10	180	45	0	4	3 carb, 1 fat
Oatmeal Raisin	1	250	9	32	2	35	170	42	2	4	3 carb
Shortbread	1	340	22	58	14	60	180	35	1	3	2 carb, 2 fat
White Chocolate Dipped in Chocolate Shortbread	1	380	21	50	15	40	135	46	2	8	3 carb, 1 1/2 fat
CROISSANTS											
Almond	1	510	25	44	10	95	440	63	3	13	4 starch, 4 fat
✔Apple	1	230	3	12	1.5	20	220	47	2	6	3 starch
Chocolate	1	380	15	36	7	20	300	61	3	8	4 starch, 1 1/2 fat
✔Cinnamon Raisin	1	340	5	13	2.5	20	350	69	3	9	4 1/2 starch
Ham & Cheese	1	340	10	26	6	35	720	46	2	17	3 starch, 2 lean meat
✔Plain	1	250	6	22	3	25	340	44	2	8	3 starch

✔ = Healthiest Bets

(*Continued*)

CROISSANTS (*Continued*)	Amount	Cal.	Fat (g)	% Cal. Fat	Sat. Fat (g)	Chol. (mg)	Sod. (mg)	Carb. (g)	Fiber (g)	Pro. (g)	Servings/Exchanges
Raspberry	1	340	11	29	6	50	370	55	2	9	3 1/2 starch, 1 1/2 fat
✓Spinach & Cheese	1	250	9	32	6	35	400	32	2	10	2 starch, 1 high-fat meat
Sweet Cheese	1	350	14	36	8	65	400	52	1	9	3 1/2 starch, 1 1/2 fat
DANISH											
Cranberry	1	370	10	24	3.5	45	390	63	2	8	4 starch, 1 fat
Cranberry Cheese	1	460	23	45	13	90	380	57	2	8	4 starch, 3 fat
Lemon	1	430	20	42	11	75	380	57	1	7	3 1/2 starch, 3 1/2 fat
Sweet Cheese	1	470	26	50	15	105	380	54	1	8	3 1/2 starch, 4 fat
DRESSINGS											
Balsamic Vinaigrette Dressing	5 T	150	12	72	1.5	0	460	9	0	0	1/2 carb, 2 1/2 fat
Blue Cheese Dressing	5 T	370	39	95	5	20	690	3	0	3	8 fat
Caesar Dressing	5 T	390	38	88	6	30	520	6	0	3	1/2 starch, 8 fat

Fat Free Raspberry Vinaigrette	5 T	80	0	0	0	0	190	19	0	0	1 carb
Lite Honey Mustard Dressing	5 T	240	15	56	2	30	560	26	0	2	1 1/2 carb, 2 1/2 fat
Lite Olive Oil Vinaigrette	5 T	150	14	84	2	0	550	7	0	0	1/2 carb, 2 1/2 fat
Lite Ranch Dressing	5 T	200	16	72	2.5	15	800	5	0	2	4 fat
Mediterranean Dressing	5 T	200	20	90	3.5	5	620	4	0	1	4 fat
Parmesan & Peppercorn Dressing	5 T	400	38	86	6	20	730	5	0	3	8 fat
Thai Peanut Dressing	5 T	180	8	40	1	0	1180	24	0	2	1 1/2 starch, 1 1/2 fat
FILLINGS											
Brie Cheese	1.5 oz	150	14	84	6	30	180	0	0	8	2 medium-fat meat
Cheddar Cheese	1.5 oz	170	14	74	9	45	260	1	0	11	2 medium-fat meat
Chicken Breast	4 oz	120	3	23	1	70	560	1	0	21	3 lean meat

✓ = Healthiest Bets

(Continued)

FILLINGS (*Continued*)	Amount	Cal.	Fat (g)	% Cal. Fat	Sat. Fat (g)	Chol. (mg)	Sod. (mg)	Carb. (g)	Fiber (g)	Pro. (g)	Servings/Exchanges
Cranberry Cheese	1 oz	110	8	65	5	25	85	6	0	7	1/2 starch, 1 1/2 fat
Genoa Salami	3 oz	300	27	81	9	75	1410	0	0	18	3 high-fat meat
Gorgonzola Cheese	2 oz	210	18	77	12	50	780	1	0	12	2 high-fat meat
Ham	3.8 oz	150	3	18	1	60	1140	2	0	21	3 lean meat
Hot Capicola	3 oz	160	10	56	3.5	55	1080	1	0	15	2 lean meat, 1 fat
Hummus	2 oz	100	6	54	0	0	210	8	2	4	1/2 starch, 1 fat
Mozzarella Cheese	2 oz	160	9	51	7	25	300	3	0	16	2 medium-fat meat
Olive Tapenade	2 oz	110	12	98	1.5	0	1170	1	1	1	2 1/2 fat
Provolone Cheese	1.5 oz	140	10	64	7	35	330	1	0	10	2 medium-fat meat
✓Roast Beef	3.75 oz	150	5	30	2	70	460	1	0	26	4 lean meat
✓Roasted Red Peppers	2 oz	45	4	80	0.5	0	190	4	1	1	1 veg, 1/2 fat
Sun - Dried Tomato Spread	1 T	70	6	77	0.5	0	85	4	0	1	1 fat

Swiss Cheese	1.5 oz	160	12	68	9	30	105	0	0	12	2 medium-fat meat
Tarragon Chicken	4 oz	210	14	60	2.5	70	590	1	0	18	3 lean meat, 1 fat
Tarragon Mayonnaise Sauce	4 T	420	45	96	7	40	420	2	0	0	9 fat
Tuna Salad Mix	4.5 oz	170	8	42	1	0	450	3	0	25	3 lean meat
Turkey Breast	4 oz	120	2	15	0	50	950	4	0	22	3 lean meat
MUFFINS											
Apple Spice	1	420	15	32	1.5	20	450	65	3	7	4 starch, 2 1/2 fat
Banana Walnut	1	440	19	39	2	20	450	60	3	9	4 starch, 2 fat
Blueberry	1	510	19	34	2	20	550	76	2	9	5 starch, 2 1/2 fat
Carrot Nut	1	550	27	44	5	60	860	71	4	9	4 1/2 starch, 2 1/2 fat
Chocolate Chunk	1	590	2	3	6	25	480	83	5	10	5 1/2 starch, 3 1/2 fat
Corn	1	440	18	37	3	70	640	64	2	8	4 starch, 2 1/2 fat

✓ = Healthiest Bets

(*Continued*)

MUFFINS (*Continued*)	Amount	Cal.	Fat (g)	% Cal. Fat	Sat. Fat (g)	Chol. (mg)	Sod. (mg)	Carb. (g)	Fiber (g)	Pro. (g)	Servings/Exchanges
Cranberry Blueberry	1	520	2	3	3	20	490	76	5	9	5 starch, 2 1/2 fat
Cranberry Walnut	1	560	26	42	2	20	530	69	5	11	4 1/2 starch, 4 1/2 fat
✓Low fat Chocolate Cake	1	320	2	6	0.5	20	590	74	4	4	4 1/2 starch
✓Low fat Triple Berry	1	290	2	6	0.5	25	310	61	2	5	3 1/2 starch
Pumpkin	1	580	20	31	4	70	390	84	3	10	5 1/2 starch, 3 fat
Raisin Bran	1	530	13	22	2.5	35	780	100	12	14	6 1/2 starch
SALAD											
✓Caesar	1	240	11	41	6	25	310	23	4	13	1 starch, 2 veg, 1 medium-fat meat, 1 fat
Chef's	1	260	13	45	7	60	890	9	4	25	2 veg, 3 medium-fat meat
✓Chicken Caesar	1	320	13	37	6	70	660	24	4	26	1 starch, 2 veg, 3 lean meat, 1/2 fat
Chicken Pesto	1	420	30	64	8	60	870	14	5	26	2 veg, 4 lean meat, 3 1/2 fat

✓Garden - large	1	110	2	16	0	0	300	19	5	5	4 veg
✓Garden - small	1	50	1	18	0	150	10	10	3	2	2 veg
Gorgonzola & Walnut	1	340	28	74	7	25	500	10	7	13	2 veg, 2 high-fat meat, 2 fat
✓Mediterranean Chicken	1	230	12	47	3	50	1090	13	5	19	3 veg, 3 lean meat
✓Thai Chicken	1	140	3	19	0.5	45	470	14	6	16	2 veg, 2 lean meat
✓Tuna Garden	1	310	21	61	3	10	670	11	5	24	2 veg, 3 lean meat, 2 fat
✓Tuna Nicoise	1	300	15	45	2.5	195	930	19	5	23	1/2 starch, 2 veg, 3 lean meat, 1 fat
Turkey Medallion Cobb Salad	1	390	21	48	9	250	1070	23	6	28	1 starch, 2 veg, 3 lean meat, 1 high-fat meat
SANDWICHES											
Chicken & Mozzarella	1	740	24	29	4.5	85	1930	73	6	55	4 1/2 starch, 4 lean meat, 2 medium-fat meat
Chicken Tarragon w/ Field Greens	1	800	42	47	7	100	1710	71	4	34	4 1/2 starch, 1 veg, 3 lean meat, 5 1/2 fat

✓ = Healthiest Bets

(Continued)

SANDWICHES (*Continued*)	Amount	Cal.	Fat (g)	% Cal. Fat	Sat. Fat (g)	Chol. (mg)	Sod. (mg)	Carb. (g)	Fiber (g)	Pro. (g)	Servings/Exchanges
Chili Dijon Chicken w/ Cheddar	1	530	17	29	7	95	1510	52	4	42	3 1/2 starch, 3 lean meat, 1 high-fat meat
Goat Cheese, Garlic Sundried Tomato Spread	1	500	19	34	5	15	1020	67	6	17	4 1/2 starch, 1 high-fat meat, 1 fat
Grilled Chicken Club w/ Chili Dressing	1	670	29	39	9	105	1240	64	4	40	4 starch, 4 lean meat, 3 fat
Honey Dijon Cordon Bleu	1	590	12	18	6	120	1560	71	3	46	4 1/2 starch, 4 lean meat
Roast Beef & Emmental Swiss	1	690	36	47	11	90	1430	67	2	33	4 1/2 starch, 2 lean meat, 1 high-fat meat, 2 1/2 fat
Roast Beef & Gorgonzola w/ Mayonnaise	1	810	31	34	13	120	2070	86	8	49	5 1/2 starch, 3 lean meat, 1 high-fat meat, 2 1/2 fat
Roasted Turkey w/ Brie	1	640	17	24	7	70	1480	82	5	38	5 1/2 starch, 3 medium-fat meat

Roasted Turkey w/ Cranberry Wensleydale Cheese & Almonds	1	640	13	18	3	50	1420	96	4	34	6 starch, 2 lean meat, 1 medium-fat meat
Roasted Turkey, Wensleydale Cheese, & Sliced Apple	1	710	35	44	9	85	1300	67	6	34	4 1/2 starch, 3 lean meat, 1 high-fat meat, 2 fat
Smoked Turkey Club w/ Cheddar & Bacon	1	710	32	41	12	95	2250	59	3	48	4 starch, 3 lean meat, 2 high-fat meat, 1 fat
The Tuscan	1	710	39	49	12	75	1560	60	3	32	4 starch, 3 medium-fat meat, 3 1/2 fat
SANDWICHES - FICELLE											
✓Grilled Tarragon Chicken Ficelle	1	330	13	35	2	45	760	35	0	16	2 starch, 2 lean meat, 1 fat
Roma Tomato & Mozzarella	1	470	24	46	13	65	1410	40	0	22	2 1/2 starch, 2 high-fat meat, 2 fat

✓ = Healthiest Bets

(*Continued*)

	Amount	Cal.	Fat (g)	% Cal. Fat	Sat. Fat (g)	Chol. (mg)	Sod. (mg)	Carb. (g)	Fiber (g)	Pro. (g)	Servings/Exchanges
SANDWICHES - PANINI											
Chicken Caesar w/ Asiago	1	700	28	36	8	80	1760	76	5	34	5 starch, 3 medium-fat meat, 1 1/2 fat
Grilled Turkey Club	1	830	37	40	12	110	2520	80	5	48	5 starch, 5 lean meat, 3 1/2 fat
Portobello Mushroom, Roasted Peppers w/ Asiago	1	520	12	21	6	25	1320	80	10	24	5 starch, 1 veg, 1 high-fat meat
SANDWICHES - WRAPS											
Chicken Caesar	1	600	25	38	8	80	930	63	5	33	4 starch, 3 medium-fat meat, 1 fat
Chopped Cobb	1	570	21	33	7	120	1280	65	6	32	4 starch, 1 veg, 2 lean meat, 1 high-fat meat
Fields & Feta	1	560	17	27	4	10	880	90	14	20	5 1/2 starch, 1 veg, 1 high-fat meat

Mediterranean	1	580	23	36	2.5	5	990	80	9	19	5 starch, 1 veg, 2 medium-fat meat
Southwest Tuna	1	650	26	36	7	30	1060	68	7	44	4 1/2 starch, 4 lean meat, 1 1/2 fat
SCONES											
Cinnamon	1	480	18	34	8	125	320	88	2	11	6 starch
Orange	1	410	14	31	8	130	350	62	2	11	4 starch, 2 fat
SOUP											
Baked Stuffed Potato Soup	12 oz	240	15	56	6	25	720	20	1	6	1 1/2 starch, 2 1/2 fat
Beef Stew	12 oz	210	11	47	2.5	35	1000	17	2	12	1 starch, 1 medium-fat meat, 1 fat
Broccoli Cheddar	12 oz	230	16	63	9	50	960	13	2	6	1 starch, 1 high-fat meat, 1 fat

✔ = Healthiest Bets

(*Continued*)

SOUP (*Continued*)	Amount	Cal.	Fat (g)	% Cal. Fat	Sat. Fat (g)	Chol. (mg)	Sod. (mg)	Carb. (g)	Fiber (g)	Pro. (g)	Servings/Exchanges
✓Chicken Chili	12 oz	210	5	21	1.5	20	580	28	5	12	2 starch, 1 lean meat
✓Chicken Florentine	12 oz	170	9	48	4.5	35	780	17	1	n/a	1 starch, 1 lean meat, 1 fat
✓Chicken Noodle	12 oz	90	2	20	0	15	670	11	0	7	1 starch
Chicken Stew	12 oz	230	12	47	3.5	40	630	17	2	12	1 starch, 2 lean meat, 1 fat
Clam Chowder	12 oz	240	16	60	7	45	670	18	0	7	1 milk, 1 medium-fat meat, 1 1/2 fat
Corn & Green Chili Bisque	12 oz	160	8	45	5	25	920	17	2	4	1 starch, 2 fat
✓Corn Chowder	12 oz	240	13	49	8	35	520	25	2	5	1 starch, 1 milk, 1 1/2 fat
Curried Rice & Lentil	12 oz	100	1	9	0	0	900	18	4	n/a	1 starch
✓French Moroccan Tomato Lentil	12 oz	110	1	8	1	0	470	19	6	6	1 1/2 starch
French Onion	12 oz	80	3	34	1.5	10	1280	11	2	3	1 starch

✔Garden Vegetable	12 oz	40	1	23	0	0	610	7	2	2	2 veg
✔Holiday Turkey Stew	12 oz	240	10	38	6	65	700	20	2	15	1 starch, 2 lean meat, 1 fat
Italian Wedding	12 oz	100	4	36	1.5	10	960	12	2	5	1 starch, 1/2 fat
✔Jamaican Black Bean	12 oz	110	1	8	0	0	260	27	14	10	1 1/2 starch
✔Mediterranean Pepper	12 oz	190	4	19	0	0	450	30	7	9	2 starch, 1 fat
✔Old Fashion Tomato Rice	12 oz	80	1	11	0	0	240	15	2	3	1 starch
✔Pasta E Fagioli	12 oz	160	4	23	1	5	510	24	5	7	1 1/2 starch, 1 fat
Potato Leek	12 oz	190	12	57	8	45	1020	17	2	4	1 starch, 2 1/2 fat
✔Red Beans, Rice, & Sausage	12 oz	180	4	20	1	10	610	28	11	10	2 starch, 1/2 fat
✔Red Lentil & Mango Stew	12 oz	150	3	18	0	0	630	25	5	8	2 starch
✔Southern Black Eyed Pea	12 oz	190	1	5	0	5	400	34	12	11	2 starch, 1 lean meat

✔ = Healthiest Bets

(*Continued*)

SOUP (*Continued*)	Amount	Cal.	Fat (g)	% Cal. Fat	Sat. Fat (g)	Chol. (mg)	Sod. (mg)	Carb. (g)	Fiber (g)	Pro. (g)	Servings/Exchanges
Southwest Tortilla Soup	12 oz	140	6	39	2.5	10	1020	17	3	3	1 starch, 1 1/2 fat
✓Southwest Vegetable	12 oz	150	3	18	0.5	0	250	23	4	6	1 starch, 1 veg, 1 lean meat
✓Split Pea w/ Ham	12 oz	140	1	6	0	5	680	23	8	10	1 starch, 1 lean meat
✓Tomato Basil Bisque	12 oz	130	4	28	3	15	400	18	3	4	1 starch, 1 fat
✓Tomato Florentine	12 oz	70	2	26	0.5	5	610	10	1	3	1/2 starch, 1/2 fat
✓Tuscan Vegetable	12 oz	130	3	21	1.5	5	680	20	3	5	1 starch, 1 veg, 1/2 fat
Vegetable Beef Barley	12 oz	80	2	23	1	10	810	11	2	5	1/2 starch, 1 lean meat
Vegetarian Chili	12 oz	170	1	5	0	0	920	30	15	9	2 starch
✓Vegetarian Minestrone	12 oz	70	1	13	0	0	620	14	3	3	1 starch
Wild Mushroom Bisque	12 oz	110	5	41	1.5	5	920	12	2	3	1 starch, 1 fat

SPREADS											
Honey Walnut Cream Cheese	4 T	140	9	58	6	30	150	12	0	3	1 starch, 1 1/2 fat
Plain Cream Cheese	4 T	120	11	83	7	35	180	4	0	4	2 1/2 fat
Smoked Salmon Cream Cheese	4 T	110	9	74	6	30	230	3	0	5	2 1/2 fat
Sundried Tomato Cream Cheese	4 T	130	10	69	7	35	380	5	0	4	1/2 starch, 2 fat
Vegetable Cream Cheese	4 T	140	12	77	7	40	380	3	0	6	3 fat
STRUDELS AND SWEET ROLLS											
Apple Strudel	1	410	18	40	0	0	140	56	1	6	4 carb, 2 fat
Cherry Strudel	1	390	19	44	0	0	135	49	1	6	3 carb, 3 1/2 fat
Cinnamon Roll	1	390	12	28	4.5	45	380	67	2	9	4 1/2 carb, 1 fat
Crème De Fleur	1	550	26	43	15	110	540	71	1	12	4 1/2 carb, 2 1/2 fat
Pecan Roll	1	750	29	35	7	15	560	112	4	14	7 1/2 carb, 3 1/2 fat

✔ = Healthiest Bets

(*Continued*)

	Amount	Cal.	Fat (g)	% Cal. Fat	Sat. Fat (g)	Chol. (mg)	Sod. (mg)	Carb. (g)	Fiber (g)	Pro. (g)	Servings/Exchanges
YOGURTS & FRUIT CUPS											
Blueberry Yogurt w/ Granola & Fruit (small)	1	310	6	17	2	10	130	56	2	10	2 starch, 1 fruit, 1 milk
✓Fruit Cup (large)	1	140	1	6	0	0	20	32	2	2	2 fruit
✓Fruit Cup (small)	1	70	0	0	0	0	10	16	1	1	1 fruit
✓Oatmeal	1	150	3	18	0.5	0	0	27	4	5	2 starch
✓Plain Low Fat Yogurt (small)	1	190	2	9	1.5	10	95	36	0	6	1 starch, 1 milk
Strawberry Yogurt w/ Granola & Fruit (small)	1	310	6	17	2	10	130	56	2	10	2 starch, 1 fruit, 1 milk
Vanilla Yogurt w/ Granola & Fruit (small)	1	310	6	17	2	10	130	56	2	10	2 starch, 1 fruit, 1 milk

✓ = Healthiest Bets

Blimpie Subs and Salads

❖ Blimpie provides nutrition information for all its menu items on its Web site at www.blimpie.com.

Light 'n Lean Choice

Grande Chili with Beans and Beef
Chef Salad
French's Honey Mustard Dressing *(2 T)*

Calories	440	Sodium (mg)	2,226
Fat (g)	16	Carbohydrate (g)	40
% calories from fat	33	Fiber (g)	21
Saturated fat (g)	8	Protein (g)	38
Cholesterol (mg)	106		

Exchanges: 2 starch, 2 veg, 4 lean meat

Healthy 'n Hearty Choice

Club Sandwich *(6 inch)*
Mustard Potato Salad

Calories	600	Sodium (mg)	2,350
Fat (g)	17	Carbohydrate (g)	71
% calories from fat	26	Fiber (g)	4
Saturated fat (g)	6.5	Protein (g)	30
Cholesterol (mg)	71		

Exchanges: 4 1/2 starch, 3 medium-fat meat

(*Continued*)

Blimpie Subs and Salads

	Amount	Cal.	Fat (g)	% Cal. Fat	Sat. Fat (g)	Chol. (mg)	Sod. (mg)	Carb. (g)	Fiber (g)	Pro. (g)	Servings/Exchanges
6″ SUBS											
Beef, Turkey & Cheddar	1	600	31	47	10	69	1836	49	3	28	3 starch, 3 medium-fat meat, 3 fat
BLIMPIE Best	1	476	16	30	7	69	1690	52	3	30	3 1/2 starch, 3 lean meat, 1 1/2 fat
BLT	1	588	32	49	10	41	1596	49	3	28	3 starch, 3 medium-fat meat
Buffalo Chicken	1	400	13	29	6.5	61	2108	50	3	32	3 1/2 starch, 2 lean meat, 1 1/2 fat
ChiliMax	1	551	13	21	2	0	1287	71	8	29	4 1/2 starch, 2 lean meat, 1 1/2 fat
Club	1	440	12	25	5.5	66	1437	50	3	28	3 1/2 starch, 2 lean meat, 1 fat

Cuban	1	462	12	23	6	67	1526	50	3	30	3 1/2 starch, 2 lean meat, 1 fat
✔Grilled Chicken	1	373	9	22	2.5	35	836	50	3	29	3 1/2 starch, 2 lean meat, 1/2 fat
Ham & Cheese	1	436	13	27	6	59	1302	52	3	28	3 1/2 starch, 2 medium-fat meat, 1/2 fat
Meatball	1	572	27	42	9.5	58	1145	55	2	28	3 1/2 starch, 2 medium-fat meat, 3 1/2 fat
MexiMax	1	425	9	19	1.5	0	1012	65	7	23	4 starch, 2 lean meat, 1/2 fat
Pastrami	1	507	17	30	7	74	1658	53	3	36	3 1/2 starch, 4 medium-fat meat
Pastrami Special	1	462	14	27	6	44	1438	52	3	32	3 1/2 starch, 3 medium-fat meat
Reuben	1	630	33	47	5.4	46	1914	55	2	31	3 1/2 starch, 4 high-fat meat, 1 fat

✔ = Healthiest Bets

(*Continued*)

6″ SUBS (*Continued*)	Amount	Cal.	Fat (g)	% Cal. Fat	Sat. Fat (g)	Chol. (mg)	Sod. (mg)	Carb. (g)	Fiber (g)	Pro. (g)	Servings/Exchanges
Roast Beef	1	468	14	27	6	71	1384	49	3	37	3 starch, 4 lean meat
Seafood	1	355	8	20	1.5	19	895	58	4	14	3 1/2 starch, 1 lean meat, 1/2 fat
Steak & Onion Melt	1	440	16	33	6	68	1056	49	3	29	3 starch, 3 lean meat, 1 1/2 fat
Tuna	1	493	23	42	3.5	50	876	50	3	24	3 1/2 starch, 2 lean meat, 2 1/2 fat
Turkey	1	424	11	23	4.5	62	1597	49	3	24	3 starch, 2 lean meat, 1 fat
Ultimate Club	1	724	42	52	12	81	1933	51	3	33	3 1/2 starch, 3 lean meat, 6 fat
VegiMax	1	395	7	16	1.5	0	982	60	8	24	3 1/2 starch, 2 veg, 2 lean meat

COOKIES											
✔Chocolate Chunk	1	200	10	45	6	15	210	26	1	2	1 1/2 carb, 2 fat
✔Macadamia White Chunk	1	210	10	43	5	20	140	26	1	2	1 1/2 carb, 2 fat
✔Oatmeal Raisin	1	190	8	38	2	10	200	27	1	3	1 1/2 carb, 1 1/2 fat
✔Peanut Butter	1	220	12	49	5	15	210	23	1	4	1 1/2 carb, 2 1/2 fat
Sugar	1	330	17	46	4.5	30	290	24	0	3	1 1/2 carb, 3 1/2 fat
POTATO CHIPS											
Cheddar & Sour Cream	1 bag	210	11	47	2	4	220	25	1	3	1 1/2 starch, 2 fat
Jalapeno	1 bag	210	11	47	2	0	250	25	2	2	1 1/2 starch, 2 fat
Lea & Perrin Barbecue	1 bag	210	10	43	2	0	270	25	2	3	1 1/2 starch, 2 fat
Regular Flavor	1 bag	210	11	47	2	0	190	25	2	3	1 1/2 starch, 2 fat
Romano & Garlic	1 bag	210	11	47	2	4	220	25	2	3	1 1/2 carb, 2 fat
Sour Cream & Onion	1 bag	210	11	47	2	4	250	25	1	2	1 1/2 carb, 2 fat

✔ = Healthiest Bets

(*Continued*)

	Amount	Cal.	Fat (g)	% Cal. Fat	Sat. Fat (g)	Chol. (mg)	Sod. (mg)	Carb. (g)	Fiber (g)	Pro. (g)	Servings/Exchanges
SALADS											
Antipasto	regular	244	13	48	6	69	1217	10	3	23	1/2 starch, 3 lean meat, 1/2 fat
Buffalo Chicken	1	390	28	65	7	85	1300	7	2	26	1 starch, 2 veg, 3 lean meat, 2 fat
Chef	regular	212	9	38	4.5	66	961	9	3	20	2 veg, 3 lean meat
Chili Ole	regular	480	27	51	11	45	1240	42	3	21	3 starch, 2 medium-fat meat, 2 fat
Grilled Chicken w/ Caesar dressing	regular	347	27	70	5	45	862	8	2	18	2 veg, 2 medium-fat meat, 4 fat
Roast Beef 'n Bleu	regular	390	16	37	10	70	1550	29	0	31	1 starch, 3 veg, 4 lean meat, 1/2 fat
✓Seafood	regular	122	4.5	33	0.5	19	418	16	3	6	3 veg, 1 lean meat

Sicilian	1	250	13	47	6	70	1970	9	2	22	2 veg, 3 lean meat, 1 fat
✓Tuna	regular	261	20	69	2.5	50	398	8	3	16	2 veg, 2 lean meat, 1 1/2 fat
Zesto Pesto Turkey	regular	370	19	46	8	40	1410	31	0	20	1 starch, 3 veg, 2 lean meat, 2 fat
SANDWICHES											
Baja Turkey & Swiss	1	330	15	41	4.5	70	1370	16	5	30	1 starch, 4 lean meat, 1/2 fat
Buffalo Chicken	1	370	18	44	6	80	1220	17	4	40	1 starch, 5 lean meat, 1/2 fat
Cable Car Club	1	300	10	30	4.5	65	1090	16	5	32	1 starch, 4 lean meat
Durango Roast Beef & Cheddar	1	390	20	46	8	85	1470	15	4	42	1 starch, 5 1/2 lean meat, 1/2 fat
Fisherman's Wharf Tuna Melt	1	300	12	36	5	65	1070	16	7	37	1 starch, 5 lean meat

✓ = Healthiest Bets

(*Continued*)

SANDWICHES (*Continued*)	Amount	Cal.	Fat (g)	% Cal. Fat	Sat. Fat (g)	Chol. (mg)	Sod. (mg)	Carb. (g)	Fiber (g)	Pro. (g)	Servings/Exchanges
Golden Gate Gourmet	1	350	16	41	5	65	1240	20	5	37	1 1/2 starch, 5 lean meat
Tuscan Ham & Swiss	1	340	13	34	6	75	1450	18	4	37	1 starch, 5 lean meat
✔Union Square Ultimate Veggie	1	280	17	55	4.5	20	480	19	6	19	1 starch, 1 veg, 2 lean meat
SIDES											
Cole Slaw	5 oz	180	13	65	2	0	230	13	1	1	1 starch, 1 veg, 2 fat
Macaroni Salad	5 oz	360	25	63	4	10	660	25	1	4	1 1/2 starch, 5 1/2 fat
Mustard Potato Salad	5 oz	160	5	28	1	5	660	21	1	2	1 1/2 starch, 1 fat
✔Potato Salad	5 oz	270	19	63	3	10	560	19	1	2	1 starch, 4 fat
SOUPS											
Chicken Soup w/ White & Wild Rice	8 oz	230	12	47	2	30	1210	21	2	10	1 1/2 starch, 1 lean meat, 2 fat

Cream of Broccoli & Cheese	8 oz	190	12	57	5	15	940	15	3	6	1 starch, 1 medium-fat meat, 1 fat
Cream of Potato	8 oz	190	9	43	2.5	0	860	24	3	5	1 1/2 starch, 2 fat
✓Garden Vegetable	8 oz	80	1	11	0	0	620	14	3	5	1/2 starch, 2 veg
Grande Chili w/ Beans & Beef	8 oz	250	7	25	3.5	40	1230	30	18	18	2 starch, 2 lean meat
Home style Chicken Noodle	8 oz	120	3	23	0.5	20	850	18	1	7	1 starch, 1 lean meat
✓Tomato Basil w/ Raviolini	8 oz	110	1	8	0	10	720	22	0	4	1 1/2 starch
Vegetable Beef	8 oz	80	2	23	0.5	5	1010	13	2	4	1 veg, 1 lean meat
TOPPINGS, SAUCES, & DRESSINGS											
Caesar Dressing	3 T	208	22	95	3.5	10	504	2	0	1	4 1/2 fat
Cheddar Cheese	1 slice	52	5	87	2.5	10	250	0	0	3	1 medium-fat meat
Cracked Peppercorn Dressing	3 T	237	25	95	4	15	386	2	0	1	5 fat

✓ = Healthiest Bets

(*Continued*)

TOPPINGS, SAUCES, & DRESSINGS (*Continued*)	Amount	Cal.	Fat (g)	% Cal. Fat	Sat. Fat (g)	Chol. (mg)	Sod. (mg)	Carb. (g)	Fiber (g)	Pro. (g)	Servings/Exchanges
Frank's Red Hot Buffalo Sauce	2 T	12.5	1	72	0	0	836	2	0	0	free
✓French's Honey Mustard Dressing	1 T	5	0	0	0	0	35	1	0	0	free
✓GourMayo Chipotle Chili Dressing	1 T	50	5	90	1	10	100	1	0	0	1 fat
✓GourMayo Sun Dried Tomato Dressing	1 T	50	5	90	1	10	100	1	0	0	1 fat
✓GourMayo Wasabi Horseradish	1 T	50	5	90	1	10	100	1	0	0	1 fat
Guacamole	3 T	194	18	84	2.5	0	468	8	2	2	1/2 starch, 3 1/2 fat
✓Oil & Vinegar	for 6" sub	36	4	100	0.5	0	0	0	0	0	1 fat
Pesto Dressing	2 T	132	13	89	2	0	236	1	0	0	2 1/2 fat

Provolone Cheese	1 slice	80	6	68	3.5	20	200	0	0	6	1 medium-fat meat
Swiss Cheese	1 slice	80	6	68	4	20	46	0	0	7	1 medium-fat meat
WRAPS											
Beef & Cheddar	1 regular	714	37	47	11	78	2183	57	3	34	3 1/2 starch, 3 high-fat meat, 3 fat
Chicken Caesar	1 regular	646	35	49	6.6	45	1635	56	3	25	3 1/2 starch, 2 lean meat, 6 fat
Southwestern	1 regular	674	35	47	8.4	56	2504	54	3	26	3 1/2 starch, 2 high-fat meat, 4 fat
Steak & Onion	1 regular	716	37	47	10	78	1716	64	3	30	4 starch, 3 high-fat meat, 2 1/2 fat
Ultimate BLT	1 regular	831	50	54	15	78	2677	60	3	34	4 starch, 3 high-fat meat, 5 fat
Zesty Italian	1 regular	638	33	47	10	62	2374	74	3	26	5 starch, 2 high-fat meat, 1 1/2 fat

✓ = Healthiest Bets

Panera Bread

❖ Panera Bread provides complete nutrition information for its foods on its Web site at www.panerabread.com.

Light 'n Lean Choice

Low-Fat Garden Vegetable Soup *(8 oz)*
Asian Sesame Chicken Salad *(dressing included)*
Artisan Multigrain Bread (1 slice)

Calories........................540
Fat (g) 19
% calories from fat..32
Saturated fat (g) 2
Cholesterol (mg) 65
Sodium (mg) 2,260
Carbohydrate (g).........75
Fiber (g).......................8
Protein (g) 39

Exchanges: 4 starch, 2 veg, 3 lean meat

Healthy 'n Hearty Choice

Low-Fat Vegetarian Autumn Tomato Basil Soup *(8 oz)*
Smoked Turkey Breast Sandwich on Sourdough Bread
Chocolate Hazelnut Macaroon *(1/2)*

Calories........................700
Fat (g) 20
% calories from fat..26
Saturated fat (g) 2
Cholesterol (mg) 25
Sodium (mg) 3,020
Carbohydrate (g).........93
Fiber (g).......................9
Protein (g) 35

Exchanges: 4 starch, 2 veg, 2 carb, 3 lean meat

Panera Bread

	Amount	Cal.	Fat (g)	% Cal. Fat	Sat. Fat (g)	Chol. (mg)	Sod. (mg)	Carb. (g)	Fiber (g)	Pro. (g)	Servings/Exchanges
BAGELS											
✓Asiago Cheese	1	330	5	14	2.5	15	480	58	2	15	3 1/2 starch, 1 fat
✓Blueberry	1	320	2	6	0	0	490	67	3	12	4 1/2 starch
✓Chocolate Raspberry	1	370	7	17	4	0	460	67	2	11	4 1/2 starch, 1 fat
Cinnamon Crunch	1	420	7	15	4.5	0	430	78	3	10	5 starch, 1 fat
✓Dutch Apple & Raisin	1	340	3	8	0	0	410	70	3	10	4 1/2 starch
✓Everything	1	290	2	6	0	0	540	58	2	11	4 starch
French Toast	1	340	5	13	1	0	610	65	2	10	4 starch
✓Low Carb Asiago Cheese	1	240	9	34	4.5	20	500	20	9	19	1 starch, 2 lean meat, 1 fat

✓ = Healthiest Bets

(*Continued*)

BAGELS (*Continued*)	Amount	Cal.	Fat (g)	% Cal. Fat	Sat. Fat (g)	Chol. (mg)	Sod. (mg)	Carb. (g)	Fiber (g)	Pro. (g)	Servings/Exchanges
✓Low Carb Plain	1	200	2	9	0.5	0	460	25	12	18	1 1/2 starch, 2 lean meat
✓Nine Grain	1	290	1	3	0	0	390	58	3	11	4 starch
✓Plain	1	280	1	3	0	0	450	57	2	11	4 starch
Pumpkin Spice	1	360	2	5	0	0	670	76	3	11	5 starch
✓Sesame Seed	1	310	3	9	0	0	460	60	3	12	4 starch
BEVERAGES											
✓Caffe Latte	8.5 oz	120	5	38	3	20	120	12	0	7	1 milk, 1 fat
Caffe Mocha	11.5 oz	360	16	40	10	55	190	47	2	11	2 carb, 1 1/2 milk, 2 1/2 fat
✓Cappuccino	8.5 oz	120	5	38	3	20	120	12	0	7	1 milk, 1 fat
Caramel Latte	11 oz	400	16	36	9	55	450	54	0	9	2 1/2 carb, 1 1/2 milk, 2 fat
Chai Tea Latte	10 oz	210	5	21	2.5	15	115	37	0	7	1 1/2 carb, 1 milk, 1/2 fat
Home style Lemonade	16 oz	150	0	0	0	0	10	36	0	0	2 1/2 carb

Hot Chocolate	11 oz	350	15	39	10	50	190	45	2	11	3 carb, 2 1/2 fat
House Latte	11 oz	320	13	37	8	50	135	43	0	8	1 1/2 carb, 1 1/2 milk, 2 fat
I.C. Cappuccino Chip	16 oz	590	35	53	26	70	125	64	0	5	2 1/2 carb, 2 milk, 4 1/2 fat
I.C. Caramel	16 oz	550	24	39	15	80	400	77	0	6	4 carb, 1 milk, 3 1/2 fat
I.C. Honeydew Green Tea	16 oz	270	13	43	9	30	140	36	0	2	2 1/2 carb, 2 fat
I.C. Mocha	16 oz	520	24	42	15	75	140	70	2	7	3 1/2 carb, 1 milk, 3 1/2 fat
I.C. Spice	16 oz	470	22	42	13	70	80	66	0	4	4 1/2 carb, 3 1/2 fat
Iced Chai Tea Latte	16 oz	170	4	21	2	15	95	29	0	6	1 carb, 1 milk, 1/2 fat
✓Iced Green Tea	16 oz	60	0	0	0	0	5	15	0	0	1 carb
BREADS											
✓Artisan Country	1 slice	120	0	0	0	0	290	25	1	5	1 1/2 starch
✓Artisan French	1 slice	110	0	0	0	0	310	23	0	4	1 1/2 starch
✓Artisan Kalamata Olive	1 slice	140	2	13	0	0	270	26	1	5	1 1/2 starch

✓ = Healthiest Bets

(*Continued*)

BREADS (*Continued*)	Amount	Cal.	Fat (g)	% Cal. Fat	Sat. Fat (g)	Chol. (mg)	Sod. (mg)	Carb. (g)	Fiber (g)	Pro. (g)	Servings/Exchanges
✔Artisan Multigrain	1 slice	120	1	8	0	0	230	24	1	4	1 1/2 starch
✔Artisan Raisin Pecan	1 slice	140	3	19	0	0	280	25	1	4	1 1/2 starch, 1/2 fat
✔Artisan Sesame Semolina	1 slice	120	0	0	0	0	300	24	1	4	1 1/2 starch
✔Artisan Stone-Milled Rye	1 slice	110	0	0	0	0	320	22	2	4	1 1/2 starch
✔Artisan Three Cheese	1 slice	120	2	15	1	5	270	21	1	5	1 1/2 starch
✔Artisan Three Seed	1 slice	130	2	14	0	0	250	23	1	5	1 1/2 starch
✔Asiago Cheese Demi Loaf	1 slice	140	4	26	2	10	310	21	0	7	1 1/2 starch
✔Asiago Cheese Focaccia	1	150	6	36	2	5	300	19	1	5	1 1/2 starch, 1 fat
✔Basil Pesto Focaccia	1	150	6	36	1.5	5	300	19	1	4	1 starch, 1 fat
Ciabatta	1 piece	430	10	21	2	0	990	70	3	14	4 1/2 starch, 1 lean meat, 1 fat
✔Cinnamon Raisin	1 slice	160	3	17	0.5	0	300	31	1	4	2 starch

✔French Baguette, Loaf, XL Loaf	1 slice	130	1	7	0	0	270	24	1	5	1 1/2 starch
✔French Croissant	1	260	15	52	9	40	190	28	1	5	1 1/2 starch, 3 fat
BROWNIES											
Caramel Pecan	1	470	24	46	5	80	150	60	2	5	4 carb, 4 fat
Chocolate Raspberry	1	440	26	53	12	55	130	46	3	6	3 carb, 5 fat
Very Chocolate	1	460	22	43	5	80	150	62	2	5	4 carb, 4 fat
CAKES, ROLLS & SCONES											
Carrot Walnut Mini Bundt Cake	1	430	21	44	3	75	340	51	2	6	3 1/2 carb, 4 fat
Cinnamon Chip Scone	1	350	14	36	7	45	440	51	3	5	2 starch, 1 1/2 carb, 2 1/2 fat
Cinnamon Roll	1	530	25	42	15	140	480	67	3	10	2 1/2 starch, 2 carb, 4 1/2 fat

✔ = Healthiest Bets

(*Continued*)

CAKES, ROLLS & SCONES (*Continued*)	Amount	Cal.	Fat (g)	% Cal. Fat	Sat. Fat (g)	Chol. (mg)	Sod. (mg)	Carb. (g)	Fiber (g)	Pro. (g)	Servings/Exchanges
Cobblestone	1	520	31	54	6	40	620	60	1	6	2 starch, 2 carb, 5 fat
✓Coffee Cake (Cherry Cheese)	1	190	10	47	5	30	130	21	1	3	1 1/2 carb, 2 fat
Lemon Poppy Seed Mini Bundt Cake	1	460	20	39	4	90	430	62	1	6	4 carb, 3 fat
Orange Scone	1	530	25	42	15	140	370	67	3	10	2 1/2 starch, 2 carb, 4 1/2 fat
Pecan Roll	1	520	31	54	6	40	260	60	2	6	2 1/2 starch, 1 1/2 carb, 5 fat
Pineapple Upside-Down Mini Bundt Cake	1	450	20	40	8	70	490	64	2	5	4 carb, 3 1/2 fat
COOKIES											
Chocolate Chipper	1	770	46	54	24	85	570	83	4	10	5 1/2 carb, 8 fat

Chocolate Duet w/ Walnuts	1	460	20	39	4	90	430	62	1	6	4 carb, 3 1/2 fat
Chocolate Hazelnut Macaroon	1	300	3	9	0.5	30	320	63	3	6	4 carb
Nutty Chocolate Chipper	1	440	26	53	12	55	300	46	3	6	3 carb, 5 fat
Nutty Oatmeal Raisin	1	350	14	36	7	45	260	51	3	5	3 1/2 carb, 2 fat
Shortbread	1	340	21	56	13	60	160	36	1	3	2 1/2 carb, 4 fat
CROISSANT											
Apple	1	260	11	38	7	30	230	34	1	4	1 starch, 1 carb, 2 fat
Cheese	1	300	16	48	10	45	220	34	1	6	2 starch, 3 fat
Chocolate	1	770	43	50	20	100	480	88	2	11	4 starch, 2 carb, 7 fat
Raspberry Cheese	1	280	13	42	8	35	190	37	1	5	1 1/2 starch, 1 carb, 2 fat
DANISH & STRUDEL											
Apple Danish	1	510	30	53	15	85	350	50	2	9	2 starch, 1 1/2 carb, 5 fat

✓ = Healthiest Bets

(Continued)

DANISH & STRUDEL (*Continued*)	Amount	Cal.	Fat (g)	% Cal. Fat	Sat. Fat (g)	Chol. (mg)	Sod. (mg)	Carb. (g)	Fiber (g)	Pro. (g)	Servings/Exchanges
Apple Raisin Strudel	1	390	22	51	6	0	330	40	1	4	1 1/2 starch, 1 1/2 carb, 4 fat
Bear Claw	1	380	21	50	11	70	310	37	1	7	1 1/2 starch, 1 carb, 4 fat
Cheese Danish	1	590	35	53	19	110	430	55	1	10	2 starch, 1 1/2 carb, 5 fat
Cherry Danish	1	520	26	45	14	85	340	60	1	8	2 starch, 2 carb, 5 fat
Cherry Strudel	1	400	24	54	6	0	290	38	1	5	2 1/2 carb, 5 fat
Georgia Peach Danish	1	580	30	47	15	85	390	67	2	9	2 1/2 starch, 2 carb, 6 fat
German Chocolate Danish	1	770	46	54	24	85	570	83	4	10	3 starch, 2 1/2 carb, 8 fat
Gooey Butter Danish	1	770	43	50	20	100	480	88	2	11	3 starch, 3 carb, 8 fat
MUFFIES & MUFFINS											
Banana Nut Muffie	1	260	12	42	2	15	250	34	3	5	2 starch, 2 1/2 fat
Banana Nut Muffin	1	470	20	38	3	30	500	67	5	9	4 1/2 starch, 3 fat

Blueberry Muffin	1	450	15	30	3	35	570	73	4	8	4 1/2 starch, 2 fat
✓Chocolate Chip Muffie	1	190	10	47	5	30	130	21	1	3	1 1/2 starch, 2 fat
Chocolate Chip Muffin	1	580	30	47	15	85	390	67	2	9	2 1/2 starch, 2 carb, 5 1/2 fat
Low Fat Triple Berry Muffin	1	300	3	9	0.5	30	320	63	3	6	4 starch
Pumpkin Muffie	1	270	6	20	2	30	270	43	1	3	3 starch, 1 fat
Pumpkin Muffin	1	510	12	21	3	60	530	80	1	6	5 starch, 2 1/2 fat
SALADS											
Asian Sesame Chicken	1	330	17	46	2	65	1170	34	5	32	1 starch, 2 veg, 4 lean meat
Bistro Steak	1	630	58	83	12	55	940	10	4	16	2 veg, 2 high-fat meat, 8 fat
Caesar	1	390	26	60	8	110	750	22	3	13	1 starch, 2 veg, 1 high-fat meat, 4 fat
Classic Cafe	1	390	37	85	5	0	350	14	4	3	3 veg, 6 1/2 fat

✓ = Healthiest Bets

(*Continued*)

SALADS (*Continued*)	Amount	Cal.	Fat (g)	% Cal. Fat	Sat. Fat (g)	Chol. (mg)	Sod. (mg)	Carb. (g)	Fiber (g)	Pro. (g)	Servings/Exchanges
Fandango	1	400	28	63	7	25	480	21	6	7	1/2 starch, 3 veg, 1 high-fat meat, 4 fat
Greek	1	520	48	83	10	20	1560	17	5	9	3 veg, 9 1/2 fat
Grilled Chicken Caesar	1	500	33	59	8	125	1530	19	3	36	1/2 starch, 2 veg, 2 lean meat, 6 fat
Tomato & Fresh Mozzarella	1	790	55	63	21	85	790	50	6	30	2 starch, 3 veg, 3 high-fat meat, 7 fat
SANDWICHES											
Asiago Roast Beef	1	730	35	43	16	115	1620	54	2	50	3 1/2 starch, 6 medium-fat meat
Bacon Turkey Bravo	1	770	28	33	9	45	2850	84	5	47	5 1/2 starch, 3 lean meat, 1 high-fat meat, 2 fat
Chicken Salad on Artisan Sesame Semolina	1	730	26	32	4	90	1750	80	6	39	5 starch, 3 lean meat, 4 fat

Chicken Salad on Nine Grain	1	640	29	41	5	90	1340	56	4	35	3 1/2 starch, 3 lean meat, 5 fat
Garden Veggie	1	570	23	36	7	15	1490	74	5	15	4 starch, 2 veg, 4 1/2 fat
Italian Combo	1	1050	54	46	18	165	3570	80	5	60	5 starch, 6 high-fat meat, 1 fat
Peanut Butter & Jelly on Artisan French	1	570	15	24	3	0	1030	90	5	18	6 starch, 1 high-fat meat
✓Peanut Butter & Jelly on French	1	450	15	30	3	0	580	63	3	15	4 starch, 1 high-fat meat, 1/2 fat
Pepperblue Steak	1	780	38	44	8	75	2070	78	4	40	5 starch, 3 high-fat meat, 2 fat
Pesto Roma Club	1	650	38	53	12	85	2440	27	11	49	2 starch, 6 lean meat, 4 fat
Sierra Turkey	1	950	55	52	13	40	2360	71	4	40	4 1/2 starch, 4 lean meat, 8 fat

✓ = Healthiest Bets

(Continued)

SANDWICHES (*Continued*)	Amount	Cal.	Fat (g)	% Cal. Fat	Sat. Fat (g)	Chol. (mg)	Sod. (mg)	Carb. (g)	Fiber (g)	Pro. (g)	Servings/Exchanges
Smoke Ham & Swiss Sandwich on Rye	1	650	34	47	11	110	2350	47	4	42	3 starch, 4 medium-fat meat, 2 1/2 fat
Smoke Turkey Breast on Artisan Country	1	590	16	24	1.5	10	2320	73	5	34	5 starch, 3 lean meat, 1 fat
Smoked Ham & Swiss on Artisan Stone-Milled Rye	1	930	31	30	10	110	3000	106	6	52	7 starch, 4 lean meat, 3 1/2 fat
Smoked Turkey Breast on Sourdough	1	440	15	31	1.5	10	1950	44	3	29	3 starch, 2 lean meat, 2 fat
Tuna Salad on Artisan Multigrain	1	830	41	44	5	65	1790	78	5	32	5 starch, 2 lean meat, 7 fat
Tuna Salad Sandwich on Honey Wheat	1	720	43	54	6	65	1570	50	4	28	3 1/2 starch, 3 lean meat, 6 1/2 fat
Tuscan Chicken	1	950	57	54	10	80	2140	75	6	35	5 starch, 3 lean meat, 9 fat

SANDWICHES - PANINI											
Cornado Carnitas	1	810	35	39	11	95	2210	77	3	47	5 starch, 5 medium-fat meat, 1 1/2 fat
Frontega Chicken	1	860	42	44	12	110	2260	71	5	49	4 1/2 starch, 5 lean meat, 7 fat
Portobello & Mozzarella	1	670	33	44	12	45	1020	69	7	27	4 starch, 1 veg, 2 high-fat meat, 4 1/2 fat
Smokehouse Turkey on Artisan Three Cheese	1	670	23	31	10	50	2320	68	4	47	4 1/2 starch, 5 lean meat, 1 1/2 fat
Smokehouse Turkey on Asiago Focaccia	1	840	38	41	15	60	2740	73	5	50	5 starch, 5 lean meat, 4 1/2 fat
Turkey Artichoke	1	810	38	42	11	25	2470	76	6	41	5 starch, 4 lean meat, 5 fat
SOUPS											
Asparagus & Chicken Florentine	8 oz	230	16	63	9	50	870	12	3	10	1 starch, 3 fat

✓ = Healthiest Bets

(*Continued*)

SOUPS (*Continued*)	Amount	Cal.	Fat (g)	% Cal. Fat	Sat. Fat (g)	Chol. (mg)	Sod. (mg)	Carb. (g)	Fiber (g)	Pro. (g)	Servings/Exchanges
Baked Potato	8 oz	260	16	55	8	35	750	23	1	6	1 1/2 starch, 3 fat
Boston Clam Chowder	8 oz	210	11	47	6	40	990	19	0	6	1 starch, 1 milk, 1 1/2 fat
Broccoli Cheddar	8 oz	230	16	63	9	45	1000	13	1	8	1 milk, 3 fat
Cream of Chicken & Wild Rice	8 oz	200	12	54	6	35	970	19	0	5	1 starch, 1/2 milk, 1 1/2 fat
French Onion	8 oz	220	10	41	5	20	1810	23	2	9	1 1/2 starch, 1 high-fat meat
Low Fat Chicken Noodle	8 oz	100	2	18	0	15	1080	15	1	5	1 starch
Low Fat Vegetarian Autumn Tomato Basil	8 oz	110	3	25	0	0	910	17	3	3	1 starch, 1 fat
Low Fat Vegetarian Black Bean	8 oz	160	1	6	0	0	820	31	11	9	2 starch
Low Fat Vegetarian Garden Vegetable	8 oz	90	1	10	0	0	860	17	2	4	1 starch

SPREADS

Plain Cream Cheese	4 T	190	18	85	12	55	210	2	0	3	4 fat
Reduced Fat Hazelnut Cream Cheese	4 T	150	11	66	7	35	210	6	0	5	1/2 starch, 2 fat
Reduced Fat Honey Walnut Cream Cheese	4 T	150	11	66	7	30	200	9	0	4	1/2 starch, 2 fat
Reduced Fat Mocha Cream Cheese	4 T	160	11	62	7	30	180	10	0	5	1/2 starch, 2 1/2 fat
Reduced Fat Plain Cream Cheese	4 T	130	12	83	8	35	230	2	0	5	3 fat
Reduced Fat Raspberry Cream Cheese	4 T	120	10	75	7	30	200	3	0	4	2 1/2 fat
Reduced Fat Sun-Dried Tomato Cream Cheese	4 T	140	11	71	7	35	220	4	0	5	3 fat
Reduced Fat Veggie Cream Cheese	4 T	130	11	76	7	35	230	4	1	5	3 fat

✔ = Healthiest Bets

Quiznos Subs

❖ Quiznos Subs provides nutrition information on its Web site for only three of its sandwiches. Quiznos was unwilling to provide other information for this book. Because minimal information is available, no sample meals or healthiest bets are provided.

Quiznos Subs

	Amount	Cal.	Fat (g)	% Cal. Fat	Sat. Fat (g)	Chol. (mg)	Sod. (mg)	Carb. (g)	Fiber (g)	Pro. (g)	Servings/Exchanges
SUBS											
Honey Bourbon Chicken	1 small	359	6	15	1	359	1494	45	3	24	3 starch, 2 lean meat
Sierra Smoked Turkey w/ Raspberry Chipotle Sauce	1 small	350	6	15	0	25	1140	53	3	23	3 1/2 starch, 2 lean meat
Turkey Lite	1 small	334	6	16	1	19	1909	52	3	24	3 1/2 starch, 2 lean meat

✓ = Healthiest Bets

Schlotzsky's Deli

❖ Schlotzsky's Deli provides nutrition information for all its menu items on its Web site at www.schlotzskys.com.

Light 'n Lean Choice

Angus Beef and Gorgonzola Cheese Oven-Toasted Sandwich *(small)*
Fruit Salad

Calories	534	Sodium (mg)	1,439
Fat (g)	11	Carbohydrate (g)	70
% calories from fat	19	Fiber (g)	5
Saturated fat (g)	n/a	Protein (g)	32
Cholesterol (mg)	n/a		

Exchanges: 3 starch, 2 fruit, 3 lean meat

Healthy 'n Hearty Choice

Mozzarella, Eggplant, and Artichoke Pesto Hot Panini
Black Bean and Rice Soup *(8 oz)*
Oatmeal Raisin Cookie

Calories	771	Sodium (mg)	2,171
Fat (g)	24	Carbohydrate (g)	108
% calories from fat	28	Fiber (g)	9
Saturated fat (g)	n/a	Protein (g)	28
Cholesterol (mg)	n/a		

Exchanges: 4 starch, 2 veg, 2 carb, 3 lean meat

Schlotzsky's Deli

	Amount	Cal.	Fat (g)	% Cal. Fat	Sat. Fat (g)	Chol. (mg)	Sod. (mg)	Carb. (g)	Fiber (g)	Pro. (g)	Servings/Exchanges
8″ PIZZA											
Baby Spinach Salad	1	420	5	11	n/a	n/a	1392	82	4	13	5 1/2 starch
Bacon, Tomato & Portobello	1	640	25	35	n/a	n/a	1978	76	4	30	5 starch, 2 high-fat meat, 1 fat
Barbecue Chicken & Jalapeno	1	677	15	20	n/a	n/a	2645	98	2	33	6 1/2 starch, 2 medium-fat meat, 1 fat
Double Cheese	1	600	23	35	n/a	n/a	1756	74	3	26	5 starch, 2 high-fat meat
Fired Roasted Eggplant, Feta, Basil Pesto	1	560	20	32	n/a	n/a	1948	75	4	22	5 starch, 1 high-fat meat, 2 fat
Fresh Tomato & Pesto	1	545	19	31	n/a	n/a	1638	73	3	23	5 starch, 1 high-fat meat, 2 fat

✔ = Healthiest Bets; n/a = not available

(*Continued*)

8″ PIZZA (*Continued*)	Amount	Cal.	Fat (g)	% Cal. Fat	Sat. Fat (g)	Chol. (mg)	Sod. (mg)	Carb. (g)	Fiber (g)	Pro. (g)	Servings/Exchanges
Grilled Chicken & Pesto	1	627	21	30	n/a	n/a	2131	74	3	36	5 starch, 2 medium-fat meat, 2 fat
Italian Deluxe	1	817	42	46	n/a	n/a	2446	75	3	34	5 starch, 2 high-fat meat
Italian Sausage	1	826	41	45	n/a	n/a	2205	76	4	37	5 starch, 3 high-fat meat, 2 fat
Kung Pao Chicken	1	636	20	28	n/a	n/a	2000	81	4	37	5 starch, 3 lean meat, 2 fat
Mediterranean	1	552	20	33	n/a	n/a	1947	73	4	22	5 starch, 1 high-fat meat, 2 fat
Original Combination	1	655	27	37	n/a	n/a	1938	79	4	25	5 starch, 1 high-fat meat, 4 fat
Pepperoni & Double Cheese	1	684	31	41	n/a	n/a	2025	74	3	28	5 starch, 2 high-fat meat, 3 fat
Portobello & Fire Roasted Vegetables	1	572	19	30	n/a	n/a	2026	78	4	23	5 starch, 1 high-fat meat, 1 1/2 fat

Smoked Turkey & Jalapenos	1	633	20	28	n/a	n/a	2512	78	3	37	5 starch, 3 medium-fat meat, 1 1/2 fat
Thai Chicken	1	622	20	29	n/a	n/a	2305	86	5	36	5 1/2 starch, 3 medium-fat meat, 1 fat
Three Cheese & Fresh Tomato	1	668	26	35	n/a	n/a	1605	74	3	30	5 starch, 2 high-fat meat, 1 fat
Vegetarian Special	1	543	18	30	n/a	n/a	1705	73	4	22	5 starch, 1 high-fat meat, 1 1/2 fat
BAKED POTATOES											
Bacon, Cheddar, & Sour Cream	1	681	30	40	n/a	n/a	282	88	8	17	6 starch, 5 fat
Barbecue Angus, Red Onion & Jalapeno	1	560	7	11	n/a	n/a	956	99	7	22	6 1/2 starch, 1 fat
✓Broccoli Cheddar	1	527	12	20	n/a	n/a	517	93	9	16	6 starch, 2 fat

✓ = Healthiest Bets; n/a = not available

(*Continued*)

BAKED POTATOES (*Continued*)	Amount	Cal.	Fat (g)	% Cal. Fat	Sat. Fat (g)	Chol. (mg)	Sod. (mg)	Carb. (g)	Fiber (g)	Pro. (g)	Servings/Exchanges
✓Chili, Cheddar & Scallions	1	513	9	16	n/a	n/a	377	93	10	16	6 starch, 1 1/2 fat
✓Fired Roasted Vegetables & Portobellos	1	439	4	8	n/a	n/a	373	91	9	12	5 1/2 starch
✓Grilled Chicken & Applewood Bacon	1	617	18	26	n/a	n/a	782	90	8	25	6 starch, 1 high-fat meat, 1 1/2 fat
BEVERAGES											
✓Iced Tea	20 oz	0	0	0	n/a	n/a	0	0	0	0	free
Schlotzsky's Lemonade	20 oz	250	0	0	n/a	n/a	0	65	0	0	4 carb
Schlotzsky's Raspberry Lemonade	20 oz	275	0	0	n/a	n/a	0	75	0	0	5 carb
BREAD/BUNS/TORTILLAS											
Aged Cheddar & Jalapeno Bun	1 regular	313	4	12	n/a	n/a	838	58	2	11	4 starch, 1 fat

Dark Rye Bun	1 regular	304	2	6	n/a	n/a	762	63	3	10	4 starch
La Brea Country White Oval Bread	1 regular	194	0	0	n/a	n/a	483	41	1	7	3 starch
✓Low Carb Tortilla	1	127	3	21	n/a	n/a	500	15	9	11	1 starch, 1 fat
Pizza Crust	1	332	2	5	n/a	n/a	1110	68	2	11	4 1/2 starch
Sourdough Bun	1 regular	303	2	6	n/a	n/a	784	62	3	10	4 starch
Spicy Red Pepper & Cilantro Tortilla	1	135	2	13	n/a	n/a	n/a	21	2	3	1 1/2 starch
Tuscan Herb Bun	1 regular	304	2	6	n/a	n/a	811	62	2	10	4 starch
Wheat Bun	1 regular	312	2	6	n/a	n/a	802	62	3	11	4 starch
Whole Wheat Tortilla	1	135	2	13	n/a	n/a	n/a	21	2	3	1 1/2 starch
CHIPS											
Average for all flavors	1 serving	210	11	47	n/a	n/a	254	26	2	3	1 1/2 starch, 2 fat

✓ = Healthiest Bets; n/a = not available

(*Continued*)

	Amount	Cal.	Fat (g)	% Cal. Fat	Sat. Fat (g)	Chol. (mg)	Sod. (mg)	Carb. (g)	Fiber (g)	Pro. (g)	Servings/Exchanges
DESSERTS - CHEESECAKE											
Cookies & Cream	1	330	18	49	n/a	n/a	320	32	1	6	2 carb, 4 fat
New York Style	1	310	18	52	n/a	n/a	230	31	0	7	2 carb, 4 fat
✓Strawberry Swirl	1	300	17	51	n/a	n/a	230	30	0	6	2 carb, 3 fat
DESSERTS - COOKIES/BROWNIES											
Chocolate Brownie w/ Walnuts	1	490	20	37	n/a	n/a	320	72	2	5	4 1/2 carb, 3 1/2 fat
✓Chocolate Chip	1	160	7	39	n/a	n/a	150	23	0	2	1 1/2 starch, 1 1/2 fat
✓Fudge Chocolate Chip	1	170	8	42	n/a	n/a	170	22	1	2	1 1/2 carb, 1 1/2 fat
✓Oatmeal Raisin	1	150	5	30	n/a	n/a	140	24	1	1	1 1/2 carb, 1 fat
✓Peanut Butter	1	170	8	42	n/a	n/a	190	21	1	2	1 1/2 carb, 1 1/2 fat
✓Sugar	1	160	6	34	n/a	n/a	180	23	0	2	1 1/2 carb, 1 fat
✓White Chocolate Macadamia	1	170	8	42	n/a	n/a	140	22	0	2	1 1/2 carb, 1 1/2 fat

FRESHLY TOSSED SALADS											
✓Baby Spinach w/ Gorgonzola	1	287	20	63	n/a	n/a	541	8	4	16	2 veg, 2 medium-fat meat, 2 fat
✓Caesar	1	101	5	45	n/a	n/a	342	10	2	5	2 veg, 1 fat
Crunchy Chicken	1	359	22	55	n/a	n/a	1088	13	4	29	1 starch, 4 lean meat, 2 fat
✓Fresh Fruit	1	103	1	9	n/a	n/a	24	26	3	2	1 1/2 fruit
✓Garden	1	50	2	36	n/a	n/a	169	8	4	3	2 veg
✓Grilled Chicken Caesar	1	169	6	32	n/a	n/a	729	11	2	18	2 veg, 2 lean meat
Ham & Turkey Chef's	1	245	13	48	n/a	n/a	1295	12	4	23	2 veg, 3 medium-fat meat
✓Honey Lime Chicken	1	240	9	34	n/a	n/a	644	24	6	19	1 1/2 starch, 2 lean meat, 1/2 fat
✓Mediterranean Eggplant & Feta	1	140	9	58	n/a	n/a	277	11	5	8	2 veg, 1 high-fat meat

✓ = Healthiest Bets; n/a = not available

(*Continued*)

FRESHLY TOSSED SALADS (*Continued*)	Amount	Cal.	Fat (g)	% Cal. Fat	Sat. Fat (g)	Chol. (mg)	Sod. (mg)	Carb. (g)	Fiber (g)	Pro. (g)	Servings/Exchanges
✓Mediterranean Feta	1	131	9	62	n/a	n/a	574	9	4	8	2 veg, 1 high-fat meat
Turkey Chef's	1	261	13	45	n/a	n/a	1129	12	3	27	1 starch, 3 lean meat, 1 fat
GOURMET SOUPS W/ TOPPINGS											
Baked Potato	8 oz	288	17	53	n/a	n/a	1357	31	3	7	1 starch, 1 milk, 3 fat
Baked Potato	12 oz	429	26	55	n/a	n/a	2005	47	4	10	2 starch, 1 milk, 5 fat
Black Beans & Rice	12 oz	271	2	7	n/a	n/a	1513	53	7	13	3 1/2 starch
Black Beans & Rice	8 oz	181	1	5	n/a	n/a	1009	35	5	8	2 starch
Boston Clam Chowder	12 oz	394	25	57	n/a	n/a	1935	42	2	9	2 starch, 1 milk, 4 fat
Boston Clam Chowder	8 oz	264	16	55	n/a	n/a	1291	28	1	6	1 starch, 1 milk, 3 fat
Broccoli & Cheddar Cheese	8 oz	264	16	55	n/a	n/a	1291	28	2	6	1 starch, 1 milk, 3 fat
Broccoli & Cheddar Cheese	12 oz	450	31	62	n/a	n/a	1877	37	2	14	1 starch, 1 1/2 milk, 5 1/2 fat

Cheddar & Chicken Tortilla	8 oz	244	11	41	n/a	n/a	1539	24	2	13	1 1/2 starch, 1 lean meat, 2 fat
Cheddar & Chicken Tortilla	12 oz	347	16	41	n/a	n/a	2318	31	2	19	2 starch, 1 lean meat, 2 fat
Chicken Gumbo	12 oz	167	7	38	n/a	n/a	1671	20	3	6	1 starch, 1 1/2 fat
Chicken Gumbo	8 oz	112	5	40	n/a	n/a	1115	13	2	4	1 starch, 1 fat
Chicken Noodle	8 oz	211	7	30	n/a	n/a	1523	25	1	11	1 1/2 starch, 1 lean meat, 1 fat
Chicken Noodle	12 oz	277	7	23	n/a	n/a	2119	35	2	15	2 starch, 2 lean meat
Chicken w/ Wild Rice	8 oz	410	30	66	n/a	n/a	1298	27	1	11	1 1/2 starch, 1 lean meat, 5 1/2 fat
Chicken w/ Wild Rice	12 oz	614	45	66	n/a	n/a	1946	40	2	16	3 starch, 1 lean meat, 7 fat
Cream of Asparagus	8 oz	263	21	72	n/a	n/a	746	22	2	5	1/2 starch, 1 milk, 4 fat
Cream of Asparagus	12 oz	361	29	72	n/a	n/a	1119	33	2	6	1 starch, 1 milk, 5 fat
French Onion	12 oz	239	14	53	n/a	n/a	2432	17	0	12	1 starch, 2 1/2 fat

✔ = Healthiest Bets; n/a = not available

(*Continued*)

GOURMET SOUPS W/ TOPPINGS (*Continued*)	Amount	Cal.	Fat (g)	% Cal. Fat	Sat. Fat (g)	Chol. (mg)	Sod. (mg)	Carb. (g)	Fiber (g)	Pro. (g)	Servings/Exchanges
French Onion	8 oz	158	9	51	n/a	n/a	1629	12	0	7	1 starch, 1 lean meat, 1 fat
Gourmet Vegetable Beef	8 oz	155	6	35	n/a	n/a	1280	15	2	9	1 starch, 1 medium-fat meat
Gourmet Vegetable Beef	12 oz	215	8	33	n/a	n/a	1825	22	3	12	1 1/2 starch, 1 high-fat meat
Minestrone	12 oz	185	5	24	n/a	n/a	1985	29	6	8	2 starch, 1 fat
Minestrone	8 oz	135	4	27	n/a	n/a	1387	20	4	6	1 1/2 starch, 1/2 fat
Monterrey Black Bean	12 oz	365	5	12	n/a	n/a	1518	64	26	17	4 starch, 1 lean meat
Monterrey Black Bean	8 oz	245	4	15	n/a	n/a	1012	43	17	22	3 starch, 1 lean meat
Pilgrim Clam Chowder	8 oz	287	17	53	n/a	n/a	1011	38	1	2	2 1/2 starch, 2 1/2 fat
Pilgrim Clam Chowder	12 oz	429	25	52	n/a	n/a	1516	57	2	4	3 1/2 starch, 4 fat
Ravioli	8 oz	160	5	28	n/a	n/a	1463	25	1	8	1 1/2 starch, 1 fat

Ravioli	12 oz	224	6	24	n/a	n/a	2100	37	2	11	2 1/2 starch, 1 fat
Stuffed Green Bell Pepper	8 oz	189	6	29	n/a	n/a	1304	26	0	7	1 1/2 starch, 1 1/2 fat
Stuffed Green Bell Pepper	12 oz	243	6	22	n/a	n/a	1788	36	0	9	2 1/2 starch, 1 fat
✓Timberline Chili	8 oz	257	10	35	n/a	n/a	923	26	8	16	1 1/2 starch, 1 high-fat meat, 1/2 fat
Timberline Chili	12 oz	398	16	36	n/a	n/a	1406	39	12	25	2 1/2 starch, 2 high-fat meat
Tuscan Tomato Basil	8 oz	353	32	82	n/a	n/a	1199	14	3	6	1 starch, 1 high-fat meat, 5 fat
Tuscan Tomato Basil	12 oz	513	46	81	n/a	n/a	1704	20	5	9	1 1/2 starch, 1 high-fat meat, 8 fat
Vegetarian Vegetable	12 oz	192	3	14	n/a	n/a	1679	38	7	5	1 1/2 starch, 1 veg
Vegetarian Vegetable	8 oz	144	3	19	n/a	n/a	1167	27	5	4	1 starch, 1 veg
Wisconsin Cheese	8 oz	358	28	70	n/a	n/a	1256	27	1	8	1 1/2 starch, 1 high-fat meat, 3 1/2 fat

✓ = Healthiest Bets; n/a = not available

(*Continued*)

GOURMET SOUPS W/ TOPPINGS (*Continued*)	Amount	Cal.	Fat (g)	% Cal. Fat	Sat. Fat (g)	Chol. (mg)	Sod. (mg)	Carb. (g)	Fiber (g)	Pro. (g)	Servings/Exchanges
Wisconsin Cheese	12 oz	520	40	69	n/a	n/a	1833	40	2	10	2 1/2 starch, 1 high-fat meat, 6 fat
HOT PANINI SANDWICHES											
Classic Gruyere & Roma Tomato	1	658	38	52	n/a	n/a	1113	47	1	36	3 starch, 3 high-fat meat, 2 1/2 fat
Grilled Chicken Romano	1	486	19	35	n/a	n/a	1123	45	1	34	3 starch, 3 lean meat, 2 fat
Italiano	1	598	30	45	n/a	n/a	1862	46	2	19	3 starch, 1 high-fat meat, 6 fat
Mozzarella, Eggplant & Artichoke Pesto	1	440	18	37	n/a	n/a	1022	49	3	19	3 starch, 1 high-fat meat, 2 fat
Prosciutto & Fresh Parmesan	1	472	22	42	n/a	n/a	2103	58	2	23	3 1/2 starch, 2 lean meat, 2 1/2 fat
Prosciutto Crostini	1	591	32	49	n/a	n/a	1611	47	1	30	3 starch, 3 lean meat, 2 1/2 fat

Smoked Turkey & Guacamole	1	581	25	39	n/a	n/a	1516	53	5	34	3 1/2 starch, 3 lean meat, 3 fat
JUST FOR KIDS											
Cheese Pizza	1	476	13	25	n/a	n/a	1364	72	3	18	4 1/2 starch, 1 high-fat meat, 1/2 fat
Cheese Sandwich	1	367	14	34	n/a	n/a	912	55	1	16	3 1/2 starch, 1 high-fat meat, 1/2 fat
Ham & Cheese Sandwich	1	397	16	36	n/a	n/a	1286	45	1	20	3 starch, 1 high-fat meat, 1 1/2 fat
Pepperoni Pizza	1	524	17	29	n/a	n/a	1533	72	3	19	4 1/2 starch, 1 high-fat meat, 2 fat
Turkey Sandwich	1	266	4	14	n/a	n/a	965	43	1	14	3 starch, 1 lean meat
OVEN-TOASTED SANDWICHES											
Albacore Tuna on Cheddar (regular)	1	628	27	39	n/a	n/a	1754	66	4	38	4 1/2 starch, 3 lean meat, 3 fat

✓ = Healthiest Bets; n/a = not available

(Continued)

OVEN-TOASTED SANDWICHES (*Continued*)	Amount	Cal.	Fat (g)	% Cal. Fat	Sat. Fat (g)	Chol. (mg)	Sod. (mg)	Carb. (g)	Fiber (g)	Pro. (g)	Servings/Exchanges
Albacore Tuna on Cheddar (small)	1	432	19	40	n/a	n/a	1196	44	3	26	3 starch, 3 lean meat, 2 fat
Angus Beef & Cheese (regular)	1	791	28	32	n/a	n/a	2536	70	3	54	6 starch, 6 lean meat, 2 fat
Angus Beef & Cheese (small)	1	538	19	32	n/a	n/a	1651	46	2	37	3 starch, 3 lean meat, 2 1/2 fat
Angus Beef & Fired Roasted Vegetables (regular)	1	921	42	41	n/a	n/a	2678	75	4	54	5 starch, 6 lean meat, 4 1/2 fat
Angus Beef & Fired Roasted Vegetables (small)	1	650	31	43	n/a	n/a	1858	51	3	38	3 1/2 starch, 3 lean meat, 2 fat
Angus Beef & Gorgonzola (regular)	1	664	17	23	n/a	n/a	2147	67	3	46	4 1/2 starch, 4 lean meat, 2 fat

Angus Beef & Gorgonzola (small)	1	431	10	21	n/a	n/a	1415	44	2	30	3 starch, 3 lean meat, 1/2 fat
Angus Corned Beef Reuben (regular)	1	957	42	39	n/a	n/a	3241	75	4	65	5 starch, 7 lean meat, 4 fat
Angus Corned Beef Reuben (small)	1	647	28	39	n/a	n/a	2552	51	3	44	3 1/2 starch, 4 lean meat, 3 fat
Angus Pastrami & Swiss (regular)	1	966	39	36	n/a	n/a	2983	79	5	67	5 starch, 7 lean meat, 4 fat
Angus Pastrami & Swiss (small)	1	644	26	36	n/a	n/a	1991	53	4	45	3 1/2 starch, 4 medium-fat meat, 1 1/2 fat
Angus Pastrami Reuben (regular)	1	972	43	40	n/a	n/a	3063	75	4	65	5 starch, 7 medium-fat meat, 1 fat
Angus Pastrami Reuben (small)	1	657	29	40	n/a	n/a	2131	51	3	44	3 1/2 starch, 5 medium-fat meat, 1 fat
Angus Roast Beef (regular)	1	565	10	16	n/a	n/a	1907	66	3	41	4 1/2 starch, 3 lean meat, 1 fat

✓ = Healthiest Bets; n/a = not available

(*Continued*)

OVEN-TOASTED SANDWICHES (*Continued*)	Amount	Cal.	Fat (g)	% Cal. Fat	Sat. Fat (g)	Chol. (mg)	Sod. (mg)	Carb. (g)	Fiber (g)	Pro. (g)	Servings/Exchanges
Angus Roast Beef (small)	1	381	7	17	n/a	n/a	1291	44	2	28	3 starch, 2 lean meat, 1 fat
Angus Steak & Provolone (regular)	1	693	18	23	n/a	n/a	2779	73	3	50	5 starch, 5 lean meat, 1/2 fat
Angus Steak & Provolone (small)	1	452	11	22	n/a	n/a	1855	49	2	33	3 starch, 2 lean meat, 2 fat
Bacon, Lettuce & Tomato (regular)	1	584	25	39	n/a	n/a	1596	60	2	28	4 starch, 2 high-fat meat, 1 1/2 fat
Bacon, Lettuce & Tomato (small)	1	379	16	38	n/a	n/a	1029	40	2	18	3 starch, 1 high-fat meat, 1 1/2 fat
Cheese Original (regular)	1	758	38	45	n/a	n/a	1928	70	3	35	4 1/2 starch, 3 high-fat meat, 2 1/2 fat
Cheese Original (small)	1	538	28	47	n/a	n/a	1340	47	2	26	3 starch, 2 high-fat meat, 2 1/2 fat

Crunchy Garden Vegetable (regular)	1	468	12	23	n/a	n/a	1209	71	6	19	4 1/2 starch, 1 veg, 2 fat
✓Crunchy Garden Vegetable (small)	1	293	7	22	n/a	n/a	742	48	48	12	3 starch, 1 veg, 1 fat
Deluxe Original (regular)	1	869	41	42	n/a	n/a	4031	74	3	50	5 starch, 5 high-fat meat, 1 fat
Deluxe Original (small)	1	657	34	47	n/a	n/a	3013	51	2	38	3 1/2 starch, 3 high-fat meat, 2 fat
Grilled Chicken & Basil Pesto (regular)	1	638	23	32	n/a	n/a	2172	68	4	41	4 1/2 starch, 4 medium-fat meat
Grilled Chicken & Basil Pesto (small)	1	402	13	29	n/a	n/a	1469	45	2	27	3 starch, 2 medium-fat meat
Grilled Chicken & Green Chilis (regular)	1	571	13	20	n/a	n/a	2176	73	4	42	4 1/2 starch, 4 lean meat
Grilled Chicken & Green Chilis (small)	1	384	9	21	n/a	n/a	1486	49	3	28	3 starch, 2 lean meat, 1/2 fat

✓ = Healthiest Bets; n/a = not available

(*Continued*)

OVEN-TOASTED SANDWICHES (*Continued*)	Amount	Cal.	Fat (g)	% Cal. Fat	Sat. Fat (g)	Chol. (mg)	Sod. (mg)	Carb. (g)	Fiber (g)	Pro. (g)	Servings/Exchanges
Grilled Chicken & Sun - Dried Tomato (regular)	1	574	15	24	n/a	n/a	2178	69	3	44	4 1/2 starch, 4 lean meat
Grilled Chicken & Sun - Dried Tomato (small)	1	364	8	20	n/a	n/a	1367	46	2	28	3 starch, 2 lean meat
Grilled Chicken & Whole Grain Dijon (regular)	1	539	8	13	n/a	n/a	2131	74	7	41	5 starch, 3 lean meat
Grilled Chicken & Whole Grain Dijon (small)	1	357	5	13	n/a	n/a	1397	49	5	27	3 starch, 2 lean meat
Grilled Chicken Carbonara (regular)	1	661	23	31	n/a	n/a	2487	69	3	48	4 1/2 starch, 5 lean meat
Grilled Chicken Carbonara (small)	1	447	15	30	n/a	n/a	1707	46	2	33	3 starch, 2 lean meat, 2 fat
Grilled Chicken Club (regular)	1	741	28	34	n/a	n/a	2354	68	4	51	4 1/2 starch, 5 lean meat, 1 1/2 fat

Grilled Chicken Club (small)	1	502	20	36	n/a	n/a	1578	45	3	34	3 starch, 4 lean meat, 1 fat
Grilled Chicken, Salsa & Cheddar (regular)	1	822	37	41	n/a	n/a	2621	72	3	50	4 1/2 starch, 5 medium-fat meat
Grilled Chicken, Salsa & Cheddar (small)	1	545	24	40	n/a	n/a	1688	48	2	35	3 starch, 4 medium-fat meat
Ham & Cheese Original (regular)	1	711	26	33	n/a	n/a	3201	72	3	41	4 1/2 starch, 4 medium-fat meat, 1 fat
Ham & Cheese Original (small)	1	491	19	35	n/a	n/a	2174	48	2	29	3 starch, 3 medium-fat meat, 1 fat
Ham, Cheddar, Jalapeno (regular)	1	710	30	38	n/a	n/a	3028	66	2	41	4 1/2 starch, 4 medium-fat meat, 1 1/2 fat
Ham, Cheddar, Jalapeno (small)	1	495	22	40	n/a	n/a	2083	44	2	29	3 starch, 3 medium-fat meat, 1 fat
Schlotzsky's Melted Caprese (regular)	1	733	36	44	n/a	n/a	1536	67	4	30	4 1/2 starch, 2 high-fat meat, 4 fat

✔ = Healthiest Bets; n/a = not available

(*Continued*)

OVEN-TOASTED SANDWICHES (*Continued*)	Amount	Cal.	Fat (g)	% Cal. Fat	Sat. Fat (g)	Chol. (mg)	Sod. (mg)	Carb. (g)	Fiber (g)	Pro. (g)	Servings/Exchanges
Schlotzsky's Melted Caprese (small)	1	463	22	43	n/a	n/a	1033	44	2	19	3 starch, 2 high-fat meat, 1 fat
Smoked Turkey & Applewood Bacon (regular)	1	755	31	37	n/a	n/a	2796	68	3	51	3 1/2 starch, 6 medium-fat meat
Smoked Turkey & Applewood Bacon (small)	1	519	22	38	n/a	n/a	1902	45	2	35	3 starch, 3 medium-fat meat, 1 fat
Smoked Turkey & Guacamole (regular)	1	509	10	18	n/a	n/a	2136	72	8	35	4 1/2 starch, 3 lean meat
Smoked Turkey & Guacamole (small)	1	329	6	16	n/a	n/a	1413	47	5	23	3 starch, 2 lean meat
Smoked Turkey Breast (regular)	1	463	7	14	n/a	n/a	2022	68	7	33	4 starch, 3 lean meat

Smoked Turkey Breast (small)	1	311	5	14	n/a	n/a	1367	45	2	22	3 starch, 2 lean meat
Smoked Turkey Reuben (regular)	1	853	36	38	n/a	n/a	2810	72	4	57	4 1/2 starch, 6 medium-fat meat, 1 fat
Smoked Turkey Reuben (small)	1	576	24	38	n/a	n/a	1959	49	3	38	3 starch, 4 medium-fat meat, 1 fat
Southwestern Turkey Club (regular)	1	835	37	40	n/a	n/a	2947	74	4	52	5 starch, 5 medium-fat meat, 2 fat
Southwestern Turkey Club (small)	1	583	27	42	n/a	n/a	2022	51	3	36	3 1/2 starch, 4 medium-fat meat, 1 fat
Spicy Chipotle Chicken (regular)	1	476	7	13	n/a	n/a	1644	66	3	36	4 starch, 3 lean meat
Spicy Chipotle Chicken (small)	1	319	5	14	n/a	n/a	1107	44	2	25	3 starch, 2 lean meat

✔ = Healthiest Bets; n/a = not available

(*Continued*)

OVEN-TOASTED SANDWICHES (*Continued*)	Amount	Cal.	Fat (g)	% Cal. Fat	Sat. Fat (g)	Chol. (mg)	Sod. (mg)	Carb. (g)	Fiber (g)	Pro. (g)	Servings/Exchanges
The Original (regular)	1	706	31	40	n/a	n/a	2717	71	3	36	4 1/2 starch, 3 high-fat meat, 1 1/2 fat
The Original (small)	1	505	24	43	n/a	n/a	1840	47	2	25	3 starch, 2 high-fat meat, 1 1/2 fat
Turkey & Cucumber (regular)	1	467	7	13	n/a	n/a	2046	69	4	34	4 1/2 starch, 3 lean meat
Turkey & Cucumber (small)	1	316	5	14	n/a	n/a	1390	46	3	23	3 starch, 2 lean meat
TOASTED WRAPS											
✓Albacore Tuna & Mozzarella	1	365	19	47	n/a	n/a	694	25	2	22	1 1/2 starch, 3 medium-fat meat
Asian Chicken w/ Almonds	1	376	7	17	n/a	n/a	2172	56	4	18	3 1/2 starch, 1 lean meat, 1 fat
Chipotle Chicken Salad	1	496	26	47	n/a	n/a	1051	32	5	30	2 starch, 3 medium-fat meat, 2 fat

✓Fresh Veggie	1	337	13	35	n/a	n/a	556	39	4	11	2 starch, 1 veg, 1 high-fat meat, 1 fat
✓Greek Feta & Portobello	1	288	9	28	n/a	n/a	727	38	3	9	2 1/2 starch, 2 fat
Grilled Chicken, Aged Cheddar, & Guacamole	1	436	22	45	n/a	n/a	953	34	7	23	2 starch, 2 high-fat meat, 1 1/2 fat
Parmesan Chicken Caesar Wrap	1	414	25	54	n/a	n/a	914	26	3	19	1 1/2 starch, 2 medium-fat meat, 3 fat
Turkey & Garden Vegetable	1	289	9	28	n/a	n/a	999	28	3	20	2 starch, 2 lean meat, 1 fat

✓ = Healthiest Bets; n/a = not available

Subway

❖ Subway provides nutrition information for most of its menu items on its Web site at www.subway.com.

Light 'n Lean Choice

Minestrone Soup *(8 oz)*
Grilled Chicken and Baby Spinach Salad
Greek Vinaigrette *(2 T, 1/2 serving)*
Oatmeal Raisin Cookie *(1)*

Calories	530	Sodium (mg)	2,090
Fat (g)	25	Carbohydrate (g)	49
% calories from fat	42	Fiber (g)	7
Saturated fat (g)	6.5	Protein (g)	37
Cholesterol (mg)	85		

Exchanges: 1 starch, 2 veg, 2 carb, 3 lean meat, 2 fat

Healthy 'n Hearty Choice

Chili Con Carne *(8 oz)*
Savory Turkey Breast and Ham Sandwich *(6 inch)*
Berry Lichus Fruizie

Calories	630	Sodium (mg)	2,120
Fat (g)	15	Carbohydrate (g)	98
% calories from fat	21	Fiber (g)	13
Saturated fat (g)	6.5	Protein (g)	36
Cholesterol (mg)	40		

Exchanges: 4 1/2 starch, 1 veg, 2 carb, 3 lean meat, 2 fat

Subway

	Amount	Cal.	Fat (g)	% Cal. Fat	Sat. Fat (g)	Chol. (mg)	Sod. (mg)	Carb. (g)	Fiber (g)	Pro. (g)	Servings/Exchanges
6″ COLD SANDWICHES											
Classic Tuna	1	530	31	53	7	45	1030	45	4	22	3 starch, 2 lean meat, 4 1/2 fat
Cold Cut Combo	1	410	17	37	7	60	1550	47	4	21	3 starch, 2 high-fat meat
Subway Seafood Sensation	1	450	22	44	6	25	1150	51	5	16	3 1/2 starch, 1 lean meat, 4 fat
6″ DOUBLE MEAT SUBS											
DM Cheese Steak	1	450	14	28	6	60	1470	50	6	37	3 starch, 4 lean meat
DM Chipotle Southwest Cheese Steak	1	540	24	40	7	70	1680	51	7	37	3 1/2 starch, 4 medium-fat meat

✓ = Healthiest Bets

(Continued)

6″ DOUBLE MEAT SUBS (*Continued*)	Amount	Cal.	Fat (g)	% Cal. Fat	Sat. Fat (g)	Chol. (mg)	Sod. (mg)	Carb. (g)	Fiber (g)	Pro. (g)	Servings/Exchanges
DM Classic tuna	1	790	55	63	11	80	1340	45	4	32	3 starch, 3 lean meat, 7 1/2 fat
DM Cold Cut Combo	1	550	28	46	10	110	2380	49	4	31	3 starch, 3 high-fat meat, 1/2 fat
DM Ham	1	380	7	17	2.5	50	2180	57	4	28	3 1/2 starch, 2 lean meat
DM Italian BMT	1	630	35	50	14	100	2890	49	4	34	3 starch, 3 high-fat meat, 2 fat
DM Meatball Marinara	1	960	42	39	18	85	2490	82	10	37	5 1/2 starch, 3 high-fat meat, 4 fat
DM Oven Roasted Chicken	1	430	8	17	2	90	1520	50	4	39	3 1/2 starch, 3 lean meat
DM Roast Beef	1	360	7	18	3.5	40	1320	46	4	29	3 starch, 3 lean meat
DM Seafood Sensation	1	640	38	53	8	40	1580	58	5	20	3 1/2 starch, 1 lean meat, 7 fat

DM Subway Club	1	420	8	17	3.5	65	2100	50	4	39	3 starch, 4 lean meat
DM Sweet Onion Chicken Teriyaki	1	490	7	13	2	100	1630	68	4	43	4 1/2 starch, 4 lean meat
DM Turkey Breast	1	340	6	16	1.5	40	1520	48	4	28	3 starch, 3 lean meat
DM Turkey Breast & Ham	1	360	7	18	2	50	1950	50	4	31	3 1/2 starch, 3 lean meat
DM Turkey Breast, Ham & Bacon Melt	1	450	14	28	6	70	2330	51	4	36	3 1/2 starch, 3 lean meat, 1 fat

6″ HOT SANDWICHES

Cheese Steak	1	360	10	25	4.5	35	1090	47	5	24	3 starch, 2 medium-fat meat
Chipotle Southwest Cheese Steak	1	450	20	40	6	45	1310	48	6	24	3 starch, 2 medium-fat meat, 2 fat
Italian LT	1	450	21	42	8	55	1790	47	4	23	3 starch, 2 high-fat meat
Meatball Marinara	1	610	24	35	11	45	1610	63	7	24	4 starch, 2 high-fat meat, 1 1/2 fat

✔ = Healthiest Bets

(*Continued*)

6″ HOT SANDWICHES (*Continued*)	Amount	Cal.	Fat (g)	% Cal. Fat	Sat. Fat (g)	Chol. (mg)	Sod. (mg)	Carb. (g)	Fiber (g)	Pro. (g)	Servings/Exchanges
Turkey Breast, Ham & Bacon Melt	1	380	12	28	5	45	1610	48	4	25	3 starch, 1 medium-fat meat, 1 1/2 fat
6″ PROMOTIONAL/REGIONAL SUBS											
Barbecue Rib Patty	1	420	19	41	6	50	830	47	4	20	3 starch, 1 high-fat meat, 2 fat
Barbeque Chicken	1	310	6	17	2	35	1110	52	5	16	3 1/2 starch, 2 lean meat
Buffalo Chicken	1	390	13	30	3	55	1510	46	5	26	3 starch, 2 lean meat, 1 1/2 fat
✓Gardenburger	1	390	7	16	2.5	5	970	66	9	19	4 starch, 1 lean meat, 1/2 fat
Pastrami	1	570	29	46	9	10	1890	49	5	32	3 starch, 3 high-fat meat, 1 fat
Spicy Italian	1	480	25	47	9	55	1670	46	4	21	3 starch, 2 high-fat meat, 2 fat

Veggi-Max	1	390	8	18	1.5	10	1040	56	7	24	3 1/2 starch, 1 veg, 2 lean meat
6″ SANDWICHES											
Honey Mustard Ham	1	320	5	14	1.5	25	1420	54	4	19	3 1/2 starch, 1 lean meat
Oven Roasted Chicken Breast	1	330	6	16	1.5	45	1020	47	4	24	3 starch, 2 lean meat
Roast Beef	1	290	5	16	2	20	920	45	4	19	3 starch, 1 lean meat
Savory Turkey Breast	1	280	5	16	1.5	20	1020	46	4	18	3 starch, 1 lean meat
Savory Turkey Breast & Ham	1	290	5	16	1.5	25	1230	47	4	20	3 starch, 1 lean meat
Subway Club	1	320	6	17	2	35	1310	47	1	24	3 starch, 2 lean meat
✔Veggie Delite	1	230	3	12	1	0	520	44	4	9	2 1/2 starch, 1 veg
BREADS											
✔6″ Wheat Bread	1	200	3	14	1	0	360	40	3	8	2 1/2 starch
✔6″ Hearty Italian Bread	1	210	3	13	1.5	0	340	41	3	8	2 1/2 starch

✔ = Healthiest Bets

(*Continued*)

BREADS (*Continued*)	Amount	Cal.	Fat (g)	% Cal. Fat	Sat. Fat (g)	Chol. (mg)	Sod. (mg)	Carb. (g)	Fiber (g)	Pro. (g)	Servings/Exchanges
✓6″ Honey Oat Bread	1	250	4	14	1	0	380	48	4	10	3 starch
✓6″ Italian White Bread	1	200	3	14	1.5	0	340	38	3	7	2 1/2 starch
✓6″ Monterey Cheddar Bread	1	240	6	23	3.5	10	400	39	3	10	2 1/2 starch, 1 fat
✓6″ Parmesan Oregano Bread	1	210	4	17	1.5	0	500	40	3	8	2 1/2 starch
✓Carb Conscious Wrap	1	120	5	38	0	0	680	13	8	14	1 starch, 1 lean meat
✓Deli Style Roll	1	170	3	16	1	0	280	32	3	6	2 starch
BREAKFAST SANDWICHES ON DELI ROUND											
✓Bacon & Egg	1	320	15	42	4.5	185	520	34	3	15	2 starch, 1 high-fat meat, 1 1/2 fat
✓Cheese & Egg	1	320	15	42	5	185	550	34	3	14	2 starch, 2 medium-fat meat, 1 fat
✓Ham & Egg	1	310	13	38	3.5	190	720	34	3	16	2 starch, 2 medium-fat meat, 1/2 fat

✓Steak & Egg	1	330	14	38	4	190	570	35	3	19	2 starch, 2 medium-fat meat, 1/2 fat
✓Vegetable & Egg	1	290	12	37	3	175	430	36	3	12	2 starch, 1 medium-fat meat, 1 1/2 fat
✓Western & Egg	1	300	12	36	3.5	180	530	36	3	14	2 starch, 1 medium-fat meat, 1 1/2 fat
BREAKFAST SANDWICHES ON ITALIAN OR WHEAT											
✓Bacon & Egg	1	450	19	38	7	570	700	42	3	28	3 starch, 3 medium-fat meat
✓Cheese & Egg	1	440	19	39	7	570	730	42	3	27	3 starch, 2 medium-fat meat, 1 1/2 fat
Ham & Egg	1	430	17	36	5	575	900	42	3	29	3 starch, 3 lean meat, 1 1/2 fat
✓Steak & Egg	1	460	18	35	6	575	750	43	4	33	3 starch, 3 medium-fat meat

✓ = Healthiest Bets

(*Continued*)

BREAKFAST SANDWICHES ON ITALIAN OR WHEAT (*Continued*)	Amount	Cal.	Fat (g)	% Cal. Fat	Sat. Fat (g)	Chol. (mg)	Sod. (mg)	Carb. (g)	Fiber (g)	Pro. (g)	Servings/Exchanges
✓Vegetable & Egg	1	410	16	35	5	560	610	44	4	25	3 starch, 2 medium-fat meat
✓Western & Egg	1	430	17	36	5	565	710	44	4	27	3 starch, 2 medium-fat meat, 1 1/2 fat
CHEESE											
✓American	for 6″ sub	40	4	90	2	10	200	1	0	2	1 fat
Monterey Cheddar	for 6″ sub	110	9	74	6	30	180	1	0	7	1 high-fat meat
✓Natural Cheddar	for 6″ sub	60	5	75	3	15	95	0	0	4	1 medium-fat meat
✓Pepperjack	for 6″ sub	50	4	72	2.5	15	140	0	0	3	1 fat
✓Provolone	for 6″ sub	50	4	72	2	10	125	0	0	4	1 fat
✓Swiss	for 6″ sub	50	5	90	2.5	15	30	0	0	4	1 fat

DELI-STYLE SANDWICHES											
✓Classic Tuna	1	350	18	46	5	30	750	35	3	14	2 starch, 1 lean meat, 3 fat
✓Ham	1	210	4	17	1.5	10	770	36	3	11	2 starch, 1 lean meat
✓Roast Beef	1	220	5	20	2	15	660	35	3	13	2 starch, 1 medium-fat meat
✓Savory Turkey Breast	1	210	4	17	1.5	15	730	36	3	13	2 starch, 1 lean meat
DESSERTS - COOKIES											
✓Chocolate Chip	1	210	10	43	4	15	160	30	1	2	2 carb, 1 1/2 fat
✓Chocolate Chunk	1	220	10	41	3.5	10	105	30	1	2	2 carb, 1 1/2 fat
✓Double Chocolate Chip	1	210	10	43	4	15	170	30	1	2	2 carb, 1 1/2 fat
✓M&M Cookie	1	210	10	43	3.5	15	105	30	1	2	2 carb, 1 1/2 fat
✓Oatmeal Raisin	1	200	8	36	2.5	15	170	30	2	3	2 carb, 1 1/2 fat
✓Peanut Butter	1	220	12	49	4	10	200	26	1	4	1 1/2 carb, 2 fat

✓ = Healthiest Bets

(Continued)

DESSERTS - COOKIES (*Continued*)	Amount	Cal.	Fat (g)	% Cal. Fat	Sat. Fat (g)	Chol. (mg)	Sod. (mg)	Carb. (g)	Fiber (g)	Pro. (g)	Servings/Exchanges
✓Sugar Cookie	1	230	12	47	3.5	15	135	28	0	2	2 carb, 2 fat
✓White Chip Macadamia Nut	1	220	11	45	3.5	15	160	28	1	2	2 carb, 2 fat
DESSERTS - PIE											
✓Apple Pie	1 serving	245	10	37	2	0	290	37	1	0	2 1/2 carb, 1 1/2 fat
FRUIT ROLL UP											
✓Fruit Roll Up	1	50	1	18	0	0	55	12	0	0	1 carb
FRUIZIE EXPRESS											
✓Berry Lishus	small	100	0	0	0	0	30	28	1	1	1 1/2 carb
Berry Lishus w/ banana	small	140	0	0	0	0	30	35	2	1	2 carb
✓Peach Pizzazz	small	100	0	0	0	0	25	26	0	0	1 1/2 carb
Pineapple Delight	small	130	0	0	0	0	25	33	1	1	2 carb
Pineapple Delight w/ banana	small	160	0	0	0	0	25	40	1	1	2 1/2 carb

✓Sunrise Refresher	small	120	0	0	0	0	20	29	1	1	2 carb
OMELETS & FRENCH TOAST											
Bacon & Egg	1 order	240	17	64	6	570	350	2	0	20	3 medium-fat meat, 1/2 fat
Cheese & Egg	1 order	240	17	64	6	570	370	2	0	19	3 medium-fat meat
✓French Toast w/ syrup	1 order	350	8	21	2.5	280	350	57	2	14	3 starch, 1 carb, 1 1/2 fat
✓Ham & Egg	1 order	230	14	55	4.5	575	550	2	0	21	3 medium-fat meat
✓Steak & Egg	1 order	250	15	54	5	580	390	3	1	24	3 medium-fat meat
✓Vegetable & Egg	1 order	210	14	60	4	560	250	4	1	17	1 veg, 2 medium-fat meat, 1/2 fat
✓Western & Egg	1 order	220	14	57	4.5	565	360	4	1	19	3 medium-fat meat
SALAD DRESSING											
Atkins Honey Mustard	4 T	200	22	99	3	0	510	1	0	1	4 1/2 fat
Greek Vinaigrette	4 T	200	21	95	3	0	590	3	0	1	4 fat

✓ = Healthiest Bets

(*Continued*)

SALAD DRESSING (*Continued*)	Amount	Cal.	Fat (g)	% Cal. Fat	Sat. Fat (g)	Chol. (mg)	Sod. (mg)	Carb. (g)	Fiber (g)	Pro. (g)	Servings/Exchanges
Kraft Fat Free Italian	4 T	35	0	0	0	0	720	7	0	1	1/2 carb
Ranch	4 T	200	22	99	3.5	10	550	1	0	1	4 1/2 fat
SALADS W/OUT DRESSING & CROUTONS											
✓Grilled Chicken & Baby Spinach	1	140	3	19	1	50	450	11	4	20	2 veg, 3 lean meat
✓Subway Club	1	160	4	23	1.5	35	880	15	4	18	3 veg, 2 lean meat
✓Tuna w/ cheese	1	360	29	73	6	45	600	12	4	16	2 veg, 2 medium-fat meat, 4 1/2 fat
✓Veggie Delite	1	60	1	15	0	0	90	12	4	3	2 veg
SANDWICH CONDIMENTS											
Bacon (2 strips)	for 6″ sub	45	4	80	1.5	10	180	0	0	3	1 fat
Chipotle Southwest Sauce	for 6″ sub	100	4	36	1.5	10	220	0	0	0	1 1/2 fat

✔Fat Free Honey Mustard	for 6″ sub	30	0	0	0	0	140	7	0	0	1/2 carb
✔Fat Free Sweet Onion Sauce	for 6″ sub	40	0	0	0	0	100	9	0	0	1/2 carb
✔Light Mayonnaise	for 6″ sub	45	5	100	1	10	100	1	0	0	1 fat
Mayonnaise	for 6″ sub	110	12	98	3	10	80	0	0	0	2 1/2 fat
✔Mustard	for 6″ sub	5	0	0	0	0	115	1	0	0	free
✔Olive Oil Blend	for 6″ sub	45	5	100	1	0	0	0	0	0	1 fat
Ranch Dressing	for 6″ sub	70	0	0	0	5	210	0	0	0	1 1/2 fat
✔Vinegar	for 6″ sub	0	0	0	0	0	0	0	0	free	
SOUP											
Brown & Wild Rice w/ Chicken	8 oz	190	11	52	4.5	20	990	17	2	6	1 starch, 2 fat

✔ = Healthiest Bets

(Continued)

SOUP (*Continued*)	Amount	Cal.	Fat (g)	% Cal. Fat	Sat. Fat (g)	Chol. (mg)	Sod. (mg)	Carb. (g)	Fiber (g)	Pro. (g)	Servings/Exchanges
Cheese w/ Ham & Bacon	8 oz	240	15	56	6	20	1160	17	1	8	1 starch, 1 high-fat meat, 1 1/2 fat
Chicken & Dumpling	8 oz	130	2	14	2.5	30	1030	16	1	7	1 starch, 1 lean meat
✔Chili Con Carne	8 oz	240	10	38	5	15	860	23	8	15	1 1/2 starch, 1 medium-fat meat, 1 fat
✔Cream of Broccoli	8 oz	130	6	42	2	10	860	15	2	5	1 milk, 1 fat
Cream of Potato w/ Bacon	8 oz	200	11	50	4	15	840	21	2	4	1/2 starch, 1 milk, 2 fat
Golden Broccoli & Cheese	8 oz	180	11	55	4	15	1120	16	2	5	1 milk, 2 fat
Minestrone	8 oz	90	4	40	1	20	1180	7	1	7	1/2 starch, 1 lean meat
✔New England Style Clam Chowder	8 oz	110	4	33	0.5	10	990	16	1	5	1 starch, 1 fat
✔Roasted Chicken Noodle	8 oz	60	2	30	0.5	10	940	7	1	6	1/2 starch, 1/2 fat

✓Spanish Style Chicken w/ Rice	8 oz	90	2	20	0.5	5	800	13	1	5	1 starch
Tomato Garden Vegetable w/ Rotini	8 oz	100	1	9	0	0	2340	20	2	3	1 starch, 1 veg
Vegetable Beef	8 oz	90	1	10	0.5	5	1050	15	3	5	1 starch
WRAPS											
Chicken & Bacon Ranch w/ cheese	1	440	27	55	10	90	1670	18	9	41	1 starch, 5 medium-fat meat
Tuna w/ cheese	1	440	32	65	6	45	1310	16	9	27	1 starch, 3 lean meat, 4 1/2 fat
Turkey Breast	1	190	6	28	1	20	1290	18	9	24	1 starch, 3 lean meat
Turkey Breast & Bacon Melt w/ chipotle sauce	1	440	28	57	10	65	1870	20	9	34	1 starch, 5 medium-fat meat

✓ = Healthiest Bets

Wienerschnitzel

❖ Wienerschnitzel provides nutrition information for all its menu items on its Web site at www.wienerschnitzel.com.

Light 'n Lean Choice

Healthy Choice Chili Dog
Onion Rings *(1/2 order)*

Calories	470	Sodium (mg)	1,410
Fat (g)	18	Carbohydrate (g)	64
% calories from fat	34	Fiber (g)	3
Saturated fat (g)	8	Protein (g)	15
Cholesterol (mg)	38		

Exchanges: 4 starch, 1 veg, 1 high fat meat, 1 fat

Healthy 'n Hearty Choice

Kraut Dog
French Fries *(1/2 regular)*
Plain Ice Cream Cone

Calories	660	Sodium (mg)	1,280
Fat (g)	33	Carbohydrate (g)	72
% calories from fat	45	Fiber (g)	4
Saturated fat (g)	14	Protein (g)	15
Cholesterol (mg)	78		

Exchanges: 3 starch, 2 carb, 1 high fat meat, 3 fat

Wienerschnitzel

	Amount	Cal.	Fat (g)	% Cal. Fat	Sat. Fat (g)	Chol. (mg)	Sod. (mg)	Carb. (g)	Fiber (g)	Pro. (g)	Servings/Exchanges
BREAKFAST											
Burrito	1	580	33	51	11	520	1280	41	1	28	3 starch, 2 high-fat meat, 3 fat
Chili Cheese Burrito	1	510	24	42	8	500	1570	44	2	27	3 starch, 2 high-fat meat, 1 1/2 fat
Country	1	630	45	64	14	520	1240	31	1	25	2 starch, 3 high-fat meat, 4 fat
Croissant	1	570	36	57	12	275	950	41	2	22	3 starch, 1 high-fat meat, 5 fat
French Toast	1	500	30	54	10	20	550	50	3	6	3 1/2 starch, 5 fat

✓ = Healthiest Bets

(Continued)

BREAKFAST (*Continued*)	Amount	Cal.	Fat (g)	% Cal. Fat	Sat. Fat (g)	Chol. (mg)	Sod. (mg)	Carb. (g)	Fiber (g)	Pro. (g)	Servings/Exchanges
Hash Browns	1	290	25	78	10	20	240	14	2	1	1 starch, 5 fat
Platter	1	680	48	64	18	520	870	42	3	24	3 starch, 2 high-fat meat, 5 fat
Sandwich	1	370	22	54	9	275	820	28	1	18	2 starch, 2 high-fat meat, 1 fat
BREAKFAST - BISCUITS											
Plain	1	200	12	54	3	0	460	19	1	4	1 starch, 2 1/2 fat
w/ Egg	1	280	18	58	5	240	530	20	1	11	1 1/2 starch, 1 medium-fat meat, 2 1/2 fat
w/ Egg, Sausage & Bacon	1	410	29	64	9	265	820	22	1	15	1 1/2 starch, 2 high-fat meat, 2 1/2 fat
w/ Egg, Sausage, Bacon & Cheese	1	460	34	67	11	275	1080	22	1	18	1 1/2 starch, 2 high-fat meat, 3 1/2 fat

w/ Gravy	1	290	18	56	5	5	750	26	1	6	1 1/2 starch, 3 1/2 fat
w/ Sausage & Bacon	1	320	23	65	7	25	750	21	1	8	1 1/2 starch, 2 high-fat meat
DESSERTS											
Apple Turnover	1	310	19	55	10	15	290	31	1	2	2 carb, 4 fat
Milk Chocolate Chunk Cookie	1	240	9	34	4	20	220	36	1	3	2 1/2 carb, 2 fat
White Chunk Macadamia Cookie	1	260	13	45	3	20	180	34	1	3	2 carb, 2 1/2 fat
FRIES & SIDES											
Chili Cheese Fries	1	540	38	63	19	55	1380	39	4	12	2 1/2 starch, 7 1/2 fat
Jalapeno Poppers	1	480	32	60	13	50	1400	37	3	12	2 1/2 starch, 6 fat
Large Fries	1	470	34	65	17	35	690	39	4	4	2 1/2 starch, 7 fat
Onion Rings	1	470	25	48	11	25	660	56	3	6	3 1/2 starch, 5 fat

✔ = Healthiest Bets

(*Continued*)

FRIES AND SIDES (*Continued*)	Amount	Cal.	Fat (g)	% Cal. Fat	Sat. Fat (g)	Chol. (mg)	Sod. (mg)	Carb. (g)	Fiber (g)	Pro. (g)	Servings/Exchanges
Ranch Dressing	1	120	12	90	2	15	290	2	0	1	2 1/2 fat
Regular Fries	1	340	25	66	12	25	460	28	3	3	2 starch, 5 fat
HEALTHY CHOICE HOT DOGS											
BBQ Bacon Dog	1	320	12	34	5	40	1050	38	1	15	2 1/2 starch, 1 high-fat meat, 1 fat
Chili Cheese Dog	1	290	10	31	4	35	1340	36	1	15	2 starch, 1 high-fat meat
Chili Dog	1	240	5	19	2	25	1080	36	1	12	2 starch, 1 medium-fat meat
Deluxe Dog	1	220	4	16	1	20	1160	35	2	10	2 starch, 1 lean meat
Kraut Dog	1	210	4	17	1	20	970	33	1	10	2 starch, 1 lean meat
✓Mustard Dog	1	210	4	17	1	20	770	33	1	10	2 starch, 1 lean meat
✓Relish Dog	1	220	4	16	1	20	800	35	1	10	2 starch, 1 lean meat

HOT DOGS											
BBQ Bacon Dog	1	370	20	49	8	45	970	33	1	14	2 starch, 1 high-fat meat, 1 1/2 fat
Chili Cheese Dog	1	340	17	45	6	40	1260	31	1	14	2 starch, 1 high-fat meat, 2 fat
Chili Dog	1	290	13	40	4	30	1000	31	1	11	2 starch, 1 high-fat meat, 1 fat
Deluxe Dog	1	270	12	40	4	25	1080	30	2	9	2 starch, 1 high-fat meat, 1 fat
Kraut Dog	1	260	12	42	4	25	890	28	1	9	2 starch, 1 high-fat meat, 1/2 fat
Kraut Dog - Pretzel Bun	1	400	15	34	5	25	950	54	2	12	3 1/2 starch, 1 high-fat meat, 1 fat
✓Mustard Dog	1	260	12	42	4	25	690	28	1	9	2 starch, 1 high-fat meat, 1/2 fat

✓ = Healthiest Bets

(*Continued*)

HOT DOGS (*Continued*)	Amount	Cal.	Fat (g)	% Cal. Fat	Sat. Fat (g)	Chol. (mg)	Sod. (mg)	Carb. (g)	Fiber (g)	Pro. (g)	Servings/Exchanges
✓Relish Dog	1	270	12	40	4	25	720	30	1	9	2 starch, 1 high-fat meat, 1/2 fat
HOT DOGS - ALL BEEF											
BBQ Bacon Dog	1	470	28	54	11	70	1570	35	1	19	2 starch, 2 high-fat meat, 2 1/2 fat
Chili Cheese Dog	1	430	25	52	10	65	1860	33	1	19	2 starch, 2 high-fat meat, 2 fat
Chili Dog	1	380	21	50	7	50	1600	33	1	16	2 starch, 1 high-fat meat, 2 1/2 fat
Deluxe Dog	1	370	20	49	7	45	1680	32	2	14	2 starch, 1 high-fat meat, 2 1/2 fat
Kraut Dog	1	360	20	50	7	45	1490	30	1	14	2 starch, 1 high-fat meat, 2 1/2 fat

Mustard Dog	1	350	20	51	7	45	1230	30	1	14	2 starch, 1 high-fat meat, 2 1/2 fat
Relish Dog	1	360	20	50	7	45	1320	32	1	14	2 starch, 1 high-fat meat, 2 1/2 fat
HOT DOGS ON PRETZEL BUN											
BBQ Bacon Dog	1	510	23	41	9	45	1040	59	1	17	4 starch, 1 high-fat meat, 3 fat
Chili Cheese Dog	1	480	20	38	7	40	1330	57	2	17	3 1/2 starch, 1 high-fat meat, 2 1/2 fat
Chili Dog	1	430	16	33	5	29	1070	57	2	14	3 1/2 starch, 1 high-fat meat, 1 1/2 fat
Deluxe Dog	1	410	15	33	5	25	1150	56	2	12	3 1/2 starch, 1 high-fat meat, 1 1/2 fat
✓Mustard Dog	1	400	15	34	5	25	750	54	1	12	3 1/2 starch, 1 high-fat meat, 1 fat

✓ = Healthiest Bets

(*Continued*)

HOT DOGS ON PRETZEL BUN (*Continued*)	Amount	Cal.	Fat (g)	% Cal. Fat	Sat. Fat (g)	Chol. (mg)	Sod. (mg)	Carb. (g)	Fiber (g)	Pro. (g)	Servings/Exchanges
✓Relish Dog	1	410	15	33	5	25	780	56	1	12	3 1/2 starch, 1 high-fat meat, 1 1/2 fat
HOT DOGS ON PRETZEL BUN - ALL BEEF											
Chili Dog	1	520	24	42	8	51	1670	59	2	19	4 starch, 1 high-fat meat, 3 fat
BBQ Bacon Dog	1	610	31	46	12	70	1640	61	1	22	4 starch, 2 high-fat meat, 2 fat
Chili Cheese Do	1	570	28	44	11	65	1930	59	2	22	3 starch, 2 high-fat meat, 2 1/2 fat
Deluxe Dog	1	510	23	41	8	45	1750	58	2	17	3 1/2 starch, 1 high-fat meat, 3 fat
Kraut Dog	1	500	23	41	8	45	1550	56	2	17	3 1/2 starch, 1 high-fat meat, 3 fat

Mustard Dog	1	490	23	42	8	45	1350	56	1	17	3 1/2 starch, 1 high-fat meat, 3 fat
Relish Dog	1	500	23	41	8	45	1380	58	1	17	4 starch, 1 high-fat meat, 3 fat
KIDS' BAGS											
✔Corn Dog	1	250	17	61	6	45	490	15	1	7	1 starch, 1 high-fat meat, 2 fat
✔Hamburger	1	290	8	25	3	20	800	31	1	20	2 starch, 2 medium-fat meat
✔Mustard Dog	1	260	12	42	4	25	690	28	1	9	2 starch, 1 high-fat meat, 1/2 fat
SANDWICHES - BURGERS											
Chili Cheeseburger	1	350	13	33	5	35	1270	32	1	25	2 starch, 3 medium-fat meat
Deluxe Cheeseburger	1	450	23	46	7	40	1250	33	2	23	2 starch, 2 high-fat meat, 1 1/2 fat

✔ = Healthiest Bets

(*Continued*)

SANDWICHES - BURGERS (*Continued*)	Amount	Cal.	Fat (g)	% Cal. Fat	Sat. Fat (g)	Chol. (mg)	Sod. (mg)	Carb. (g)	Fiber (g)	Pro. (g)	Servings/Exchanges
Deluxe Hamburger	1	400	19	43	4	30	990	33	2	21	2 starch, 2 high-fat meat, 1/2 fat
Double Chili Cheeseburger	1	560	24	39	10	70	2270	35	2	45	2 1/2 starch, 5 medium-fat meat
SANDWICHES											
Bacon Ranch Chicken Sandwich	1	530	31	53	10	75	1480	41	2	24	3 starch, 4 medium-fat meat, 2 fat
Chili Cheese Tamale	1	450	27	54	10	55	1580	33	4	18	2 starch, 1 high-fat meat, 4 fat
✓Fish Sandwich	1	390	17	39	2	30	640	48	1	12	3 starch, 3 fat
SANDWICHES - SAUSAGES											
Bratwurst Sandwich	1	340	17	45	5	45	1020	30	1	16	2 starch, 2 high-fat meat
Cheddar Sausage Melt	1	460	27	53	10	60	1030	35	2	19	2 1/2 starch, 2 high-fat meat, 2 fat

Italian Sausage Sandwich	1	350	17	44	4	35	940	31	2	17	2 starch, 2 high-fat meat
Polish Sausage Sandwich	1	480	28	53	10	70	2030	39	3	22	2 1/2 starch, 2 high-fat meat, 2 1/2 fat
Southwest Smoky Sausage Sandwich	1	460	27	53	10	60	1030	35	2	19	2 1/2 starch, 2 high-fat meat, 2 fat
TASTEE-FREEZ DESSERTS											
Banana Split	1	780	23	27	11	65	300	141	8	11	9 1/2 carb, 4 1/2 fat
Cone, chocolate dipped	1	420	26	56	22	40	180	45	2	5	3 carb, 5 fat
Cone, plain	1	230	8	31	4	40	160	36	1	4	2 1/2 carb, 1 1/2 fat
TASTEE-FREEZ DESSERTS - FREEZEE											
Butterfinger	1	590	22	34	13	95	400	92	3	10	6 carb, 4 1/2 fat
M&M	1	600	24	36	14	100	360	92	2	11	6 carb, 5 fat
Oreo	1	590	23	35	11	90	350	92	3	10	6 carb, 4 1/2 fat

✔ = Healthiest Bets

(*Continued*)

	Amount	Cal.	Fat (g)	% Cal. Fat	Sat. Fat (g)	Chol. (mg)	Sod. (mg)	Carb. (g)	Fiber (g)	Pro. (g)	Servings/Exchanges
TASTEE-FREEZ DESSERTS - SHAKE											
Chocolate	1	580	20	31	12	100	450	97	3	10	4 carb, 4 fat
Strawberry	1	590	19	29	11	95	380	98	2	10	4 carb, 4 fat
Vanilla	1	580	19	29	11	95	370	98	2	10	6 1/2 carb, 4 fat
TASTEE-FREEZ DESSERTS - SUNDAE											
Caramel	1	370	12	29	8	55	220	60	1	5	4 carb, 2 1/2 fat
Chocolate	1	360	12	30	8	55	220	58	2	5	3 1/2 carb, 2 1/2 fat
Hot Fudge	1	370	15	36	10	55	330	56	1	5	3 1/2 carb, 3 fat
Pineapple	1	340	12	32	8	55	190	53	1	5	3 1/2 carb, 2 1/2 fat
Strawberry	1	340	12	32	8	55	190	53	1	5	3 1/2 carb, 2 1/2 fat

✓ = Healthiest Bets

Chinese Fare

RESTAURANTS

Panda Express

P. F. Chang's China Bistro

Note: This is a new chapter for the 3rd edition. When it comes to Chinese fare, most restaurants in the U.S. are independently owned single store operations. However, over the past few years two national chains have expanded, and they willingly provide nutrition information. This is good news because Chinese food can make blood glucose management difficult due to the extra grams of carbohydrate that raise blood glucose without being seen, including sugar, sauces, and corn starch. Panda Express is typically found in food courts. P. F. Chang's China Bistro is a sit-down eatery.

NUTRITION PROS

- A Chinese restaurant meal has the potential to be healthy if you choose soup, an entrée with lots of vegetables, no fried items, and you eat your entrée with steamed white rice. Oh yes, go ahead and enjoy the fortune cookie.
- If you order well, you can get a bounty of vegetables.
- Eating family style is common. Order jointly and put the dishes in the middle for all to share. You can take advantage of this to both control portions and get plenty of healthy items.

- It's reasonably easy to control the saturated fat and cholesterol count. Just stay away from shrimp, calamari (squid), and red meats. Chinese cooking uses little milk, cream, cheese, or eggs.
- Liquid peanut oil, which is mainly made of the healthy monounsaturated fats, is the main oil used in Chinese stir-frying. It is not only healthy but also has a high smoking point and can withstand the high temperature of stir-frying.
- It's easy to fill up first on a low-calorie soup. Try hot and sour or sizzling rice with vegetables. These are especially helpful if your dining mates are downing the high-fat and high-calorie fried appetizers.

NUTRITION CONS

- Chinese food tends to contain more carbohydrate than meets the eye. Sugar and sugar-containing ingredients can be in the marinades and sauces. Corn starch is commonly used to thicken sauces.
- Chinese food can contain more fat than you might think from the oil used to stir-fry and deep-fry. Read about the preparation in the menu descriptions to find out about the fat level.
- You might want to opt for soup and skip the appetizers. Most of them—egg rolls, spring rolls, fried dumplings, and spareribs—are fried or are high in fat.
- It's easy to eat a lot of carbohydrate from rice and noodles.
- Chinese food can be high in sodium due to the ingredients in marinades and sauces, such as soy sauce and MSG (monosodium glutamate).

Healthy Tips

- ★ To keep sodium low, don't dip appetizers in sauces. Go for the lighter white sauces. Choose steamed white rice rather than fried rice. And request no MSG.
- ★ You'll be better able to control what you get if you choose a sit-down Chinese restaurant rather than one in a food court or an all-you-can-eat buffet.
- ★ The hot mustard sauce can add some zing without much sodium, sugar, or fat.
- ★ If you eat family style, order fewer dishes than the number of people at the table. This controls portions from the start. And make at least one of the dishes you order vegetables only.
- ★ Use chopsticks. They will slow down your eating, particularly if you haven't mastered using them.

Get it Your Way

- ★ Try to order dishes with meats sautéed instead of fried.
- ★ Ask to have one or two more vegetables added to a dish to make it chock full of vegetables. You might have to pay a bit more.
- ★ Because dishes are made to order in a sit-down Chinese restaurant, feel free to ask that one item be left out or another added in.
- ★ You may want to order a sauce on the side and use the dipping technique to limit the amount you eat. This will help decrease both sodium and sugar intake.

Panda Express

❖ Panda Express provides nutrition information for many of its menu items at www.pandaexpress.com.

Light 'n Lean Choice

Veggie Spring Roll *(1)*
Beef with Broccoli *(1 serving)*
Spicy Chicken with Peanuts *(1 serving)*
Steamed White Rice *(1/2 order, 4 oz)*

Calories....................595
Fat (g)........................18
% calories from fat..27
Saturated fat (g).....3.5
Cholesterol (mg).........85
Sodium (mg)..........1,810
Carbohydrate (g).........77
Fiber (g).....................6
Protein (g)...................35

Exchanges: 4 starch, 2 veg, 3 medium-fat meat

Healthy 'n Hearty Choice

Veggie Spring Roll *(1)*
String Beans with Fried Tofu *(1 serving)*
Chicken with Mushrooms *(1 serving)*
Vegetable Fried Rice *(1 serving)*

Calories....................780
Fat (g)........................32
% calories from fat..37
Saturated fat (g)........6
Cholesterol (mg).......134
Sodium (mg)..........2,250
Carbohydrate (g).........93
Fiber (g).....................7
Protein (g)...................32

Exchanges: 5 starch, 3 veg, 3 medium-fat meat, 2 fat

(Continued)

Panda Express

	Amount	Cal.	Fat (g)	% Cal. Fat	Sat. Fat (g)	Chol. (mg)	Sod. (mg)	Carb. (g)	Fiber (g)	Pro. (g)	Servings/Exchanges
APPETIZERS											
Chicken Egg Roll	1	190	8	38	1.5	25	450	21	3	8	1 1/2 starch, 1 lean meat, 1 fat
Fried Shrimp	6 pcs.	260	12	42	2.5	65	730	26	0	12	1 1/2 starch, 1 lean meat, 2 fat
✓Veggie Spring Roll	1	80	3	34	0	0	270	14	0	2	1 starch
BEEF											
✓Beef w/ Broccoli	5.5 oz	150	8	48	2	15	730	9	1	11	1/2 starch, 1 medium-fat meat, 1/2 fat
✓Beef w/ String Beans	5.5 oz	170	9	48	2	20	640	11	2	12	1/2 starch, 2 medium-fat meat

CHICKEN

✓Black Pepper Chicken	5.5 oz	180	10	50	2	40	630	10	2	13	1/2 starch, 2 lean meat, 1 fat
✓Chicken w/ Mushrooms	5.5 oz	130	7	48	1.5	50	590	7	2	11	1/2 starch, 2 lean meat
Chicken w/ Potato	5.5 oz	220	11	45	2	55	920	17	1	12	1 starch, 2 lean meat, 1 fat
✓Chicken w/ String Beans	5.5 oz	170	8	42	1.5	30	560	12	3	11	1 starch, 2 lean meat
Mandarin Chicken	5.5 oz	250	9	32	2.5	125	960	8	2	34	1/2 starch, 5 lean meat
Orange Flavored Chicken	5.5 oz	480	21	39	4.5	80	820	50	2	21	3 1/2 starch, 2 lean meat, 2 1/2 fat
✓Spicy Chicken w/ Peanuts	5.5 oz	200	7	32	1.5	70	800	17	4	18	1 starch, 2 lean meat
✓Sweet & Sour Chicken	4 oz	310	14	41	2	50	330	28	2	18	2 starch, 2 lean meat, 1 1/2 fat

✓ = Healthiest Bets

(*Continued*)

	Amount	Cal.	Fat (g)	% Cal. Fat	Sat. Fat (g)	Chol. (mg)	Sod. (mg)	Carb. (g)	Fiber (g)	Pro. (g)	Servings/Exchanges
PORK											
BBQ Pork	4.5 oz	350	19	49	7	85	970	13	0	32	1 starch, 4 medium-fat meat
Sweet & Sour Pork	4 oz	410	30	66	7	55	350	17	3	19	1 starch, 2 medium-fat meat, 4 1/2 fat
RICE & NOODLES											
✓Steamed Rice	8 oz	330	1	3	0	0	20	74	2	7	5 starch
Vegetable Chow Mein	8 oz	330	11	30	2	0	810	48	4	10	2 1/2 starch, 2 veg, 2 fat
Vegetable Fried Rice	8 oz	390	12	28	2.5	85	740	61	2	9	4 starch, 2 fat
SAUCES											
✓Hot Mustard Sauce	2.5 t	18	0	0	0	0	90	1	0	0	free

✓Hot Sauce	2 t	10	1	90	0	0	130	2	0	0	free
Mandarin Sauce	3 T	70	0	0	0	0	670	16	0	0	1 starch
Soy Sauce	1 T	16	0	0	0	0	660	2	0	2	free
Sweet & Sour Sauce	3 T	60	0	0	0	0	120	15	0	0	1 starch
TOFU											
✓String Beans w/ Fried Tofu	5.5 oz	180	11	55	2	0	650	11	3	10	1/2 starch, 1 lean meat, 1 fat
VEGETABLES											
✓Mixed Vegetables	5.5 oz	70	3	39	0.5	0	420	8	1	3	2 veg

✓ = Healthiest Bets

P. F. Chang's China Bistro

❖ P. F. Chang's China Bistro provides nutrition information for its menu items on its Web site, www.pfchangs.com. It also provides the ingredients for each dish. Note that the nutrition information for most menu items is provided per order, not per serving. Order cautiously and split items. The healthiest bets are not based on the criteria on page 48 because the nutrition information is provided per order. They are based on the nutrition information and contents of the dish. In addition, no sodium information is provided. As the sodium content of Chinese food is often high, you can assume that the sodium content of these items is high as well.

Light 'n Lean Choice

Hot and Sour Soup *(1 cup/8 oz)*
Cantonese Shrimp *(1/2 dish)*
Buddha's Feast, Stir-fried *(1/2 dish)*
Vegetable Fried Rice *(1/4 dish, about 2/3 cup)*

Calories....................630
Fat (g)........................19
% calories from fat..27
Saturated fat (g)........3
Cholesterol (mg)........n/a
Sodium (mg)..............n/a
Carbohydrate (g).........80
Fiber (g)..................n/a
Protein (g)...................41

Exchanges: 4 starch, 3 veg, 3 lean meat, 2 fat

Healthy 'n Hearty Choice

Vegetable Dumplings, Steamed *(1/3 order)*
Wonton Soup *(1 cup/8 oz)*
Ginger Chicken with Broccoli *(1/3 dish)*
Vegetable Lo Mein *(1/2 dinner size)*
Shanghai Cucumbers *(1/2 dish)*

Calories	740	Sodium (mg)	n/a
Fat (g)	23	Carbohydrate (g)	85
% calories from fat	28	Fiber (g)	n/a
Saturated fat (g)	4	Protein (g)	48
Cholesterol (mg)	n/a		

Exchanges: 4 1/2 starch, 3 veg, 4 lean meat, 2 fat

(Continued)

P. F. Chang's China Bistro

	Amount	Cal.	Fat (g)	% Cal. Fat	Sat. Fat (g)	Chol. (mg)	Sod. (mg)	Carb. (g)	Fiber (g)	Pro. (g)	Servings/Exchanges
APPETIZERS											
✓Banana Spring Rolls	1 order	1860	97	47	43	n/a	n/a	235	n/a	26	13 starch, 2 fruit, 19 fat
✓Chang's Chicken Lettuce Wraps	1 order	630	8	11	2	n/a	n/a	92	n/a	44	5 starch, 2 veg, 3 lean meat
Chang's Spare Ribs	1 order	1410	109	70	32	n/a	n/a	47	n/a	59	3 starch, 1 veg, 7 medium-fat meat, 14 fat
✓Chang's Vegetarian Lettuce Wraps	1 order	370	4	10	1	n/a	n/a	71	n/a	14	4 starch, 3 veg
Crab Wontons	1 order	520	26	45	8	n/a	n/a	51	n/a	19	3 starch, 1 veg, 1 lean meat, 4 fat
✓Harvest Spring Rolls	1 order	640	17	24	1.5	n/a	n/a	106	n/a	15	5 starch, 4 veg, 3 fat

Northern Style Spare Ribs	1 order	1090	95	78	27	n/a	n/a	6	n/a	49	1/2 starch, 7 medium-fat meat, 12 fat
✓Peking Dumplings, pan fried	1 order	420	22	47	7	n/a	n/a	31	n/a	20	1 1/2 starch, 1 veg, 2 medium-fat meat, 3 fat
✓Peking Dumplings, steamed	1 order	400	20	45	7	n/a	n/a	31	n/a	20	1 1/2 starch, 1 veg, 2 medium-fat meat, 2 fat
Salt & Pepper Calamari	1 order	590	37	56	3.5	n/a	n/a	35	n/a	26	2 starch, 3 very lean meat, 7 fat
Shanghai Street Dumplings	1 order	860	46	48	4	n/a	n/a	90	n/a	18	6 starch, 1 veg, 8 fat
Shrimp Dumplings, pan fried	1 order	360	17	43	1.5	n/a	n/a	26	n/a	24	1 1/2 starch, 1 veg, 2 very lean meat, 3 fat
✓Shrimp Dumplings, steamed	1 order	320	12	34	1	n/a	n/a	26	n/a	24	1 1/2 starch, 1 veg, 2 very lean meat, 2 fat

✓ = Healthiest Bets; n/a = not available

(*Continued*)

APPETIZERS (*Continued*)	Amount	Cal.	Fat (g)	% Cal. Fat	Sat. Fat (g)	Chol. (mg)	Sod. (mg)	Carb. (g)	Fiber (g)	Pro. (g)	Servings/Exchanges
✓Vegetable Dumplings, pan fried	1 order	340	12	32	1	n/a	n/a	47	n/a	9	2 starch, 3 veg, 2 fat
✓Vegetable Dumplings, steamed	1 order	300	8	24	1	n/a	n/a	47	n/a	9	2 starch, 3 veg, 1 fat
CHICKEN & DUCK DISHES											
Almond & Cashew Chicken	1 order, lunch	740	30	36	5	n/a	n/a	51	n/a	62	3 starch, 3 veg, 7 lean meat
Almond & Cashew Chicken	1 order, dinner	850	33	35	6	n/a	n/a	57	n/a	77	3 starch, 3 veg, 9 lean meat
Cantonese Roasted Duck	1 order	1160	59	46	19	n/a	n/a	109	n/a	45	7 carb, 1 veg, 3 medium-fat meat, 8 fat
Cantonese Roasted Duck	1 order	1730	103	54	34	n/a	n/a	123	n/a	76	7 1/2 carb, 2 veg, 7 medium-fat meat, 12 fat

Chang's Spicy Chicken	1 order	990	51	46	5	n/a	n/a	70	n/a	61	4 starch, 2 veg, 7 lean meat, 7 fat
✓Chicken w/ black bean sauce	1 order	640	22	31	3	n/a	n/a	31	n/a	73	1 1/2 starch, 1 veg, 10 very lean meat, 3 fat
Crispy Honey Chicken	1 order, lunch	860	36	38	3	n/a	n/a	84	n/a	43	5 carb, 2 veg, 3 lean meat, 5 fat
Crispy Honey Chicken	1 order, dinner	960	37	35	3.5	n/a	n/a	90	n/a	56	5 1/2 carb, 2 veg, 4 lean meat, 6 fat
✓Ginger Chicken w/ Broccoli	1 order	620	21	30	3	n/a	n/a	43	n/a	63	2 starch, 2 veg, 8 very lean meat, 3 fat
Kung Pao Chicken	1 order	930	50	48	7	n/a	n/a	38	n/a	81	2 starch, 1 veg, 11 very lean meat, 8 fat
✓Mango Chicken	1 order	730	19	23	2	n/a	n/a	63	n/a	64	3 starch, 2 veg, 1 fruit, 7 very lean meat, 3 fat

✓ = Healthiest Bets; n/a = not available

(*Continued*)

CHICKEN & DUCK DISHES (*Continued*)	Amount	Cal.	Fat (g)	% Cal. Fat	Sat. Fat (g)	Chol. (mg)	Sod. (mg)	Carb. (g)	Fiber (g)	Pro. (g)	Servings/Exchanges
✓Moo Goo Gai Pan	1 order	610	25	37	4	n/a	n/a	32	n/a	61	1 starch, 3 veg, 8 very lean meat, 4 fat
Mu Shu Chicken	1 order	750	31	37	6	n/a	n/a	55	n/a	63	2 1/2 starch, 3 veg, 7 lean meat, 2 fat
Orange Peel Chicken	1 order	1090	60	50	5	n/a	n/a	73	n/a	65	3 1/2 carb, 1 veg, 8 lean meat, 10 fat
Philip's Better Lemon Chicken	1 order	810	21	23	2.5	n/a	n/a	94	n/a	62	5 1/2 starch, 2 veg, 6 very lean meat, 2 fat
Spicy Ground Chicken & Eggplant	1 order	890	43	43	6	n/a	n/a	70	n/a	53	4 starch, 2 veg, 5 lean meat, 5 fat
Sweet & Sour Chicken	1 order	800	31	35	2.5	n/a	n/a	89	n/a	43	4 starch, 2 veg, 1 fruit, 4 lean meat, 3 fat

CHOW MEIN											
Beef	1 order	770	24	28	7	n/a	n/a	90	n/a	47	5 starch, 3 veg, 3 medium-fat meat, 2 fat
✓Chicken	1 order	670	16	21	2.5	n/a	n/a	92	n/a	42	5 starch, 3 veg, 2 lean meat, 2 fat
Pork	1 order	800	27	30	6	n/a	n/a	92	n/a	48	5 starch, 3 veg, 3 medium-fat meat, 2 fat
✓Shrimp	1 order	750	20	24	2.5	n/a	n/a	94	n/a	50	5 starch, 3 veg, 3 lean meat, 2 fat
✓Vegetable	1 order	520	7	12	1.5	n/a	n/a	95	n/a	22	5 starch, 3 veg, 1 fat
Combo	1 order	1130	28	22	6	n/a	n/a	150	n/a	61	5 starch, 3 veg, 4 medium-fat meat, 8 fat

✓ = Healthiest Bets; n/a = not available

(*Continued*)

	Amount	Cal.	Fat (g)	% Cal. Fat	Sat. Fat (g)	Chol. (mg)	Sod. (mg)	Carb. (g)	Fiber (g)	Pro. (g)	Servings/Exchanges
DESSERTS											
Great Wall of Chocolate	1 order	1883	71	34	17	n/a	n/a	325	n/a	18	insufficient info. to calculate
New York Style Cheesecake	1 order	870	58	60	34	n/a	n/a	72	n/a	15	5 carb, 11 fat
MEAT DISHES											
Beef a La Sichuan	1 order	990	55	50	15	n/a	n/a	55	n/a	69	2 1/2 carb, 3 veg, 8 medium-at meat, 3 fat
Beef w/ Broccoli	1 order, lunch	760	49	58	12	n/a	n/a	23	n/a	56	1 carb, 2 veg, 8 medium-fat meat, 1 fat
Beef w/ Broccoli	1 order, dinner	910	59	58	15	n/a	n/a	24	n/a	70	1 carb, 2 veg, 10 medium-fat meat, 1 fat

Mongolian Beef	1 order	1080	72	60	19	n/a	n/a	18	n/a	85	1 starch, 12 medium-fat meat, 4 1/2 fat
Mu Shu Pork	1 order	780	38	44	9	n/a	n/a	53	n/a	57	3 starch, 2 veg, 6 medium-at meat, 1 fat
Orange Peel Beef	1 order	1330	82	55	18	n/a	n/a	69	n/a	77	4 starch, 1 veg, 9 medium-fat meat, 5 fat
Sichuan Style Pork	1 order	910	47	46	10	n/a	n/a	43	n/a	71	2 carb, 3 veg, 8 medium-fat meat, 2 fat
Sweet & Sour Pork	1 order	910	43	43	7	n/a	n/a	89	n/a	42	4 carb, 2 veg, 1 fruit, 4 medium-fat meat, 4 fat
Wok-Seared Lamb	1 order	1270	95	67	34	n/a	n/a	22	n/a	80	1 carb, 2 veg, 10 medium-fat meat, 9 fat

✔ = Healthiest Bets; n/a = not available

(*Continued*)

	Amount	Cal.	Fat (g)	% Cal. Fat	Sat. Fat (g)	Chol. (mg)	Sod. (mg)	Carb. (g)	Fiber (g)	Pro. (g)	Servings/Exchanges
NOODLES & RICE											
Cantonese Chow Fun, Beef	1 order	1080	48	40	12	n/a	n/a	101	n/a	56	6 1/2 starch, 1 veg, 5 medium-fat meat, 4 fat
Cantonese Chow Fun, Chicken	1 order	930	34	33	3	n/a	n/a	105	n/a	48	6 1/2 starch, 1 veg, 4 lean meat, 4 fat
Dan Dan	1 order	1070	30	25	4.5	n/a	n/a	128	n/a	65	8 starch, 2 veg, 5 lean meat, 2 fat
Double Pan-Fried, Beef	1 order	1240	61	44	13	n/a	n/a	111	n/a	57	6 1/2 starch, 3 veg, 4 medium-fat meat, 8 fat
Double Pan-Fried, Chicken	1 order	1140	53	42	8	n/a	n/a	113	n/a	52	6 1/2 starch, 3 veg, 3 lean meat, 8 fat

Double Pan-Fried, Pork	1 order	1170	57	44	10	n/a	n/a	113	n/a	48	6 1/2 starch, 3 veg, 3 medium-fat meat, 8 fat
Double Pan-Fried, Shrimp	1 order	1130	53	42	8	n/a	n/a	114	n/a	49	6 1/2 starch, 3 veg, 3 lean meat, 8 fat
Double Pan-Fried, Vegetable	1 order	980	44	40	7	n/a	n/a	114	n/a	30	6 1/2 starch, 3 veg, 8 fat
Double Pan-Fried, Combo	1 order	1390	70	45	13	n/a	n/a	116	n/a	71	6 1/2 starch, 3 veg, 6 medium-fat meat, 8 fat
Fried Rice, Beef	1 order	1080	28	23	9	n/a	n/a	144	n/a	53	9 starch, 1 veg, 3 medium-at meat, 2 fat
Fried Rice, Chicken	1 order	960	17	16	3	n/a	n/a	145	n/a	48	9 starch, 1 veg, 3 lean meat, 1 fat

✓ = Healthiest Bets; n/a = not available

(Continued)

NOODLES & RICE (*Continued*)	Amount	Cal.	Fat (g)	% Cal. Fat	Sat. Fat (g)	Chol. (mg)	Sod. (mg)	Carb. (g)	Fiber (g)	Pro. (g)	Servings/Exchanges
Fried Rice, Pork	1 order	990	22	20	5	n/a	n/a	145	n/a	45	9 starch, 1 veg, 2 medium-at meat, 2 fat
Fried Rice, Shrimp	1 order	950	17	16	3	n/a	n/a	146	n/a	45	9 starch, 1 veg, 2 lean meat, 2 fat
✓Fried Rice, Vegetable	1 order	820	12	13	2.5	n/a	n/a	147	n/a	25	9 starch, 1 veg, 2 fat
Fried Rice, Combo	1 order	1130	61	49	6	n/a	n/a	150	n/a	61	9 starch, 1 veg, 4 medium-fat meat, 2 fat
Garlic Noodles	1 order	610	12	18	3	n/a	n/a	107	n/a	19	6 1/2 starch, 2 veg, 1 fat
Lo Mein, Beef	1 order, lunch	850	34	36	8	n/a	n/a	90	n/a	47	5 starch, 2 veg, 4 medium-fat meat, 2 fat

Lo Mein, Beef	1 order, dinner	990	42	38	11	n/a	n/a	90	n/a	61	5 starch, 2 veg, 6 medium-fat meat, 2 fat
Lo Mein, Chicken	1 order, lunch	720	20	25	2.5	n/a	n/a	92	n/a	42	5 starch, 2 veg, 4 lean meat, 1 fat
Lo Mein, Chicken	1 order, dinner	810	25	28	3	n/a	n/a	93	n/a	54	5 starch, 2 veg, 6 lean meat, 1 fat
Lo Mein, Pork	1 order, lunch	740	25	30	4.5	n/a	n/a	91	n/a	39	5 starch, 2 veg, 3 medium-at meat, 3 fat
Lo Mein, Pork	1 order, dinner	840	31	33	6	n/a	n/a	92	n/a	48	5 starch, 2 veg, 4 medium-fat meat, 4 fat
Lo Mein, Shrimp	1 order, lunch	700	20	26	2.5	n/a	n/a	92	n/a	39	5 starch, 2 veg, 3 lean meat, 2 fat

✓ = Healthiest Bets; n/a = not available

(*Continued*)

NOODLES & RICE (*Continued*)	Amount	Cal.	Fat (g)	% Cal. Fat	Sat. Fat (g)	Chol. (mg)	Sod. (mg)	Carb. (g)	Fiber (g)	Pro. (g)	Servings/Exchanges
Lo Mein, Shrimp	1 order, dinner	790	24	27	3	n/a	n/a	94	n/a	50	5 starch, 2 veg, 5 lean meat, 1 fat
✔Lo Mein, Vegetable	1 order, lunch	550	12	20	1.5	n/a	n/a	93	n/a	21	5 starch, 2 veg, 2 fat
✔Lo Mein, Vegetable	1 order, dinner	560	12	19	1.5	n/a	n/a	95	n/a	22	5 starch, 2 veg, 2 fat
Lo Mein, Combo	1 order, lunch	900	35	35	6	n/a	n/a	94	n/a	51	5 starch, 2 veg, 5 medium-fat meat, 2 fat
Lo Mein, Combo	1 order, dinner	960	37	35	7	n/a	n/a	94	n/a	62	5 starch, 2 veg, 6 medium-fat meat, 2 fat
✔Sichuan Chicken Chow Fun	1 order	690	19	25	2	n/a	n/a	97	n/a	31	6 starch, 1 veg, 2 lean meat, 2 fat

Singapore Street Noodles	1 order	600	24	36	3	n/a	n/a	67	n/a	29	3 1/2 starch, 3 veg, 2 lean meat, 3 fat
SALADS											
Oriental Chicken	1 order	940	56	54	6	n/a	n/a	49	n/a	60	2 starch, 3 veg, 7 lean meat, 7 fat
Peanut Chicken	1 order	1080	69	58	9	n/a	n/a	47	n/a	73	2 starch, 3 veg, 8 lean meat, 9 fat
✓Sockeye Salmon Salad	1 order	470	30	57	4	n/a	n/a	18	n/a	33	3 veg, 4 lean meat, 4 fat
Warm Duck Spinach	1 order	940	66	63	15	n/a	n/a	44	n/a	45	1 1/2 starch, 2 veg, 1 fruit, 5 medium-fat meat, 8 fat
SEAFOOD DISHES											
Alaskan Sockeye Salmon Lemon Pepper	1 order	670	36	48	5	n/a	n/a	32	n/a	53	1 1/2 starch, 1 veg, 7 lean meat, 3 fat

✓ = Healthiest Bets; n/a = not available

(*Continued*)

SEAFOOD DISHES (*Continued*)	Amount	Cal.	Fat (g)	% Cal. Fat	Sat. Fat (g)	Chol. (mg)	Sod. (mg)	Carb. (g)	Fiber (g)	Pro. (g)	Servings/Exchanges
✓Cantonese Scallops	1 order	370	13	32	2	n/a	n/a	20	n/a	42	1/2 starch, 2 veg, 6 very lean meat, 2 fat
✓Cantonese Shrimp	1 order	380	15	36	2	n/a	n/a	17	n/a	44	1/2 starch, 2 veg, 6 very lean meat, 2 fat
Chang's Lemon Scallops	1 order	720	18	23	1.5	n/a	n/a	96	n/a	44	6 starch, 1 veg, 3 lean meat, 1 fat
Crispy Honey Shrimp	1 order	860	37	39	3	n/a	n/a	85	n/a	38	5 starch, 1 veg, 3 lean meat, 6 fat
Hot Fish	1 order	960	42	39	7	n/a	n/a	86	n/a	59	5 starch, 3 veg, 5 very lean meat, 8 fat
Kung Pao Scallops	1 order	1180	76	58	8	n/a	n/a	56	n/a	70	3 1/2 carb, 1 veg, 8 lean meat, 10 fat

Kung Pao Shrimp	1 order	1230	79	58	8	n/a	n/a	52	n/a	80	3 1/2 carb, 1 veg, 9 lean meat, 10 fat
Kung Pao Shrimp	1 order	1230	79	58	8	n/a	n/a	52	n/a	80	3 starch, 2 veg, 10 lean meat, 9 fat
Lemon Pepper Shrimp	1 order	520	25	43	2.5	n/a	n/a	31	n/a	44	1 1/2 starch, 2 veg, 5 lean meat, 2 fat
Oolong Marinated Sea Bass	1 order	740	30	36	4	n/a	n/a	39	n/a	78	2 starch, 2 veg, 10 very lean meat, 4 fat
Orange Peel Shrimp	1 order	1070	60	50	5	n/a	n/a	74	n/a	58	4 1/2 carb, 1 veg, 6 lean meat, 8 fat
✓Seared Ahi Tuna	1 order	220	5	20	1	n/a	n/a	18	n/a	25	1/2 starch, 2 veg, 3 lean meat
✓Shrimp w/ lobster sauce	1 order, lunch	490	24	44	4	n/a	n/a	21	n/a	44	1 starch, 2 veg, 5 very lean meat, 4 fat

✓ = Healthiest Bets; n/a = not available

(*Continued*)

SEAFOOD DISHES (*Continued*)	Amount	Cal.	Fat (g)	% Cal. Fat	Sat. Fat (g)	Chol. (mg)	Sod. (mg)	Carb. (g)	Fiber (g)	Pro. (g)	Servings/Exchanges
✓Shrimp w/ lobster sauce	1 order, dinner	560	27	43	5	n/a	n/a	22	n/a	54	1 starch, 2 veg, 7 very lean meat, 4 fat
Sichuan from the Sea, Calamari	1 order	720	21	26	2	n/a	n/a	88	n/a	45	5 1/2 carb, 1 veg, 4 lean meat, 1 fat
✓Sichuan from the Sea, Scallops	1 order	630	19	27	1.5	n/a	n/a	66	n/a	47	4 carb, 1 veg, 5 lean meat
✓Sichuan from the Sea, Shrimp	1 order	630	21	30	2	n/a	n/a	52	n/a	55	3 carb, 1 veg, 6 lean meat, 1 fat
Spicy Salt & Pepper Prawns	1 order	770	50	58	4	n/a	n/a	28	n/a	53	1 1/2 starch, 1 veg, 6 lean meat, 7 fat
✓Wild Alaskan Sockeye Salmon Steamed w/ Ginger	1 order	478	28	53	7	n/a	n/a	5	n/a	51	1 veg, 7 lean meat, 1 fat

SOUPS											
✓Hot and Sour	1 cup/ 8 oz	56	4	64	1	n/a	n/a	2	n/a	3	1 fat
✓Pin Rice Noodle	1 cup/ 8 oz	270	2	7	1	n/a	n/a	55	n/a	12	3 starch, 1 veg, 1/2 lean meat
✓Wonton	1 cup/ 8 oz	52	3	52	1	n/a	n/a	4	n/a	3	1 veg, 1/2 fat
VEGETARIAN DISHES											
✓Buddha's Feast, Steamed	1 order	200	2	9	0	n/a	n/a	44	n/a	10	1 starch, 4 veg
✓Buddha's Feast, Stir-Fried	1 order	370	7	17	1	n/a	n/a	64	n/a	21	3 starch, 4 veg, 1 lean meat
Coconut-Curry Vegetables	1 order	950	63	60	40	n/a	n/a	79	n/a	36	4 carb, 4 veg, 2 medium-fat meat, 8 fat
✓Garlic Snap Peas	1 order	220	7	29	0.5	n/a	n/a	20	n/a	6	4 veg, 2 fat

✓ = Healthiest Bets; n/a = not available

(*Continued*)

VEGETARIAN DISHES (*Continued*)	**Amount**	**Cal.**	**Fat (g)**	**% Cal. Fat**	**Sat. Fat (g)**	**Chol. (mg)**	**Sod. (mg)**	**Carb. (g)**	**Fiber (g)**	**Pro. (g)**	**Servings/Exchanges**
Ma Po Tofu	1 order	760	52	62	6	n/a	n/a	40	n/a	45	2 starch, 2 veg, 5 lean meat, 6 fat
✔Sichuan Style Asparagus	1 order	170	4	21	0.5	n/a	n/a	29	n/a	11	1/2 starch, 4 veg, 1/2 fat
✔Sichuan Style Long Beans	1 order	190	4	19	0.5	n/a	n/a	36	n/a	9	1 starch, 4 veg
✔Shanghai Cucumbers	1 order	120	6	45	1	n/a	n/a	8	n/a	10	2 veg, 1 medium-fat meat
Stir-Fried Eggplant	1 order	510	29	51	2	n/a	n/a	60	n/a	8	3 carb, 4 veg, 5 fat
✔Vegetable Chow Fun	1 order	440	2	4	0	n/a	n/a	100	n/a	10	6 starch, 2 veg

✔ = Healthiest Bets; n/a = not available

Pizza, Pasta, and All Else Italian

RESTAURANTS

Chuck E. Cheese's
Domino's Pizza
Fazoli's
Godfather's Pizza
Little Caesars
Olive Garden Italian Restaurant
Papa John's Pizza
Papa Murphy's Take 'N' Bake
Pizza Hut
Round Table Pizza
Sbarro

NUTRITION PROS

- Surprisingly, pizza and pasta—as long as you top them wisely—can be healthy restaurant choices.
- Pizza and pasta can hold the line on fat and calories better than some burger and french fry meals.
- Pizza and pasta meals can match today's diabetes nutrition goals: low in fat, moderate in protein and carbohydrate.
- You can eat vegetables, both raw and cooked, in most pizza and pasta restaurants. That's an accomplishment in a fast-food restaurant. Raw vegetables come as salads. Cooked vegetables come as pizza sauce and toppings, or as tomato-based sauces and toppings on pasta.

- Splitting and sharing is the way to go in most pizza restaurants.
- You can design your own pizza with healthier toppings (see list on page 531). Pizza parlors are used to made-for-you orders.
- Most pizza chains offer a veggie combination pizza.
- Pizza chains are slowly but surely divulging their nutrition information, so you can pick and choose with nutrition facts in hand.
- Several pizza chains have gone uptown. That's good news for health-focused pizza lovers. They bake their pizzas in brick ovens, and they offer novel and healthy toppings. Pineapple, spinach, feta cheese, roasted red peppers, and grilled chicken are just a few.
- Taking home leftovers is a snap. Boxes are ready.

NUTRITION CONS

- It's hard to eat just two or three slices. There's always just one more piece of pizza begging you to eat it.
- High-fat pizza toppings—extra cheese, three kinds of cheese, pepperoni, and sausage—can quickly add fat and calories.
- These high-fat toppings also add more sodium.
- Some pizza chains now promote more toppings, extra cheese, and bigger pizzas. That all adds up to more fat and calories.
- Restaurant combination pizzas often add high-fat and high-calorie toppers.

- Pasta with high-fat and high-calorie toppings—cream sauce, creamy cheese sauce, butter sauce—is easy to find.
- Pasta portions are often heavy-handed.
- Breadsticks and garlic bread sound healthy, but they are often drenched in fat. Check their nutrition numbers.

HEALTHY PIZZA TOPPINGS

part-skim cheese	sliced tomatoes	chicken
green peppers	spinach	ham
onions	broccoli	Canadian bacon
mushrooms	pineapple	

NOT-SO-HEALTHY PIZZA TOPPINGS

extra cheese	pepperoni	anchovies
several types of cheese	sausage	bacon

Get It Your Way

★ Ask your pizza maker to go light on the cheese and heavy on the veggies.

★ Request a half-order of pasta if you don't have someone to split it with.

★ Remember to order your salad dressing on the side.

Healthy Tips

- ★ If you count calories carefully, stick with the thin crust and load up on the veggies.
- ★ If your favorite chain does not publish nutrition information, check the nutrition information for similar items from two other pizza chains. That gives you ballpark figures to base your choice on.
- ★ If your dining partner wants not-so-healthy pizza toppings, order healthier toppings on one half and let your partner handle the other.
- ★ If you count grams of carbohydrate, make sure the slices you eat are average. If they are bigger or smaller, change your carbohydrate estimate based on the carbohydrate information.
- ★ Order just enough for everyone at the table, to avoid that just-one-more-piece syndrome.
- ★ If you know a few extra pieces will be left over, package them up before you take your first bite.
- ★ Try an appetizer side portion of pasta, split an order with your dining partner, or stash a portion in a take-home container before you lift your fork to your mouth.
- ★ Along with pizza or pasta, crunch on a healthy garden salad to fill you up and not out.
- ★ The red pepper flakes you'll probably find sitting right on your table add zip to your pizza, pasta, or salad without adding calories.

Chuck E. Cheese's

❖ Chuck E. Cheese's provides nutrition information for all its menu items on its Web site at www.chuckecheeses.com.

Light 'n Lean Choice

Medium BBQ Chicken Pizza *(2 slices)*

Calories	410	Sodium (mg)	640
Fat (g)	13	Carbohydrate (g)	51
% calories from fat	29	Fiber (g)	3
Saturated fat (g)	7	Protein (g)	22
Cholesterol (mg)	50		

Exchanges: 3 1/2 starch, 1 high-fat meat, 1 fat

Healthy 'n Hearty Choice

Cheese Pizza *(4 slices)*

Calories	660	Sodium (mg)	920
Fat (g)	26	Carbohydrate (g)	86
% calories from fat	35	Fiber (g)	6
Saturated fat (g)	6	Protein (g)	30
Cholesterol (mg)	46		

Exchanges: 5 1/2 starch, 2 high-fat meat

(Continued)

Chuck E. Cheese's

	Amount	Cal.	Fat (g)	% Cal. Fat	Sat. Fat (g)	Chol. (mg)	Sod. (mg)	Carb. (g)	Fiber (g)	Pro. (g)	Servings/Exchanges
APPETIZERS											
✓Blended Pizza Sauce	4 T	35	0	0	0	0	380	7	1	1	1/2 starch
Bread Sticks	3	370	12	29	4	5	480	51	3	14	3 1/2 starch, 2 fat
Buffalo Wings	4	220	15	61	3.5	110	560	1	0	20	3 medium-fat meat
French Fries	1	283	10	32	2.5	0	433	43	3	5	3 starch, 2 fat
Mozzarella Sticks	2	380	24	57	7	40	380	26	2	13	1 1/2 starch, 3 high-fat meat
BREAKFAST ITEMS											
Banana Loaf Cake	1	350	11	28	4.5	30	320	50	2	5	3 starch, 2 fat
✓Cinnamon Blast Cereal	1	140	5	32	1	0	210	24	1	2	1 starch, 1/2 carb, 1 fat

Cinnamon Crumb Pound Cake	1	386	17	40	3	38	236	55	1	4	1 1/2 starch, 2 carb, 3 fat
✓Fruit Loops	1	120	1	8	1	0	160	28	1	2	1 starch, 1 carb
✓Rice Krispies	1	130	1	7	1	0	200	26	0	2	1 starch, 1 carb
CAKES											
✓Chocolate Cake w/ whipped cream	1 slice	208	11	48	8	21	200	25	1	2	1 1/2 carb, 2 fat
✓White Cake w/ whipped cream	1 slice	208	11	48	8	25	167	26	0	2	1 1/2 carb, 2 fat
OTHER DESSERTS											
Brownie	1	382	18	42	4.5	60	143	n/a	2	4	insufficient info. to calculate
Chocolate Chunk Cookie	1	410	19	42	6	20	390	56	0	5	3 1/2 carb, 4 fat
Original Krispy Treat	1	340	9	24	2	0	250	50	1	3	3 carb, 2 fat

✓ = Healthiest Bets; n/a = not available

(Continued)

	Amount	Cal.	Fat (g)	% Cal. Fat	Sat. Fat (g)	Chol. (mg)	Sod. (mg)	Carb. (g)	Fiber (g)	Pro. (g)	Servings/Exchanges
PIZZA-MEDIUM SIZE											
✓BBQ Chicken	2 slices	410	13	29	7	50	640	51	3	22	3 1/2 starch, 2 lean meat, 1 1/2 fat
✓Beef	2 slices	411	17	37	9	36	607	43	3	18	3 starch, 1 medium-fat meat, 2 1/2 fat
✓Cheese	2 slices	330	10	27	6	20	460	43	3	15	3 starch, 1 medium-fat meat, 1 fat
✓Pepperoni	2 slices	371	14	34	7	28	619	43	3	17	3 starch, 1 high-fat meat, 1 fat
✓Sausage	2 slices	387	15	35	8	31	662	44	3	18	3 starch, 1 high-fat meat, 1 fat
SALAD BAR DRESSINGS											
Bleu Cheese	2 T	170	18	95	3	15	120	1	0	1	3 1/2 fat

Catalina Dressing	2 T	35	0	0	0	0	320	8	0	0	1/2 starch
Lite Ranch	2 T	80	8	90	1	5	240	2	0	1	2 fat
Olive Oil & Vinegar	2 T	90	9	90	1	0	170	2	0	0	2 fat
Thousand Island	2 T	110	10	82	2	10	170	4	0	0	2 fat
SANDWICHES											
Grilled Chicken Sub	1	740	39	47	12	110	1080	57	5	41	3 1/2 starch, 4 medium-fat meat, 3 fat
Ham & Cheese	1	770	41	48	9	85	1490	60	6	39	4 starch, 4 high-fat meat, 1 fat
Hot Dog	1	430	29	61	13	50	710	27	2	15	1 1/2 starch, 2 high-fat meat, 2 1/2 fat
Italian Sub	1	770	47	55	16	80	1560	52	4	35	3 1/2 starch, 4 high-fat meat, 2 fat

✓ = Healthiest Bets; n/a = not available

Domino's Pizza

❖ Domino's provides nutrition information for all its menu items on its Web site at www.dominos.com.

Light 'n Lean Choice

14″ Crunchy Thin-Crust Green Pepper, Onion, and Mushroom Pizza *(3 slices)*

Calories	603	Sodium (mg)	1,213
Fat (g)	30	Carbohydrate (g)	63
% calories from fat	42	Fiber (g)	6
Saturated fat (g)	10.5	Protein (g)	24
Cholesterol (mg)	39		

Exchanges: 3 starch, 3 veg, 1 medium-fat meat, 5 fat

Healthy 'n Hearty Choice

12″ Classic Hand-Tossed Vegi Feast Pizza *(4 slices)*

Calories	872	Sodium (mg)	1,956
Fat (g)	32	Carbohydrate (g)	116
% calories from fat	33	Fiber (g)	8
Saturated fat (g)	14	Protein (g)	36
Cholesterol (mg)	52		

Exchanges: 6 1/2 starch, 3 veg, 2 medium-fat meat, 3 fat

Domino's Pizza

	Amount	Cal.	Fat (g)	% Cal. Fat	Sat. Fat (g)	Chol. (mg)	Sod. (mg)	Carb. (g)	Fiber (g)	Pro. (g)	Servings/Exchanges
12" CLASSIC HAND-TOSSED											
America's Favorite Feast	1 slice	257	12	42	4.5	22	626	29	2	10	2 starch, 1 medium-fat meat, 1/2 fat
Bacon Cheeseburger Feast	1 slice	273	13	43	5.5	27	634	28	2	12	2 starch, 1 medium-fat meat, 2 fat
Barbecue Feast	1 slice	252	10	36	4.5	20	600	31	1	11	2 starch, 1 high-fat meat
Beef	1 slice	225	9	36	3.5	16	493	28	2	9	2 starch, 1 medium-fat meat
✔Cheese	1 slice	186	6	29	2	9	385	28	1	7	1 1/2 starch, 1 medium-fat meat

✔ = Healthiest Bets

(*Continued*)

12" CLASSIC HAND-TOSSED (*Continued*)	Amount	Cal.	Fat (g)	% Cal. Fat	Sat. Fat (g)	Chol. (mg)	Sod. (mg)	Carb. (g)	Fiber (g)	Pro. (g)	Servings/Exchanges
Deluxe Feast	1 slice	234	10	38	3.5	17	542	29	2	9	2 starch, 1 medium-fat meat
Extravaganzza	1 slice	289	14	44	5.5	28	764	30	2	13	2 starch, 1 high-fat meat, 1/2 fat
✓Green Pepper, Onion, & Mushroom	1 slice	191	6	28	2	9	385	29	2	8	1 1/2 starch, 1 medium-fat meat
Ham	1 slice	198	6	27	2.5	13	492	28	1	9	1 1/2 starch, 1 medium-fat meat
Ham & Pineapple	1 slice	200	6	27	2.5	12	467	29	2	9	1 1/2 starch, 1 medium-fat meat
Hawaiian Feast	1 slice	223	8	32	3.5	16	547	30	2	10	2 starch, 1 medium-fat meat
Meatzza Feast	1 slice	281	14	45	5.5	28	740	29	2	13	2 starch, 1 high-fat meat, 1/2 fat

Pepperoni	1 slice	223	9	36	3.5	16	522	28	2	9	2 starch, 1 medium-fat meat
Pepperoni & Sausage	1 slice	255	12	42	4.5	22	625	28	2	10	2 starch, 1 medium-fat meat, 1/2 fat
Pepperoni Feast	1 slice	265	13	44	5	24	670	28	2	11	2 starch, 1 high-fat meat
Sausage	1 slice	231	10	39	3.5	17	530	28	1	9	2 starch, 1 medium-fat meat
Vegi Feast	1 slice	218	8	33	3.5	13	489	29	2	9	1 1/2 starch, 1 veg, 1 medium-fat meat
12″ CRUNCHY THIN CRUST											
✓Beef	1 slice	175	11	57	4	17	400	14	1	7	1 starch, 1 high-fat meat
✓Cheese	1 slice	137	7	46	2.5	10	293	14	1	5	1 starch, 1 medium-fat meat
✓Green Pepper, Onion, & Mushroom	1 slice	142	8	51	2.5	10	293	15	1	6	1 starch, 1 medium-fat meat

✓ = Healthiest Bets

(Continued)

12" CRUNCHY THIN CRUST (*Continued*)	Amount	Cal.	Fat (g)	% Cal. Fat	Sat. Fat (g)	Chol. (mg)	Sod. (mg)	Carb. (g)	Fiber (g)	Pro. (g)	Servings/Exchanges
✓Ham	1 slice	148	8	49	3	14	400	14	1	7	1 starch, 1 medium-fat meat
✓Ham & Pineapple	1 slice	150	8	48	3	13	374	15	1	7	1 starch, 1 medium-fat meat
✓Pepperoni	1 slice	174	11	57	4	17	429	14	1	7	1 starch, 1 high-fat meat
Pepperoni & Sausage	1 slice	206	14	61	5	23	533	14	1	8	1 starch, 1 high-fat meat, 1/2 fat
Pepperoni Feast	1 slice	216	14	58	5.5	26	577	14	1	9	1 starch, 1 high-fat meat, 1 fat
✓Sausage	1 slice	181	11	55	4	18	438	14	1	7	1 starch, 1 high-fat meat
12" ULTIMATE DEEP DISH											
America's Favorite Feast	1 slice	309	17	50	6	25	797	29	2	12	2 starch, 2 high-fat meat
Bacon Cheeseburger Feast	1 slice	325	19	53	7	30	805	28	2	14	2 starch, 2 high-fat meat, 1/2 fat

Barbecue Feast	1 slice	304	15	44	6	23	771	32	2	12	2 starch, 2 high-fat meat
Beef	1 slice	277	15	49	5	19	664	28	2	11	2 starch, 1 high-fat meat
Cheese	1 slice	238	11	42	3.5	11	556	28	2	9	2 starch, 1 medium-fat meat
Deluxe Feast	1 slice	287	15	47	5	17	712	29	2	11	2 starch, 1 high-fat meat, 1/2 fat
Extravaganzza	1 slice	341	20	53	7	31	935	30	2	14	2 starch, 2 high-fat meat, 1/2 fat
Green Pepper, Onion, & Mushroom	1 slice	244	11	41	3.5	11	556	30	2	9	2 starch, 1 medium-fat meat
Ham	1 slice	250	12	43	4	16	663	28	2	11	2 starch, 1 medium-fat meat, 1/2 fat
Ham & Pineapple	1 slice	252	12	43	4	15	637	30	2	10	2 starch, 1 medium-fat meat, 1/2 fat
Hawaiian Feast	1 slice	275	13	43	5	19	717	30	2	12	2 starch, 1 medium-fat meat, 1 fat

✔ = Healthiest Bets

(*Continued*)

12" ULTIMATE DEEP DISH (*Continued*)	Amount	Cal.	Fat (g)	% Cal. Fat	Sat. Fat (g)	Chol. (mg)	Sod. (mg)	Carb. (g)	Fiber (g)	Pro. (g)	Servings/Exchanges
Meatzza Feast	1 slice	333	19	51	7	31	911	29	2	14	2 starch, 2 high-fat meat, 1/2 fat
Pepperoni	1 slice	275	14	46	5	19	692	28	2	11	2 starch, 1 high-fat meat, 1/2 fat
Pepperoni & Sausage	1 slice	307	17	50	6	25	796	29	2	12	2 starch, 2 medium-fat meat, 1/2 fat
Pepperoni Feast	1 slice	317	18	51	6.5	27	841	29	2	13	2 starch, 2 medium-fat meat
Sausage	1 slice	283	15	48	5	19	701	29	2	11	2 starch, 1 high-fat meat, 1 fat
Vegi Feast	1 slice	270	14	47	5	15	660	30	2	11	1 starch, 1 veg, 1 high-fat meat, 1 fat
14" CLASSIC HAND-TOSSED											
America's Favorite Feast	1 slice	353	16	41	6	31	864	39	2	14	2 1/2 starch, 1 medium-fat meat, 2 fat

Bacon Cheeseburger Feast	1 slice	379	18	43	8	38	900	38	2	17	2 1/2 starch, 2 high-fat meat
Barbecue Feast	1 slice	344	14	37	6	27	832	43	2	14	3 starch, 1 high-fat meat, 1/2 fat
Beef	1 slice	312	13	38	5	23	690	38	2	13	2 1/2 starch, 1 high-fat meat, 1/2 fat
✔Cheese	1 slice	256	8	28	3	12	534	38	2	10	2 starch, 1 high-fat meat
Deluxe Feast	1 slice	316	12	34	5	23	728	39	2	13	2 1/2 starch, 1 medium-fat meat, 1 fat
Extravaganzza Feast	1 slice	388	19	44	7.5	37	1014	40	3	17	2 1/2 starch, 2 high-fat meat
✔Green Pepper, Onion, & Mushroom	1 slice	263	8	27	3	12	537	39	2	11	2 1/2 starch, 1 medium-fat meat
Ham	1 slice	272	9	30	3.5	18	682	38	2	12	2 1/2 starch, 1 medium-fat meat, 1/2 fat

✔ = Healthiest Bets

(*Continued*)

14" CLASSIC HAND-TOSSED (*Continued*)	Amount	Cal.	Fat (g)	% Cal. Fat	Sat. Fat (g)	Chol. (mg)	Sod. (mg)	Carb. (g)	Fiber (g)	Pro. (g)	Servings/Exchanges
Ham & Pineapple	1 slice	275	9	29	3.5	17	653	40	2	13	2 1/2 starch, 1 medium-fat meat, 1/2 fat
Hawaiian Feast	1 slice	309	11	32	4.5	23	765	41	2	14	2 1/2 starch, 1 medium-fat meat, 1 fat
Meatzza Feast	1 slice	378	18	43	7.5	37	938	39	2	17	2 1/2 starch, 2 high-fat meat
Pepperoni	1 slice	305	12	35	5	22	718	38	2	12	2 starch, 1 high-fat meat, 1 fat
Pepperoni & Sausage	1 slice	350	16	41	6	31	863	39	2	14	2 starch, 2 high-fat meat
Pepperoni Feast	1 slice	363	17	42	7	33	920	39	2	16	2 starch, 2 high-fat meat
Sausage	1 slice	320	14	39	5	24	744	39	2	13	2 starch, 1 high-fat meat, 1 fat
Vegi Feast	1 slice	300	11	33	4.5	18	678	40	3	13	2 starch, 1 veg, 1 medium-fat meat, 1 fat

14" CRUNCHY THIN CRUST											
America's Favorite Feast	1 slice	285	19	60	7	32	736	20	2	11	1 starch, 2 high-fat meat
Bacon Cheeseburger Feast	1 slice	311	21	61	8.5	40	773	19	1	14	1 starch, 2 high-fat meat, 1 fat
Barbecue Feast	1 slice	276	16	52	6.5	29	704	24	1	11	1 1/2 starch, 2 high-fat meat
Beef	1 slice	243	15	56	5.5	24	563	19	1	10	1 starch, 2 high-fat meat
✓Cheese	1 slice	188	10	48	3.5	13	409	19	1	7	1 starch, 1 high-fat meat
Deluxe Feast	1 slice	248	15	54	25.5	24	601	20	2	10	1 starch, 1 high-fat meat, 1 1/2 fat
Extravaganzza Feast	1 slice	320	21	59	8	38	886	21	2	14	1 1/2 starch, 2 high-fat meat, 1/2 fat
✓Green Pepper, Onion, & Mushroom	1 slice	201	10	45	3.5	13	410	21	2	8	1 starch, 1 veg, 1 high-fat meat

✓ = Healthiest Bets

(Continued)

14" CRUNCHY THIN CRUST (*Continued*)	Amount	Cal.	Fat (g)	% Cal. Fat	Sat. Fat (g)	Chol. (mg)	Sod. (mg)	Carb. (g)	Fiber (g)	Pro. (g)	Servings/Exchanges
Ham	1 slice	204	11	49	4	20	555	19	1	9	1 starch, 1 medium-fat meat, 1 fat
Ham & Pineapple	1 slice	207	11	48	4	18	526	21	1	9	1 1/2 starch, 1 medium-fat meat, 1/2 fat
Hawaiian Feast	1 slice	240	13	49	5	24	638	21	2	11	1 1/2 starch, 1 medium-fat meat, 1 fat
Meatzza Feast	1 slice	310	20	58	8	38	856	20	2	14	1 starch, 2 high-fat meat, 1 fat
Pepperoni	1 slice	237	15	57	5.5	24	591	19	1	10	1 starch, 1 high-fat meat, 2 fat
Pepperoni & Sausage	1 slice	282	19	61	7	32	736	19	2	11	1 starch, 2 high-fat meat
Pepperoni Feast	1 slice	295	19	58	7.5	35	792	20	1	13	1 starch, 2 high-fat meat, 1/2 fat

Sausage	1 slice	252	16	57	5.5	25	616	20	2	10	1 starch, 1 high-fat meat, 1 1/2 fat
Vegi Feast	1 slice	231	14	55	5	19	550	21	2	10	1 starch, 1 veg, 1 medium-fat meat, 1 1/2 fat
14″ ULTIMATE DEEP DISH											
America's Favorite Feast	1 slice	433	24	50	8	34	1110	42	3	17	2 1/2 starch, 2 high-fat meat, 1 fat
Bacon Cheeseburger Feast	1 slice	459	16	31	10	42	1146	41	2	20	3 starch, 2 high-fat meat, 1 fat
Barbecue Feast	1 slice	424	21	45	8	31	1078	46	2	17	3 starch, 2 high-fat meat, 1 fat
Beef	1 slice	392	20	46	7	26	937	41	2	15	2 1/2 starch, 2 high-fat meat
Cheese	1 slice	336	15	40	5	16	782	41	2	13	2 1/2 starch, 1 high-fat meat, 1 fat

✔ = Healthiest Bets

(*Continued*)

14" ULTIMATE DEEP DISH (*Continued*)	Amount	Cal.	Fat (g)	% Cal. Fat	Sat. Fat (g)	Chol. (mg)	Sod. (mg)	Carb. (g)	Fiber (g)	Pro. (g)	Servings/Exchanges
Deluxe Feast	1 slice	396	20	45	7	26	974	42	3	15	2 1/2 starch, 2 high-fat meat
Extravaganzza Feast	1 slice	468	26	50	9.5	40	1260	43	3	20	2 1/2 starch, 2 high-fat meat, 1 1/2 fat
Green Pepper, Onion, & Mushroom	1 slice	343	15	39	5	16	783	42	3	13	2 1/2 starch, 1 veg, 1 medium-fat meat, 1 1/2 fat
Ham	1 slice	352	15	38	5.5	22	929	41	2	15	2 1/2 starch, 1 medium-fat meat, 1 1/2 fat
Ham & Pineapple	1 slice	335	16	43	5.5	21	900	42	2	14	3 starch, 1 medium-fat meat, 1 fat
Hawaiian Feast	1 slice	389	18	42	6.5	26	1011	43	3	17	3 starch, 2 medium-fat meat, 1/2 fat

Meatzza Feast	1 slice	458	25	49	9.5	40	1230	42	3	19	3 starch, 2 high-fat meat, 1 fat
Pepperoni	1 slice	385	20	47	7	26	964	41	2	15	3 starch, 1 high-fat meat, 1 fat
Pepperoni & Sausage	1 slice	430	23	48	8	34	1109	41	3	17	3 starch, 2 high-fat meat
Pepperoni Feast	1 slice	443	24	49	9	37	1166	42	3	18	3 starch, 2 high-fat meat
Sausage	1 slice	400	21	47	7	27	990	42	3	15	3 starch, 1 high-fat meat, 1 1/2 fat
Vegi Feast	1 slice	380	18	43	6.5	21	934	43	3	15	2 1/2 starch, 1 veg, 1 high-fat meat, 1 fat
SIDE DISHES											
Blue Cheese Dipping Sauce	3 T	223	24	97	4	20	417	2	0	1	5 fat
Breadsticks	1	115	6	47	1.1	0	122	12	0	2	1 starch

✓ = Healthiest Bets

(*Continued*)

SIDE DISHES (*Continued*)	Amount	Cal.	Fat (g)	% Cal. Fat	Sat. Fat (g)	Chol. (mg)	Sod. (mg)	Carb. (g)	Fiber (g)	Pro. (g)	Servings/Exchanges
Buffalo Chicken Kickers	1 piece	47	2	38	0.5	9	162	3	0	4	1 lean meat
Cheesy Bread	1	123	7	51	1.9	6	163	13	0	4	1 starch, 1 fat
Cinna Stix	1	123	6	44	1.1	0	111	15	1	2	1 starch, 1 fat
Garlic Sauce	3 T	440	49	100	10	0	380	0	0	0	10 fat
Hot Buffalo Wings	1 piece	50	3	54	0.5	26	176	2	0	6	1 lean meat
Hot Dipping Sauce	3 T	15	0	0	0	0	1820	4	0	0	free
Marinara Dipping Sauce	3 T	25	0	0	0	0	262	5	0	1	1 veg
Ranch Dipping Sauce	3 T	197	21	96	3	9	380	2	0	1	4 fat
Sweet Icing	4 T	250	3	11	2.5	0	0	57	0	0	4 carb

✓ = Healthiest Bets

Fazoli's

❖ Fazoli's provides some nutrition information for its menu items on its Web site at www.fazolis.com. Fazoli's provided additional information for this book.

Light 'n Lean Choice

Spaghetti and Meat Balls *(small)*
Garden Salad *(dressing not included)*

Calories	485	Sodium (mg)	930
Fat (g)	8	Carbohydrate (g)	88
% calories from fat	15	Fiber (g)	9
Saturated fat (g)	2	Protein (g)	19
Cholesterol (mg)	5		

Exchanges: 5 starch, 2 veg, 1 medium-fat meat

Healthy 'n Hearty Choice

Cheese Ravioli with Meat Sauce
Caesar Salad *(dressing not included)*

Calories	770	Sodium (mg)	1,621
Fat (g)	27	Carbohydrate (g)	97
% calories from fat	32	Fiber (g)	9
Saturated fat (g)	9	Protein (g)	31
Cholesterol (mg)	65		

Exchanges: 6 starch, 1 veg, 1 high-fat meat, 1 fat

(*Continued*)

Fazoli's

	Amount	Cal.	Fat (g)	% Cal. Fat	Sat. Fat (g)	Chol. (mg)	Sod. (mg)	Carb. (g)	Fiber (g)	Pro. (g)	Servings/Exchanges
BREADSTICKS											
✓Breadstick	1	140	6	39	1	0	250	18	0	3	1 starch, 1 1/2 fat
✓Dry Breadstick	1	100	2	18	0	0	150	18	0	3	1 starch
BRICK-OVEN-STYLE PIZZAS											
Italian Meat	1 whole	970	46	43	19	85	2880	92	6	42	6 starch, 3 high-fat meat, 4 1/2 fat
Kids' Cheese Round	6″ round	380	15	36	8	30	990	43	2	17	3 starch, 2 medium-fat meat
Kids' Pepperoni Round	6″ round	450	21	42	10	45	1260	43	2	20	3 starch, 2 high-fat meat

Mediterranean	1 whole	890	43	43	17	90	2420	85	5	39	3 starch, 4 high-fat meat, 5 1/2 fat
Pepperoni	1 whole	870	39	40	16	70	2410	89	4	34	6 starch, 4 high-fat meat
Spicy Southwest Chicken	1 whole	830	32	35	13	85	2340	89	4	86	6 starch, 4 medium-fat meat, 1 fat
Ultimate Cheese	1 whole	800	32	36	16	60	1970	89	4	35	6 starch, 4 medium-fat meat, 1/2 fat
DESSERTS											
Freezi - Strawberry	1	510	6	11	6	0	260	115	0	0	7 carb
Freezi - Strawberry Banana	1	530	6	10	6	0	230	118	0	0	7 carb
Freezi - Triple Berry	1	520	6	10	6	0	200	116	0	0	7 carb
Fresh Baked Chocolate Chunk Cookie	1	590	28	43	12	60	410	77	3	7	5 carb, 4 fat

✔ = Healthiest Bets

(*Continued*)

DESSERTS (*Continued*)	Amount	Cal.	Fat (g)	% Cal. Fat	Sat. Fat (g)	Chol. (mg)	Sod. (mg)	Carb. (g)	Fiber (g)	Pro. (g)	Servings/Exchanges
Lemon Ice	1	190	0	0	0	0	95	45	0	0	3 carb
✓Plain Cheesecake	1	290	22	68	14	95	220	17	0	6	1 carb, 4 1/2 fat
✓Strawberry Topping	1	35	0	0	0	0	40	8	0	0	1/2 carb
Turtle Cheesecake	1	420	34	73	17	100	220	24	2	8	1 1/2 carb, 6 1/2 fat
ITALIAN SPECIALTIES											
Baked Chicken Parmesan	1	760	16	19	4	65	1720	110	7	41	7 starch, 3 medium-fat meat
Baked Spaghetti Parmesan	1	700	25	32	13	60	770	76	5	38	5 starch, 4 medium-fat meat
Baked Spaghetti w/ Meatballs	1	970	42	39	22	120	2010	91	6	46	6 starch, 4 high-fat meat, 2 fat
Broccoli 6 Layer Lasagna	1	680	28	37	12	55	2290	38	6	30	2 1/2 starch, 2 veg, 3 high-fat meat, 3 fat

Cheese Ravioli w/ Marinara Sauce	1	580	15	23	7	60	1350	85	6	26	6 starch, 1 medium-fat meat, 2 fat
Cheese Ravioli w/ Meat Sauce	1	610	16	24	8	65	1480	85	7	29	6 starch, 2 medium-fat meat, 2 fat
Chicken Broccoli Bake	1	560	27	43	14	170	3590	13	3	67	1/2 starch, 2 veg, 9 lean meat
Classic Meaty Ziti - Regular	1	760	37	44	21	95	2790	58	8	41	4 starch, 4 medium-fat meat, 3 fat
Classic Meaty Ziti w/ Meat Sauce	1	500	24	43	14	60	1820	37	5	26	2 1/2 starch, 3 high-fat meat
Classic Sampler w/ 6 Layer Lasagna	1	790	18	21	8	35	1880	99	7	30	6 1/2 starch, 2 high-fat meat, 1 1/2 fat
Six Layer Lasagna w/ Meat Sauce	1	620	23	33	11	50	2020	33	4	28	2 starch, 3 medium-fat meat, 1 high-fat meat, 3 fat

✓ = Healthiest Bets

(Continued)

ITALIAN SPECIALTIES (*Continued*)	Amount	Cal.	Fat (g)	% Cal. Fat	Sat. Fat (g)	Chol. (mg)	Sod. (mg)	Carb. (g)	Fiber (g)	Pro. (g)	Servings/Exchanges
Tuscan Chicken Bake	1	660	29	40	14	125	1800	53	3	43	3 1/2 starch, 5 lean meat, 2 1/2 fat
Twice Baked Lasagna	1	890	43	43	24	110	2770	36	4	48	2 starch, 6 medium-fat meat, 2 fat
Twice Baked Ziti w/ Meat Sauce	1	1340	81	54	49	235	4250	60	8	94	4 starch, 12 medium-fat meat, 4 fat
Ultimate Sampler Platter	1	1010	29	26	13	60	2700	116	9	42	8 starch, 5 medium-fat meat, 1 fat
PASTAS											
Broccoli Fettuccine Alfredo, regular	1	840	22	24	6	25	1740	129	9	27	8 starch, 4 1/2 fat
Broccoli Fettuccine Alfredo, small	1	590	17	26	4	15	1320	89	7	19	6 starch, 2 1/2 fat
Fettuccine Alfredo, regular	1	740	15	18	5	20	1290	122	5	24	8 starch, 2 fat

Fettuccine Alfredo, small	1	500	11	20	4	15	870	81	4	16	5 starch, 2 fat
Garden Style Chicken Penne, regular	1	830	28	30	2	40	1040	100	7	35	6 1/2 starch, 4 lean meat, 2 fat
Garden Style Chicken Penne, small	1	770	24	28	4	40	2550	102	10	37	6 1/2 starch, 3 lean meat, 1 fat
Peppery Chicken Alfredo, regular	1	820	17	19	5	60	1610	122	5	40	8 starch, 3 lean meat, 1 fat
Peppery Chicken Alfredo, small	1	570	12	19	4	55	1190	81	4	32	5 starch, 3 lean meat
Roasted Garlic Alfredo	1	710	17	22	5	60	2210	101	7	38	6 1/2 starch, 3 lean meat, 1 fat
Spaghetti w/ Marinara Sauce, regular	1	650	3	4	0	0	1140	126	9	21	8 starch
✔Spaghetti w/ Marinara Sauce, small	1	440	2	4	0	0	770	84	6	14	5 1/2 starch

✔ = Healthiest Bets

(Continued)

PASTAS (*Continued*)	Amount	Cal.	Fat (g)	% Cal. Fat	Sat. Fat (g)	Chol. (mg)	Sod. (mg)	Carb. (g)	Fiber (g)	Pro. (g)	Servings/Exchanges
Spaghetti w/ Meat Sauce, regular	1	690	6	8	2	5	1340	125	9	26	8 starch, 1 lean meat
✓Spaghetti w/ Meat Sauce, small	1	460	4	8	2	5	900	84	6	17	5 1/2 starch, 1 lean meat
Spaghetti w/ Meatballs, regular	1	980	27	25	10	75	2080	135	10	38	9 starch, 2 high-fat meat, 1 1/2 fat
Spaghetti w/ Meatballs, small	1	690	20	26	8	55	1470	91	6	27	6 starch, 1 high-fat meat
Spicy Marinara Penne w/ Chicken	1	990	13	12	2	40	2420	178	13	36	11 starch, 3 lean meat
PIZZA											
Cheese Pizza	2 slices	460	15	29	8	40	970	58	2	24	4 starch, 2 medium-fat meat

Combination Pizza	2 slices	570	25	39	12	60	1360	63	3	29	4 starch, 3 medium-fat meat, 1 fat
Pepperoni Pizza	2 slices	530	22	37	11	55	1230	61	2	27	4 starch, 2 high-fat meat
SOUPS & SALADS											
Caesar Side	1	190	12	57	2	5	270	12	3	6	1/2 starch, 1 veg, 1 high-fat meat, 1/2 fat
Chicken & Pasta Caesar	1	520	27	47	7	90	1670	27	4	27	1 starch, 3 veg, 3 medium-fat meat, 3 fat
Chicken Caesar	1	520	14	24	2	45	520	14	4	21	3 veg, 3 medium-fat meat, 5 fat
✓Garden	1	25	0	0	0	0	30	4	3	2	1 veg
✓Grilled Chicken	1	110	6	49	0	40	370	6	4	19	1 veg, 2 lean meat
Italian Market Salad	1	620	32	46	13	90	2910	32	4	26	1 starch, 3 veg, 3 medium-fat meat, 5 1/2 fat

✓ = Healthiest Bets

(*Continued*)

SOUPS & SALADS (*Continued*)	Amount	Cal.	Fat (g)	% Cal. Fat	Sat. Fat (g)	Chol. (mg)	Sod. (mg)	Carb. (g)	Fiber (g)	Pro. (g)	Servings/Exchanges
Minestrone Soup	1	90	2	20	0	0	960	19	2	2	1 starch
Side Pasta Salad	1	240	22	83	4	15	1030	22	1	6	1 1/2 starch, 2 1/2 fat
SUBMARINOS & PANINIS											
Chicken Caesar Club Panini	1	740	41	50	16	135	1730	47	3	50	3 starch, 5 lean meat, 3 fat
Chicken Pesto Panini	1	580	28	43	8	65	1400	50	3	35	3 starch, 4 lean meat, 1 fat
Four Cheese & Tomato Panini	1	820	52	57	21	105	1290	51	4	39	3 1/2 starch, 3 high-fat meat, 5 1/2 fat
Grilled Chicken Panini	1	380	7	17	3	50	1360	50	3	30	3 starch, 3 lean meat
Smoked Turkey Panini	1	710	40	51	12	100	2110	51	4	35	3 starch, 3 medium-fat meat, 5 1/2 fat
Submarino Club	1	1040	44	38	12	105	2630	117	6	45	7 1/2 starch, 3 high-fat meat, 4 fat

Submarino Ham & Swiss	1	980	38	35	10	95	2240	117	6	41	7 1/2 starch, 3 medium-fat meat, 3 1/2 fat
Submarino Meatball	1	1110	44	36	20	125	2750	124	7	51	8 starch, 4 high-fat meat, 1 1/2 fat
Submarino Original	1	1390	78	51	22	135	3320	116	8	48	7 1/2 starch, 5 high-fat meat, 6 1/2 fat
Submarino Turkey	1	940	36	34	9	80	2500	114	6	40	7 1/2 starch, 3 medium-fat meat, 2 1/2 fat

✔ = Healthiest Bets

Godfather's Pizza

❖ Godfather's Pizza provides nutrition information for its menu on its Web site at www.godfathers.com.

Light 'n Lean Choice

Large Veggie Thin Crust Pizza *(3 slices)*

Calories	681	Sodium (mg)	792
Fat (g)	30	Carbohydrate (g)	63
% calories from fat	40	Fiber (g)	3
Saturated fat (g)	n/a	Protein (g)	26
Cholesterol (mg)	48		

Exchanges: 3 1/2 starch, 2 veg, 2 high-fat meat, 3 fat

Healthy 'n Hearty Choice

Medium Golden Crust Veggie Pizza *(1 slice)*

Calories	928	Sodium (mg)	1,664
Fat (g)	32	Carbohydrate (g)	108
% calories from fat	31	Fiber (g)	8
Saturated fat (g)	n/a	Protein (g)	40
Cholesterol (mg)	52		

Exchanges: 6 starch, 2 veg, 3 high-fat meat, 2 fat

Godfather's Pizza

	Amount	Cal.	Fat (g)	% Cal. Fat	Sat. Fat (g)	Chol. (mg)	Sod. (mg)	Carb. (g)	Fiber (g)	Pro. (g)	Servings/Exchanges
GOLDEN CRUST PIZZA											
Large All Meat Combo	1 slice	325	15	42	n/a	31	8751	29	2	16	2 starch, 2 high-fat meat, 1 1/2 fat
Large Cheese	1 slice	252	9	32	n/a	15	425	28	1	11	2 starch, 1 high-fat meat
Large Veggie	1 slice	264	10	34	n/a	15	480	30	2	11	2 starch, 1 high-fat meat
Medium All Meat Combo	1 slice	285	13	41	n/a	27	654	27	1	14	1 1/2 starch, 2 medium-fat meat, 1/2 fat
✓Medium Cheese	1 slice	221	8	33	n/a	13	371	26	1	10	1 1/2 starch, 1 high-fat meat
✓Medium Veggie	1 slice	232	8	31	n/a	13	416	27	2	10	1 1/2 starch, 1 high-fat meat

✓ = Healthiest Bets; n/a = not available

(*Continued*)

	Amount	Cal.	Fat (g)	% Cal. Fat	Sat. Fat (g)	Chol. (mg)	Sod. (mg)	Carb. (g)	Fiber (g)	Pro. (g)	Servings/Exchanges
INDIVIDUAL DESSERTS											
✓Chocolate Chip Cookie	1	195	8	37	n/a	21	157	30	0	2	2 carb, 1 fat
✓Golden Apple Dessert	1	139	2	13	n/a	0	142	28	1	3	1 carb, 1 fruit
✓Golden Cherry Dessert	1	142	2	13	n/a	0	135	29	1	3	1 carb, 1 fruit
✓Golden Cinnamon Streusel	1	161	3	17	n/a	0	150	30	1	3	2 carb
Golden M&M Streusel	1	173	4	21	n/a	0	152	31	1	4	2 carb
ORIGINAL CRUST PIZZA											
Jumbo All Meat Combo	1 slice	566	23	37	n/a	57	1352	56	3	29	3 1/2 starch, 3 high-fat meat

Jumbo Cheese	1 slice	431	13	27	n/a	27	759	53	2	20	3 1/2 starch, 2 medium-fat meat
Jumbo Veggie	1 slice	456	14	28	n/a	27	869	56	3	21	3 1/2 starch, 2 medium-fat meat, 1/2 fat
Large All Meat Combo	1 slice	383	16	38	n/a	38	911	38	2	19	2 1/2 starch, 2 high-fat meat
Large Cheese	1 slice	366	15	37	n/a	40	870	37	2	18	2 1/2 starch, 2 medium-fat meat
Large Veggie	1 slice	310	8	23	n/a	17	543	45	3	14	3 starch, 1 medium-fat meat
Medium All Meat Combo	1 slice	373	16	39	n/a	39	905	35	2	19	2 starch, 2 high-fat meat
Medium Cheese	1 slice	260	7	24	n/a	15	455	34	1	12	2 starch, 1 high-fat meat
Medium Veggie	1 slice	275	8	26	n/a	15	524	36	2	12	2 1/2 starch, 1 medium-fat meat

✓ = Healthiest Bets; n/a = not available

(*Continued*)

ORIGINAL CRUST PIZZA (*Continued*)	Amount	Cal.	Fat (g)	% Cal. Fat	Sat. Fat (g)	Chol. (mg)	Sod. (mg)	Carb. (g)	Fiber (g)	Pro. (g)	Servings/Exchanges
Mini All Meat Combo	1 slice	201	8	36	n/a	19	459	21	1	10	1 1/2 starch, 1 high-fat meat
✓Mini Cheese	1 slice	150	4	24	n/a	9	242	20	0	7	1 starch, 1 medium-fat meat
✓Mini Veggie	1 slice	161	5	28	n/a	9	287	21	1	7	1 starch, 1 medium-fat meat
SIDES											
✓Breadstick	1	80	2	23	n/a	0	71	14	1	2	1 starch
✓Cheesesticks	1 serving	132	4	27	n/a	6	197	18	1	5	1 starch, 1 fat
Potato Wedges	4 oz	192	9	42	n/a	0	342	24	4	3	1 1/2 starch, 1 1/2 fat
THIN CRUST PIZZA											
Large All Meat Combo	1 slice	311	17	49	n/a	37	697	20	1	15	1 1/2 starch, 2 high-fat meat

✔Large Cheese	1 slice	215	10	42	n/a	16	308	19	0	9	1 starch, 1 high-fat meat, 1 fat
✔Large Veggie	1 slice	227	10	40	n/a	16	264	21	1	10	1 1/2 starch, 1 high-fat meat
Medium All Meat Combo	1 slice	282	15	48	n/a	31	607	20	1	13	1 starch, 2 high-fat meat
✔Medium Cheese	1 slice	200	9	41	n/a	14	271	19	0	8	1 starch, 1 high-fat meat
✔Medium Veggie	1 slice	209	9	39	n/a	14	317	20	1	9	1 1/2 starch, 1 high-fat meat

✔ = Healthiest Bets; n/a = not available

Little Caesars

❖ Little Caesars provides nutrition information for all its menu items on its Web site at www.littlecaesars.com.

Light 'n Lean Choice

14″ Cheese Thin-Crust Pizza *(3 slices)*
Greek Salad
Fat-Free Italian Dressing *(3 T)*

Calories	625	Sodium (mg)	1,043
Fat (g)	29	Carbohydrate (g)	42
% calories from fat	42	Fiber (g)	0
Saturated fat (g)	15	Protein (g)	24
Cholesterol (mg)	70		

Exchanges: 3 starch, 2 veg, 2 high-fat meat, 3 fat

Healthy 'n Hearty Choice

14″ Round Veggie Pizza *(3 slices)*
Tossed Salad
Fat-Free Italian Dressing *(3 T)*

Calories	845	Sodium (mg)	2,710
Fat (g)	26	Carbohydrate (g)	116
% calories from fat	28	Fiber (g)	12
Saturated fat (g)	12	Protein (g)	38
Cholesterol (mg)	45		

Exchanges: 7 starch, 2 veg, 2 high-fat meat, 1 fat

Little Caesars

	Amount	Cal.	Fat (g)	% Cal. Fat	Sat. Fat (g)	Chol. (mg)	Sod. (mg)	Carb. (g)	Fiber (g)	Pro. (g)	Servings/Exchanges
DEEP DISH PIZZA											
Large Cheese	1 slice	320	12	34	5	20	460	37	2	15	2 1/2 starch, 1 high-fat meat, 1 fat
Large Pepperoni	1 slice	350	14	36	6	25	610	38	2	17	2 1/2 starch, 1 high-fat meat, 1 fat
✓Medium Cheese	1 slice	230	9	35	1	2	340	27	1	11	1 1/2 starch, 1 high-fat meat
Medium Pepperoni	1 slice	260	11	38	4.5	20	450	27	1	12	1 1/2 starch, 1 high-fat meat, 1 fat
DELI SANDWICHES											
Ham & Cheese	1	680	29	38	3	50	1540	66	3	32	4 1/2 starch, 3 high-fat meat, 1 fat
Italian	1	800	45	51	10.0	90	1950	66	3	35	4 1/2 starch, 3 high-fat meat, 3 fat
Veggie	1	600	28	42	2.5	30	980	67	3	24	4 carb, 1 veg, 2 high-fat meat, 1 fat

✓ = Healthiest Bets

(*Continued*)

	Amount	Cal.	Fat (g)	% Cal. Fat	Sat. Fat (g)	Chol. (mg)	Sod. (mg)	Carb. (g)	Fiber (g)	Pro. (g)	Servings/Exchanges
INDIVIDUAL SIDE SALADS											
Antipasto	1	140	8	51	1.5	20	560	6	2	9	1/2 starch, 1 high-fat meat
✓Caesar	1	90	3	30	1	0	190	12	3	4	2 veg, 1 fat
Greek	1	120	7	53	4.5	25	590	11	3	6	2 veg, 1 medium-fat meat
✓Tossed	1	100	3	27	1	0	190	15	3	2	3 veg, 1/2 fat
OTHER ITEMS											
Baby Pan Pan	1 piece	360	16	40	7	30	630	34	2	17	2 starch, 2 high-fat meat
Chicken Wings	1	71	5	63	1.5	25	210	0	0	5	1 medium-fat meat
✓Cinnamon Crazy Bread	2 sticks	100	2	18	0	0	95	19	0	3	1 starch
✓Crazy Bread	1 stick	90	3	30	0	0	140	15	0	3	1 starch

✓Crazy Sauce	4 oz	45	0	0	0	0	380	9	3	0	1/2 starch
Italian Cheese Bread	1 piece	130	6	42	2.5	10	310	13	0	7	1 starch, 1 medium-fat meat
PIZZA BY THE SLICE											
Cheese	1 slice	330	11	30	5	25	530	42	2	17	3 starch, 1 medium-fat meat, 1/2 fat
Pepperoni	1 slice	390	14	32	7	35	750	42	2	20	3 starch, 2 medium-fat meat
ROUND PIZZA											
✓12″ Cheese	1 slice	180	6	30	3	15	280	23	1	10	1 1/2 starch, 1 lean meat
✓12″ Pepperoni	1 slice	210	7	30	4	20	400	23	1	11	1 1/2 starch, 1 high-fat meat
✓14″ Cheese	1 slice	200	7	32	3	15	310	25	1	10	1 1/2 starch, 1 medium-fat meat
14″ Meatsa	1 slice	280	13	42	6	30	630	36	2	15	2 starch, 1 high-fat meat
14″ Pepperoni	1 slice	230	8	31	4	20	430	25	1	12	1 1/2 starch, 1 high-fat meat

✓ = Healthiest Bets

(Continued)

ROUND PIZZA (*Continued*)	Amount	Cal.	Fat (g)	% Cal. Fat	Sat. Fat (g)	Chol. (mg)	Sod. (mg)	Carb. (g)	Fiber (g)	Pro. (g)	Servings/Exchanges
14″ Supreme	1 slice	270	11	37	5	25	510	31	3	13	2 starch, 1 high-fat meat
14″ Veggie	1 slice	240	7	26	3.5	15	710	32	3	12	2 starch, 1 medium-fat meat
✓16″ Cheese	1 slice	220	7	29	3.5	15	340	27	1	11	1 1/2 starch, 1 high-fat meat
16″ Pepperoni	1 slice	240	9	34	4.5	20	450	27	1	12	1 1/2 starch, 1 high-fat meat
✓18″ Cheese	1 slice	230	7	27	3.5	15	350	30	1	12	2 starch, 1 medium-fat meat
18″ Pepperoni	1 slice	260	9	31	4.5	20	480	30	1	13	2 starch, 1 high-fat meat
SALAD DRESSING											
Caesar	3 T	230	25	98	4	55	360	1	0	1	5 fat
Fat Free Italian	3 T	25	0	0	0	0	390	5	0	0	free
Greek	3 T	270	29	97	5	0	200	0	0	0	6 fat
Italian	3 T	220	23	94	3.5	0	370	2	0	0	5 fat
Ranch	3 T	230	24	94	3.5	10	380	2	0	1	5 fat

THIN CRUST											
✔12″ Cheese	1 slice	140	7	45	3	15	190	13	0	8	1 starch, 1 medium-fat meat
✔12″ Pepperoni	1 slice	170	8	42	4	20	290	13	0	9	1 starch, 1 high-fat meat
✔14″ Cheese	1 slice	160	7	39	3.5	15	210	14	0	8	1 starch, 1 high-fat meat
✔14″ Pepperoni	1 slice	180	9	45	4.5	20	320	14	0	9	1 starch, 1 high-fat meat

✔ = Healthiest Bets

Olive Garden Italian Restaurant

❖ Olive Garden gives nutrition information only for its "Garden Fare" menu items on its Web site, www.olivegarden.com. No meals or healthiest bets are provided due to the minimal information available.

Olive Garden Italian Restaurant

	Amount	Cal.	Fat (g)	% Cal. Fat	Sat. Fat (g)	Chol. (mg)	Sod. (mg)	Carb. (g)	Fiber (g)	Pro. (g)	Servings/Exchanges
GARDEN FARE DINNER ENTRÉES											
Capellini Pomodoro	1	611	13	19	n/a	n/a	n/a	n/a	8	n/a	insufficient info. to calculate
Chicken Giardino	1	612	18	26	n/a	n/a	n/a	n/a	8	n/a	insufficient info. to calculate
Linguine alla Marinara	1	514	8	14	n/a	n/a	n/a	n/a	7	n/a	insufficient info. to calculate
Shrimp Primavera	1	738	24	29	n/a	n/a	n/a	n/a	8	n/a	insufficient info. to calculate
GARDEN FARE LUNCH ENTRÉES											
Capellini Pomodoro	1	387	9	21	n/a	n/a	n/a	n/a	6	n/a	insufficient info. to calculate
Chicken Giardino	1	447	15	30	n/a	n/a	n/a	n/a	5	n/a	insufficient info. to calculate

✓ = Healthiest Bets; n/a = not available

(Continued)

GARDEN FARE LUNCH ENTRÉES (*Continued*)	Amount	Cal.	Fat (g)	% Cal. Fat	Sat. Fat (g)	Chol. (mg)	Sod. (mg)	Carb. (g)	Fiber (g)	Pro. (g)	Servings/Exchanges
Linguine alla Marinara	1	316	5	14	n/a	n/a	n/a	n/a	5	n/a	insufficient info. to calculate
Shrimp Primavera	1	497	14	25	n/a	n/a	n/a	n/a	7	n/a	insufficient info. to calculate
SOUP AND SALAD DRESSINGS											
Low Fat Italian Dressing	2 T	37	2	49	n/a	n/a	n/a	n/a	0	n/a	insufficient info. to calculate
Low Fat Parmesan Peppercorn Dressing	2 T	45	2	40	n/a	n/a	n/a	n/a	1	n/a	insufficient info. to calculate
Minestrone	1	158	1	6	n/a	n/a	n/a	n/a	6	n/a	insufficient info. to calculate

✔ = Healthiest Bets; n/a = not available

Papa John's Pizza

❖ Papa John's provides nutrition information for all its pizzas and side items on its Web site at www.papajohns.com.

Light 'n Lean Choice

14″ Original-Crust Garden Fresh Pizza *(3 slices)*

Calories....................570
Fat (g)........................18
% calories from fat..28
Saturated fat (g).....4.5
Cholesterol (mg).........30
Sodium (mg)..........1,410
Carbohydrate (g).........84
Fiber (g).....................6
Protein (g)..................24

Exchanges: 5 starch, 2 veg, 2 high-fat meat, 1/2 fat

Healthy 'n Hearty Choice

14″ Thin-Crust Spinach Alfredo Chicken Tomato Pizza *(3 slices)*

Calories....................750
Fat (g)........................39
% calories from fat..47
Saturated fat (g)......13
Cholesterol (mg).........75
Sodium (mg)..........1,350
Carbohydrate (g).........66
Fiber (g).....................3
Protein (g)..................33

Exchanges: 3 1/2 starch, 2 veg, 3 medium-fat meat, 4 fat

(*Continued*)

Papa John's Pizza

	Amount	Cal.	Fat (g)	% Cal. Fat	Sat. Fat (g)	Chol. (mg)	Sod. (mg)	Carb. (g)	Fiber (g)	Pro. (g)	Servings/Exchanges
12" ORIGINAL CRUST PIZZA											
BBQ Chicken & Bacon	1 slice	230	7	27	2	20	670	31	1	11	2 starch, 1 high-fat meat
Cheese	1 slice	210	8	34	2	15	530	27	1	9	1 1/2 starch, 1 high-fat meat
✓Garden Fresh	1 slice	190	6	28	1.5	10	470	28	2	8	2 starch, 1/2 fat
Grilled Chicken Alfredo	1 slice	210	7	30	2.5	20	510	26	1	11	1 1/2 starch, 1 lean meat, 1 fat
Grilled Chicken Club	1 slice	220	8	33	2	20	580	29	2	11	2 starch, 1 lean meat, 1/2 fat
Hawaiian BBQ Chicken	1 slice	240	7	26	20	20	670	33	1	11	2 starch, 1 lean meat, 1 fat
Pepperoni	1 slice	230	9	35	3	15	580	27	1	10	1 1/2 starch, 1 high-fat meat

Sausage	1 slice	260	13	45	4	20	640	27	2	10	1 1/2 starch, 1 high-fat meat, 1 fat
Spicy Italian	1 slice	270	8	27	8	20	690	27	3	10	1 1/2 starch, 1 high-fat meat, 1 fat
✓Spinach Alfredo	1 slice	190	7	33	3	15	420	25	1	8	1 1/2 starch, 1 medium-fat meat
Spinach Alfredo Chicken Tomato	1 slice	210	8	34	3	20	470	26	2	9	1 1/2 starch, 1 medium-fat meat, 1/2 fat
The Meats w/ Beef	1 slice	270	13	43	4	25	710	27	2	12	1 1/2 starch, 2 medium-fat meat, 1 fat
The Meats w/out Beef	1 slice	250	11	40	3.5	20	670	27	2	11	1 1/2 starch, 1 medium-fat meat, 1 fat
The Works	1 slice	250	9	32	5	20	710	28	2	11	2 starch, 1 high-fat meat
14" ORIGINAL CRUST PIZZA											
BBQ Chicken & Bacon	1 slice	330	11	30	3	30	960	44	2	16	3 starch, 1 high-fat meat

✓ = Healthiest Bets

(*Continued*)

14" ORIGINAL CRUST PIZZA (*Continued*)	Amount	Cal.	Fat (g)	% Cal. Fat	Sat. Fat (g)	Chol. (mg)	Sod. (mg)	Carb. (g)	Fiber (g)	Pro. (g)	Servings/Exchanges
Cheese	1 slice	300	11	33	3.5	20	770	39	2	13	2 1/2 starch, 1 high-fat meat
Garden Fresh	1 slice	270	9	30	2.5	10	680	40	2	11	2 1/2 starch, 1 medium-fat meat
Grilled Chicken Alfredo	1 slice	300	10	30	3.5	30	720	36	2	15	2 starch, 1 lean meat, 1 1/2 fat
Grilled Chicken Club	1 slice	320	11	31	3	30	850	40	2	16	2 1/2 starch, 1 medium-fat meat, 1 fat
Hawaiian BBQ Chicken	1 slice	340	11	29	3	30	960	46	2	16	3 starch, 1 medium-fat meat, 1 fat
Pepperoni	1 slice	330	14	38	4.5	25	860	39	2	14	2 1/2 starch, 1 high-fat meat, 1 fat
Sausage	1 slice	360	18	45	5	25	910	38	3	14	2 1/2 starch, 1 high-fat meat, 1 1/2 fat
Spicy Italian	1 slice	390	11	25	12	35	1020	39	4	15	2 1/2 starch, 1 high-fat meat, 2 fat

Spinach Alfredo	1 slice	280	10	32	4	20	600	36	2	11	2 starch, 1 medium-fat meat, 1 fat
Spinach Alfredo Chicken Tomato	1 slice	300	11	33	4	25	670	37	2	13	2 1/2 starch, 1 medium-fat meat, 1 fat
The Meats w/ Beef	1 slice	380	18	43	6	35	1010	38	3	17	2 1/2 starch, 1 high-fat meat, 2 fat
The Meats w/out Beef	1 slice	350	16	41	5	30	950	38	2	15	2 1/2 starch, 1 high-fat meat, 1 fat
The Works	1 slice	360	13	33	7	30	990	40	3	16	2 1/2 starch, 1 medium-fat meat, 2 fat

14″ THIN CRUST PIZZA

BBQ Chicken & Bacon	1 slice	280	13	42	3.5	30	710	29	0	13	2 starch, 1 medium-fat meat, 1 1/2 fat
Cheese	1 slice	260	14	48	3.5	20	550	24	1	11	1 1/2 starch, 1 high-fat meat, 1/2 fat

✔ = Healthiest Bets

(*Continued*)

14" THIN CRUST PIZZA (*Continued*)	Amount	Cal.	Fat (g)	% Cal. Fat	Sat. Fat (g)	Chol. (mg)	Sod. (mg)	Carb. (g)	Fiber (g)	Pro. (g)	Servings/Exchanges
Garden Fresh	1 slice	230	11	43	2.5	10	460	25	2	8	1 1/2 starch, 1 high-fat meat
Grilled Chicken Alfredo	1 slice	250	13	47	4	30	500	21	1	13	1 1/2 starch, 1 lean meat, 2 fat
Grilled Chicken Club	1 slice	270	14	47	3.5	30	620	25	2	14	1 1/2 starch, 1 lean meat, 2 fat
Hawaiian BBQ Chicken	1 slice	290	13	40	3.5	30	740	21	1	13	1 1/2 starch, 1 medium-fat meat, 2 fat
Pepperoni	1 slice	280	16	51	4.5	25	640	24	1	11	1 1/2 starch, 1 high-fat meat, 1 fat
Sausage	1 slice	310	20	58	6	25	690	23	2	11	1 1/2 starch, 1 high-fat meat, 2 fat
Spicy Italian	1 slice	340	14	37	12	35	800	24	3	13	1 1/2 starch, 1 high-fat meat, 2 fat
Spinach Alfredo	1 slice	230	13	51	4.5	20	380	21	1	8	1 1/2 starch, 1 medium-fat meat, 1 fat

Spinach Alfredo Chicken Tomato	1 slice	250	13	47	4.5	25	450	22	1	11	1 1/2 starch, 1 lean meat, 1 1/2 fat
The Meats w/ Beef	1 slice	330	20	55	6	35	790	23	2	14	1 1/2 starch, 2 high-fat meat
The Meats w/out Beef	1 slice	300	18	54	5	30	730	23	2	13	1 1/2 starch, 1 medium-fat meat, 2 1/2 fat
The Works	1 slice	310	15	44	7	30	780	25	2	13	1 1/2 starch, 1 medium-fat meat, 2 1/2 fat
SIDE ITEMS											
✓BBQ Dipping Sauce	2 T	40	0	0	0	0	240	11	0	0	1/2 starch
Blue Cheese Dipping Sauce	2 T	170	18	95	3.5	20	240	1	0	1	3 1/2 fat
✓Breadsticks	1 stick	140	2	13	0	0	260	26	1	4	1 1/2 starch
Buffalo Dipping Sauce	2 T	15	1	60	0	0	890	2	0	0	free
Cheese Dipping Sauce	2 T	70	6	77	1.5	0	150	1	0	1	1 1/2 fat

✓ = Healthiest Bets

(*Continued*)

SIDE ITEMS (*Continued*)	Amount	Cal.	Fat (g)	% Cal. Fat	Sat. Fat (g)	Chol. (mg)	Sod. (mg)	Carb. (g)	Fiber (g)	Pro. (g)	Servings/Exchanges
Cheesesticks	2 sticks	360	16	40	4.5	25	830	42	2	15	3 starch, 1 high-fat meat, 1 fat
Garlic Dipping Sauce	2 T	150	17	100	3	n/a	310	n/a	0	0	3 fat
Honey Mustard Dipping Sauce	2 T	150	15	90	2	10	120	5	0	1	3 fat
Papa's Chicken Strips	2 strips	160	8	45	2	25	350	10	0	10	1/2 starch, 1 lean meat, 1 1/2 fat
Papa's Cinnapple	2 slices	200	8	36	1.5	n/a	320	29	0	3	1 carb, 1 fruit, 1 1/2 fat
Papa's Mild Chipotle Barbecue Wings	2 wings	160	10	56	3	85	n/a	5	0	13	2 lean meat, 1 fat
Papa's Spicy Buffalo Wings	2 wings	160	11	62	3.5	90	n/a	1	0	14	2 lean meat, 1 fat
✔Pizza Dipping Sauce	2 T	20	0	0	0	0	140	3	0	0	free
Ranch Dipping Sauce	2 T	110	11	90	2	10	250	1	0	1	2 fat

✔ = Healthiest Bets; n/a = not available

Papa Murphy's Take 'N' Bake

❖ Papa Murphy's provides nutrition information for all its menu items on its Web site at www.papamurphys.com.

Light 'n Lean Choice

Veggie Calzone
Family Club Salad
(1 serving, no dressing included)

Calories	540	Sodium (mg)	1,150
Fat (g)	26	Carbohydrate (g)	51
% calories from fat	43	Fiber (g)	5
Saturated fat (g)	10.5	Protein (g)	28
Cholesterol (mg)	50		

Exchanges: 3 starch, 1 veg, 3 medium-fat meat, 1 fat

Healthy 'n Hearty Choice

Gourmet Veggie Pizza *(2 slices)*
Family Club Salad
(1 serving, no dressing included)

Calories	730	Sodium (mg)	1,570
Fat (g)	37	Carbohydrate (g)	67
% calories from fat	46	Fiber (g)	6
Saturated fat (g)	15.5	Protein (g)	39
Cholesterol (mg)	70		

Exchanges: 4 starch, 2 veg, 3 high-fat meat, 3 fat

(*Continued*)

Papa Murphy's Take 'N' Bake

	Amount	Cal.	Fat (g)	% Cal. Fat	Sat. Fat (g)	Chol. (mg)	Sod. (mg)	Carb. (g)	Fiber (g)	Pro. (g)	Servings/Exchanges
CALZONES - FAMILY SIZE											
Combo Calzone	1/8	450	20	40	9	45	870	45	2	22	3 starch, 2 high-fat meat
Italian Calzone	1/8	480	23	43	9	45	970	46	2	23	3 starch, 2 high-fat meat, 1/2 fat
✓Veggie Calzone	1/8	410	17	37	7	30	720	46	3	19	3 starch, 1 high-fat meat, 1 1/2 fat
DEEP DISH PIZZAS - FAMILY SIZE											
Traditional DD	1/8	440	24	49	10	40	900	34	2	23	2 starch, 2 medium-fat meat, 3 fat
DESSERTS											
Apple Dessert Pizza	1 slice	240	5	19	1	0	280	47	2	4	2 starch, 1 fruit, 1 fat
Cherry Dessert Pizza	1 slice	230	5	20	1	0	270	44	2	4	2 starch, 1 fruit, 1 fat
Chocolate Chip Cookies	2	250	11	40	3.5	10	220	34	0	2	2 1/2 carb, 1 1/2 fat

GOURMET PIZZAS - FAMILY SIZE											
Chicken Garlic	1 slice	320	15	42	6	35	600	30	1	18	2 starch, 2 lean meat, 1 1/2 fat
Classic Italian	1 slice	360	19	48	8	35	730	30	2	18	2 starch, 2 high-fat meat
Gourmet Veggie	1 slice	300	14	42	6	25	570	31	2	15	2 starch, 1 high-fat meat, 1 fat
PAPA'S PIZZAS - FAMILY SIZE											
All Meat	1/12	370	19	46	8	40	860	31	2	20	2 starch, 2 high-fat meat
BBQ Chicken	1/12	320	13	37	6	35	780	32	2	19	2 starch, 1 lean meat, 2 fat
Cheese	1/12	270	10	33	5	20	470	29	2	14	2 starch, 1 high-fat meat
Cowboy	1/12	370	19	46	7	35	850	31	2	18	2 starch, 1 high-fat meat, 2 fat
Hawaiian	1/12	290	11	34	5	25	580	34	2	16	2 starch, 1 medium-fat meat, 1 fat
Murphy's Combo	1/12	380	20	47	7	35	910	32	2	18	2 starch, 2 high-fat meat
Papa's Favorite	1/12	380	20	47	8	35	860	32	2	18	2 starch, 2 high-fat meat
Pepperoni	1/12	310	15	44	7	30	650	29	2	16	2 starch, 1 high-fat meat, 1 fat

✔ = Healthiest Bets

(Continued)

PAPA'S PIZZAS - FAMILY SIZE (*Continued*)	Amount	Cal.	Fat (g)	% Cal. Fat	Sat. Fat (g)	Chol. (mg)	Sod. (mg)	Carb. (g)	Fiber (g)	Pro. (g)	Servings/Exchanges
Perfect	1/12	300	13	39	6	25	620	32	2	16	2 starch, 1 high-fat meat, 1/2 fat
Rancher	1/12	330	15	41	7	30	720	31	2	18	2 starch, 1 medium-fat meat, 2 fat
Specialty	1/12	340	17	45	6	30	740	31	2	17	2 starch, 1 medium-fat meat, 2 1/2 fat
Veggie Combo	1/12	300	13	39	5	20	570	32	2	14	2 starch, 1 medium-fat meat, 2 fat
SALADS W/OUT DRESSING											
✓Family Club	1	130	9	62	3.5	20	430	5	2	9	1 veg, 2 fat
Individual Club	1	290	21	65	8	50	930	11	4	21	2 veg, 3 lean meat, 2 1/2 fat
SIDES											
Cheesy Bread	2 pieces	180	7	35	2	5	290	23	0	7	1 1/2 starch, 1 1/2 fat
STUFFED PIZZAS - FAMILY SIZE											
Big Murphy	1/16	380	17	40	7	30	800	39	2	18	2 1/2 starch, 2 medium-fat meat, 1 1/2 fat

Chicago - Style	1/16	370	16	39	7	30	770	39	2	17	2 1/2 starch, 2 medium-fat meat, 1 fat
Chicken & Bacon	1/16	370	16	39	6	35	750	38	2	19	2 1/2 starch, 1 lean meat, 1 high-fat meat, 1/2 fat
THIN CRUST DELITES - LARGE SIZE											
✔BBQ Chicken deLite	1 slice	160	8	45	3.5	25	360	12	0	11	1 starch, 1 medium-fat meat
✔Cheese deLite	1 slice	130	6	42	3.5	15	240	11	0	8	1 starch, 1 lean meat, 1/2 fat
✔Hawaiian deLite	1 slice	140	7	45	3.5	15	300	14	1	9	1 starch, 1 medium-fat meat
Meat deLite	1 slice	190	12	57	5	25	430	11	0	11	1 starch, 1 high-fat meat
✔Pepperoni deLite	1 slice	160	9	51	4.5	20	350	11	0	9	1 starch, 1 high-fat meat
✔Veggie deLite	1 slice	150	8	48	3.5	15	200	11	0	8	1 starch, 1 medium-fat meat

✔ = Healthiest Bets

Pizza Hut

❖ Pizza Hut provides nutrition information for all its menu items on its Web site at www.pizzahut.com.

Light 'n Lean Choice

12″ Medium Thin 'N Crispy Chicken Lover's Pizza *(3 slices)*

Calories	600	Sodium (mg)	1,560
Fat (g)	21	Carbohydrate (g)	66
% calories from fat	32	Fiber (g)	3
Saturated fat	10.5	Protein (g)	36
Cholesterol (mg)	75		

Exchanges: 4 starch, 1 veg, 3 medium-fat meat, 1 fat

Healthy 'n Hearty Choice

14″ Large Thin 'N Crispy Supreme Pizza *(3 slices)*

Calories	750	Sodium (mg)	1,860
Fat (g)	30	Carbohydrate (g)	84
% calories from fat	36	Fiber (g)	6
Saturated fat (g)	15	Protein (g)	39
Cholesterol (mg)	75		

Exchanges: 5 starch, 2 veg, 3 high-fat meat

Pizza Hut

	Amount	Cal.	Fat (g)	% Cal. Fat	Sat. Fat (g)	Chol. (mg)	Sod. (mg)	Carb. (g)	Fiber (g)	Pro. (g)	Servings/Exchanges
12″ MEDIUM HAND-TOSSED-STYLE PIZZAS											
Cheese Only	1 slice	240	8	30	1.5	25	520	30	22	12	2 starch, 1 medium-fat meat
Chicken Supreme	1 slice	230	6	23	3	25	550	30	2	14	2 starch, 1 medium-fat meat
Meat Lover's	1 slice	300	13	39	6	35	760	29	2	15	2 starch, 1 high-fat meat, 1 fat
Pepperoni	1 slice	250	9	32	4.5	25	570	29	2	12	2 starch, 1 high-fat meat
Pepperoni Lover's	1 slice	300	13	39	7	40	710	30	2	15	2 starch, 1 high-fat meat, 1 fat
Quartered Ham	1 slice	220	6	25	3	20	550	29	2	12	2 starch, 1 lean meat, 1/2 fat
Super Supreme	1 slice	300	13	39	6	35	780	31	2	15	2 starch, 1 high-fat meat, 1 fat
Supreme	1 slice	270	11	37	5	25	660	30	2	13	2 starch, 1 high-fat meat

✓ = Healthiest Bets

(Continued)

12" MEDIUM HAND-TOSSED-STYLE PIZZAS (*Continued*)	Amount	Cal.	Fat (g)	% Cal. Fat	Sat. Fat (g)	Chol. (mg)	Sod. (mg)	Carb. (g)	Fiber (g)	Pro. (g)	Servings/Exchanges
✓Veggie Lover's	1 slice	220	6	25	3	15	490	31	2	10	2 starch, 1 medium-fat meat
Sausage Lover's	1 slice	280	12	39	5	30	650	30	2	13	2 starch, 1 high-fat meat, 1/2 fat
12" MEDIUM PAN PIZZAS											
Cheese Only	1 slice	280	13	42	5	25	500	29	1	11	2 starch, 1 high-fat meat
Chicken Supreme	1 slice	280	12	39	4	25	530	30	2	13	2 starch, 1 high-fat meat, 1/2 fat
Meat Lover's	1 slice	340	19	50	7	35	750	29	2	15	2 starch, 1 high-fat meat, 2 fat
Pepperoni	1 slice	290	15	47	5	25	560	29	12	11	2 starch, 1 high-fat meat, 1 fat
Pepperoni Lover's	1 slice	340	19	50	7	40	700	29	2	15	2 starch, 1 high-fat meat, 2 fat
Quartered Ham	1 slice	260	11	38	4	20	540	29	1	11	2 starch, 1 high-fat meat
Sausage Lover's	1 slice	330	17	46	6	30	640	29	2	13	2 starch, 1 high-fat meat, 1 1/2 fat
Super Supreme	1 slice	340	18	48	6	35	760	30	2	14	2 starch, 1 high-fat meat, 2 fat

Supreme	1 slice	320	16	45	6	25	650	30	2	13	2 starch, 1 high-fat meat, 1 1/2 fat
Veggie Lover's	1 slice	260	12	42	4	15	570	30	2	10	2 starch, 1 high-fat meat
12" MEDIUM THIN 'N CRISPY PIZZAS											
✔Cheese Only	1 slice	200	8	36	4.5	25	490	21	1	10	1 1/2 starch, 1 medium-fat meat
Chicken Supreme	1 slice	200	7	32	3.5	25	520	22	1	12	1 1/2 starch, 1 medium-fat meat
Meat Lover's	1 slice	270	14	47	6	35	740	21	2	13	1 1/2 starch, 1 high-fat meat, 1 fat
Pepperoni	1 slice	210	10	43	4.5	25	550	21	1	10	1 1/2 starch, 1 high-fat meat
Pepperoni Lover's	1 slice	260	14	48	7	40	690	21	2	13	1 1/2 starch, 1 high-fat meat, 1 fat
Quartered Ham	1 slice	180	6	30	3	20	530	21	1	9	1 1/2 starch, 1 lean meat
Sausage Lover's	1 slice	240	13	49	6	30	630	21	2	11	1 1/2 starch, 1 high-fat meat, 1/2 fat

✔ = Healthiest Bets

(*Continued*)

12" MEDIUM THIN 'N CRISPY PIZZAS (*Continued*)	Amount	Cal.	Fat (g)	% Cal. Fat	Sat. Fat (g)	Chol. (mg)	Sod. (mg)	Carb. (g)	Fiber (g)	Pro. (g)	Servings/Exchanges
Super Supreme	1 slice	260	13	45	6	35	760	23	2	13	1 1/2 starch, 1 high-fat meat, 1 fat
Supreme	1 slice	240	11	41	5	25	640	22	2	11	1 1/2 starch, 1 high-fat meat
✓Veggie Lover's	1 slice	180	7	35	3	15	480	23	2	8	1 1/2 starch, 1 medium-fat meat
14" LARGE HAND-TOSSED-STYLE PIZZAS											
Cheese Only	1 slice	220	8	33	4.5	25	480	27	1	11	1 1/2 starch, 1 high-fat meat
14" LARGE PAN PIZZAS											
Cheese Only	1 slice	270	13	43	5	25	470	27	1	11	1 1/2 starch, 1 high-fat meat, 1/2 fat
Chicken Supreme	1 slice	260	11	38	4	20	490	27	1	12	1 1/2 starch, 1 medium-fat meat, 1 1/2 fat
Meat Lover's	1 slice	320	18	51	6	35	690	27	2	14	1 1/2 starch, 2 high-fat meat

Pepperoni	1 slice	280	14	45	5	25	530	26	1	11	1 1/2 starch, 1 high-fat meat, 1 fat
Pepperoni Lover's	1 slice	330	18	49	7	35	670	27	2	14	1 1/2 starch, 1 high-fat meat, 1 1/2 fat
Quartered Ham	1 slice	250	11	40	4	20	510	26	1	11	1 1/2 starch, 1 lean meat, 1 1/2 fat
Sausage Lover's	1 slice	300	17	51	6	30	590	27	2	12	1 1/2 starch, 1 high-fat meat, 1 1/2 fat
Super Supreme	1 slice	320	17	48	6	30	700	28	2	13	2 starch, 1 high-fat meat, 2 fat
Supreme	1 slice	300	16	48	6	25	600	27	2	12	1 1/2 starch, 1 medium-fat meat, 2 fat
✓Veggie Lover's	1 slice	250	11	40	4	15	440	28	2	9	2 starch, 1 high-fat meat
14" LARGE THIN 'N CRISPY PIZZAS											
Cheese Only	1 slice	190	8	38	4.5	25	460	20	1	9	1 starch, 1 high-fat meat
✓Chicken Supreme	1 slice	180	6	30	3	20	480	21	1	11	1 1/2 starch, 1 lean meat

✓ = Healthiest Bets

(*Continued*)

14" LARGE THIN 'N CRISPY PIZZAS (*Continued*)	Amount	Cal.	Fat (g)	% Cal. Fat	Sat. Fat (g)	Chol. (mg)	Sod. (mg)	Carb. (g)	Fiber (g)	Pro. (g)	Servings/Exchanges
Meat Lover's	1 slice	250	13	47	6	35	700	20	2	12	1 starch, 1 high-fat meat, 1 1/2 fat
Pepperoni	1 slice	200	9	41	4.5	25	520	19	1	9	1 starch, 1 high-fat meat
Pepperoni Lover's	1 slice	250	14	50	6	35	660	20	1	12	1 starch, 1 high-fat meat, 1 1/2 fat
Quartered Ham	1 slice	170	6	32	3	20	500	19	1	9	1 starch, 1 lean meat, 1/2 fat
Sausage Lover's	1 slice	230	12	47	5	30	580	20	1	10	1 starch, 1 high-fat meat, 1/2 fat
Super Supreme	1 slice	240	12	45	5	30	710	21	2	12	1 1/2 starch, 1 high-fat meat
Supreme	1 slice	220	11	45	5	25	600	21	2	11	1 1/2 starch, 1 high-fat meat
✓Veggie Lover's	1 slice	170	7	37	3	15	450	21	2	8	1 1/2 starch, 1 medium-fat meat
14" STUFFED CRUST PIZZAS											
Cheese Only	1 slice	360	13	33	8	40	920	43	2	18	3 starch, 1 high-fat meat, 1/2 fat

Chicken Supreme	1 slice	380	13	31	7	40	1020	44	3	20	3 starch, 1 lean meat, 1 high-fat meat
Meat Lover's	1 slice	450	21	42	10	55	1250	43	3	21	3 starch, 2 high-fat meat
Pepperoni	1 slice	370	15	36	8	45	970	42	3	18	3 starch, 1 high-fat meat, 1 fat
Pepperoni Lover's	1 slice	420	19	41	40	55	1120	43	3	21	3 starch, 2 high-fat meat
Quartered Ham	1 slice	340	11	29	6	40	960	42	2	18	3 starch, 1 lean meat, 1 fat
Sausage Lover's	1 slice	430	19	40	9	50	1130	43	3	19	3 starch, 2 high-fat meat
Super Supreme	1 slice	440	20	41	9	50	1270	45	3	21	3 starch, 2 high-fat meat
Supreme	1 slice	400	16	36	8	45	1070	44	3	20	3 starch, 2 medium-fat meat
Veggie Lover's	1 slice	360	14	35	7	35	980	45	3	16	3 starch, 1 high-fat meat, 1/2 fat
16″ EXTRA LARGE PIZZAS											
Cheese Only	1 slice	420	15	32	8	45	1080	51	3	20	3 1/2 starch, 2 medium-fat meat
Chicken Supreme	1 slice	400	12	27	63	40	1070	52	3	22	3 1/2 starch, 1 lean meat, 1 medium-fat meat

✓ = Healthiest Bets

(*Continued*)

16" EXTRA LARGE PIZZAS (*Continued*)	Amount	Cal.	Fat (g)	% Cal. Fat	Sat. Fat (g)	Chol. (mg)	Sod. (mg)	Carb. (g)	Fiber (g)	Pro. (g)	Servings/Exchanges
Meat Lover's	1 slice	500	22	40	10	60	1400	51	3	24	3 1/2 starch, 2 high-fat meat
Pepperoni	1 slice	430	17	36	8	45	1130	50	3	19	3 1/2 starch, 1 high-fat meat, 1 1/2 fat
Pepperoni Lover's	1 slice	520	24	42	11	65	1370	51	3	25	3 1/2 starch, 2 high-fat meat, 1 fat
Quartered Ham	1 slice	380	12	28	6	4	1110	50	3	19	3 1/2 starch, 1 lean meat, 1 medium-fat meat
Sausage Lover's	1 slice	510	23	41	10	55	1330	51	3	23	3 1/2 starch, 2 high-fat meat, 1/2 fat
Super Supreme	1 slice	490	21	39	9	55	1430	53	4	23	3 1/2 starch, 2 high-fat meat
Supreme	1 slice	460	19	37	9	45	1250	52	4	22	3 1/2 starch, 2 high-fat meat
Veggie Lover's	1 slice	390	12	28	6	30	1030	53	4	17	3 1/2 starch, 1 high-fat meat

6" PERSONAL PAN PIZZAS											
✓Cheese Only	1 slice	160	7	39	3	15	310	18	0	7	1 starch, 1 medium-fat meat
✓Chicken Supreme	1 slice	160	6	34	2.5	15	320	19	0	8	1 starch, 1 lean meat, 1/2 fat
Meat Lover's	1 slice	200	10	45	4	20	470	18	1	9	1 starch, 1 high-fat meat
✓Pepperoni	1 slice	170	8	42	3	15	340	18	0	7	1 starch, 1 high-fat meat
Pepperoni Lover's	1 slice	200	10	45	4.5	25	440	18	1	9	1 starch, 1 high-fat meat
✓Quartered Ham	1 slice	150	6	36	2	15	330	18	0	7	1 starch, 1 medium-fat meat
✓Sausage Lover's	1 slice	190	10	47	4	20	400	18	1	8	1 starch, 1 high-fat meat
Super Supreme	1 slice	200	10	45	4	20	480	19	1	9	1 starch, 1 high-fat meat
Supreme	1 slice	190	9	43	3.5	20	420	19	1	8	1 starch, 1 high-fat meat
✓Veggie Lover's	1 slice	150	6	36	2	10	280	19	1	6	1 starch, 1 medium-fat meat

✓ = Healthiest Bets

(*Continued*)

	Amount	Cal.	Fat (g)	% Cal. Fat	Sat. Fat (g)	Chol. (mg)	Sod. (mg)	Carb. (g)	Fiber (g)	Pro. (g)	Servings/Exchanges
APPETIZERS											
✓Breadsticks	1	150	6	36	1	0	220	20	0	4	1 1/2 starch, 1 fat
✓Breadsticks Dipping Sauce	6 T	50	0	0	0	0	370	11	2	1	1/2 starch
Cheese Breadsticks	1	200	10	45	3.5	15	340	21	0	7	1 1/2 starch, 2 fat
Hot Wings	2 pieces	110	6	49	2	70	450	1	0	11	2 lean meat
Mild Wings	2 pieces	110	7	57	2	70	320	0	0	11	2 lean meat
Wing Blue Cheese Dipping Sauce	3 T	230	24	94	5	25	550	2	0	2	5 fat
Wing Ranch Dipping Sauce	3 T	210	22	94	3.5	10	340	4	0	2	4 1/2 fat
DESSERTS											
Apple Dessert Pizza	1 slice	260	4	14	0.5	0	250	53	1	4	3 1/2 carb, 1 fat

Cherry Dessert Pizza	1 slice	240	4	15	0.5	0	250	47	1	4	3 carb, 1 fat
✓Cinnamon Sticks	2 pieces	170	5	26	1	0	170	27	0	4	1 1/2 carb, 1 fat
White Icing Dipping Cup	4 T	190	0	0	0	0	0	46	0	0	3 carb
DRESSINGS											
Caesar Dressing	2 T	150	16	96	3	5	380	1	0	0	3 fat
French Dressing	2 T	140	11	71	2	0	220	11	0	0	1/2 carb, 2 fat
Italian Dressing	2 T	140	15	96	2.5	0	360	2	0	0	3 fat
Lite Italian Dressing	2 T	60	5	75	1	0	410	5	0	0	1 fat
Lite Ranch Dressing	2 T	70	7	90	1.5	10	200	0	0	0	1 1/2 fat
Ranch Dressing	2 T	100	10	90	2	5	240	2	0	0	2 fat
Thousand Island Dressing	2 T	110	9	74	1.5	10	300	6	0	0	1/2 carb, 2 fat

✓ = Healthiest Bets

(*Continued*)

	Amount	Cal.	Fat (g)	% Cal. Fat	Sat. Fat (g)	Chol. (mg)	Sod. (mg)	Carb. (g)	Fiber (g)	Pro. (g)	Servings/Exchanges
FIT 'N DELICIOUS 12" MEDIUM											
Diced Chicken, Mushroom, Jalapeno	1 slice	170	5	26	2	15	690	22	2	10	1 1/2 starch, 1 lean meat
✓Diced Chicken, Red Onion & Green Pepper	1 slice	170	5	26	2	15	460	23	2	10	1 1/2 starch, 1 lean meat
✓Green Pepper, Red Onion, & Diced Tomato	1 slice	150	4	24	1.5	10	360	24	2	6	1 1/2 starch, 1/2 fat
✓Ham, Pineapple, & Diced Tomato	1 slice	160	4	23	2	15	470	24	2	8	1 1/2 starch, 1 fat
✓Ham, Red Onion, & Mushroom	1 slice	160	5	28	2	15	470	22	2	8	1 1/2 starch, 1 fat

Tomato, Mushroom, & Jalapeno	1 slice	150	4	24	2	10	590	22	2	6	1 1/2 starch, 1 lean meat
FIT 'N DELICIOUS 14″ MEDIUM											
Diced Chicken, Mushroom, Jalapeno	1 slice	160	5	28	2	15	630	20	2	9	1 1/2 starch, 1 lean meat
✔Diced Chicken, Red Onion & Green Pepper	1 slice	160	4	23	2	15	420	22	2	9	1 1/2 starch, 1 lean meat
✔Green Pepper, Red Onion, & Diced Tomato	1 slice	140	4	26	1.5	10	330	22	2	6	1 1/2 starch, 1 lean meat
✔Ham, Pineapple, & Diced Tomato	1 slice	150	4	24	2	15	440	22	1	7	1 1/2 starch, 1 lean meat

✔ = Healthiest Bets

(*Continued*)

FIT 'N DELICIOUS 14" MEDIUM (*Continued*)	Amount	Cal.	Fat (g)	% Cal. Fat	Sat. Fat (g)	Chol. (mg)	Sod. (mg)	Carb. (g)	Fiber (g)	Pro. (g)	Servings/Exchanges
✓Ham, Red Onion, & Mushroom	1 slice	150	4	24	2	15	440	21	2	8	1 lean meat
Tomato, Mushroom, & Jalapeno	1 slice	140	4	26	1.5	10	540	21	2	6	1 1/2 starch, 1 lean meat
P'ZONE											
Classic	1/2	610	21	31	11	50	1210	71	3	33	4 1/2 starch, 3 medium-fat meat, 1 fat
Marinara Dipping Sauce	1/2	85	0	0	0	0	380	9	2	2	1 starch
Meat Lover's	1/2	680	28	37	14	65	1540	70	3	38	4 1/2 starch, 3 high-fat meat
Pepperoni	1/2	610	22	32	11	55	1280	69	3	34	4 1/2 starch, 3 medium-fat meat, 1 fat

✓ = Healthiest Bets

Round Table Pizza

❖ Round Table Pizza provides nutrition information for all its menu items on its Web site at www.roundtablepizza.com.

Light 'n Lean Choice

Guinevere's Garden Delight Pizza, Large Pan *(2 slices)*

Calories	580	Sodium (mg)	1,380
Fat (g)	18	Carbohydrate (g)	76
% calories from fat	28	Fiber (g)	4
Saturated fat (g)	10	Protein (g)	22
Cholesterol (mg)	50		

Exchanges: 4 1/2 starch, 2 veg, 4 medium-fat meat, 2 fat

Healthy 'n Hearty Choice

Western BBQ Chicken Supreme, Large Skinny Crust *(3 slices)*
Caesar Salad *(small, no dressing included)*

Calories	740	Sodium (mg)	2,310
Fat (g)	34	Carbohydrate (g)	62
% calories from fat	41	Fiber (g)	5
Saturated fat (g)	16	Protein (g)	39
Cholesterol (mg)	121		

Exchanges: 4 starch, 3 veg, 3 medium-fat meat, 3 fat

(Continued)

Round Table Pizza

	Amount	Cal.	Fat (g)	% Cal. Fat	Sat. Fat (g)	Chol. (mg)	Sod. (mg)	Carb. (g)	Fiber (g)	Pro. (g)	Servings/Exchanges
APPETIZERS											
Buffalo Wings	6 pieces	420	28	60	7	210	1060	2	0	38	5 lean meat, 3 fat
Buffalo Wings	12 pieces	860	62	65	17	310	3530	10	0	67	1/2 starch, 9 lean meat, 7 fat
Garlic Bread	1 serving	470	21	40	4.5	5	910	59	2	11	4 starch, 4 fat
Garlic Bread w/ Cheese	1 serving	630	33	47	13	45	1240	59	2	21	4 starch, 1 high-fat meat, 4 1/2 fat
Garlic Parmesan Twists	6 pieces	880	22	23	9	40	2380	135	5	31	9 starch, 4 fat
Garlic Parmesan Twists	3 pieces	510	14	25	5	25	1350	76	3	17	5 starch, 3 fat

Honey BBQ Wings	6 pieces	390	25	58	7	205	740	8	0	35	1/2 starch, 5 lean meat, 2 fat
Honey BBQ Wings	12 pieces	930	55	53	16	275	2130	27	0	71	1 1/2 starch, 10 lean meat, 4 fat
ORIGINAL CRUST PERSONAL PIZZA											
Cheese	1 pizza	580	24	37	315	70	1410	60	3	26	4 starch, 2 high-fat meat, 1 fat
Chicken & Garlic Gourmet	1 pizza	620	25	36	13	85	1600	64	3	29	4 starch, 2 medium-fat meat, 4 fat
Chicken Rostadoro	1 pizza	680	29	38	15	85	2040	66	4	35	4 1/2 starch, 3 lean meat, 4 fat
Gourmet Veggie	1 pizza	590	23	35	12	60	1270	67	5	25	4 1/2 starch, 2 high-fat meat, 1/2 fat
Guinevere's Garden Delight	1 pizza	550	20	33	11	50	1440	66	5	23	4 1/2 starch, 1 high-fat meat, 2 fat

✓ = Healthiest Bets

(*Continued*)

ORIGINAL CRUST PERSONAL PIZZA (*Continued*)	Amount	Cal.	Fat (g)	% Cal. Fat	Sat. Fat (g)	Chol. (mg)	Sod. (mg)	Carb. (g)	Fiber (g)	Pro. (g)	Servings/Exchanges
Hearty Bacon Supreme	1 pizza	700	35	45	16	85	1790	59	3	32	4 starch, 3 high-fat meat, 1 fat
Italian Garlic Supreme	1 pizza	760	41	49	18	95	1780	63	3	30	4 starch, 3 high-fat meat, 3 1/2 fat
King Arthur Supreme	1 pizza	750	39	47	16	105	2110	64	4	33	4 starch, 3 high-fat meat, 3 fat
Maui Zaui	1 pizza	590	22	34	12	70	1680	66	1	29	4 1/2 starch, 3 medium-fat meat
Montague's All Meat Marvel	1 pizza	780	44	51	17	110	2150	61	3	33	4 starch, 3 high-fat meat, 4 fat
Pepperoni	1 pizza	640	31	44	15	80	1780	60	3	27	4 starch, 2 high-fat meat, 3 fat
Pepperoni Rostadoro	1 pizza	740	35	43	17	85	2130	70	4	33	4 1/2 starch, 3 high-fat meat, 2 fat

Roastin' Toastin' Chicken Club	1 pizza	710	33	42	15	90	1790	66	3	33	4 starch, 3 medium-fat meat, 3 1/2 fat
Western BBQ Chicken	1 pizza	610	23	34	12	85	1780	61	3	28	4 starch, 2 lean meat, 4 fat
ORIGINAL CRUST, LARGE											
Cheese	1 slice	210	8	34	5	25	530	25	1	11	1 1/2 starch, 1 high-fat meat
Chicken & Garlic Gourmet	1 slice	240	10	38	4.5	35	590	26	1	12	1 1/2 starch, 1 high-fat meat
Chicken Rostadoro	1 slice	250	10	36	5	30	750	26	2	13	1 1/2 starch, 1 medium-fat meat, 1 fat
Gourmet Veggie	1 slice	220	9	37	1.5	20	480	26	2	10	1 1/2 starch, 1 high-fat meat
Guinevere's Garden Delite	1 slice	210	7	30	4	20	550	26	2	10	1 1/2 starch, 1 high-fat meat

✓ = Healthiest Bets

(*Continued*)

ORIGINAL CRUST, LARGE (*Continued*)	Amount	Cal.	Fat (g)	% Cal. Fat	Sat. Fat (g)	Chol. (mg)	Sod. (mg)	Carb. (g)	Fiber (g)	Pro. (g)	Servings/Exchanges
Hawaiian	1 slice	210	7	30	4	25	620	26	1	11	1 1/2 starch, 1 high-fat meat
Hearty Bacon Supreme	1 slice	290	16	50	6	35	730	24	1	13	1 1/2 starch, 1 high-fat meat, 1 1/2 fat
Italian Garlic Supreme	1 slice	270	14	47	6	30	630	25	1	12	1 1/2 starch, 1 high-fat meat, 1 fat
King Arthur's Supreme	1 slice	270	14	47	6	35	730	26	2	12	1 1/2 starch, 1 high-fat meat, 1 fat
Maui Zaui (Polynesian Sauce)	1 slice	250	9	32	5	25	670	28	1	12	1 1/2 starch, 1 medium-fat meat, 1 fat
Maui Zaui (Zesty Red Sauce)	1 slice	240	9	34	4.5	25	700	27	1	12	1 1/2 starch, 1 high-fat meat
Montague's All Meat Marvel	1 slice	300	17	51	6	40	820	25	1	13	1 1/2 starch, 2 high-fat meat

Pepperoni	1 slice	240	11	41	6	30	670	24	1	11	1 1/2 starch, 1 high-fat meat, 1/2 fat
Pepperoni Rostadoro	1 slice	270	12	40	6	30	770	28	1	13	2 starch, 1 high-fat meat
Roastin' Toastin' Chicken Club	1 slice	260	12	42	6	30	650	26	1	13	1 1/2 starch, 1 lean meat, 2 fat
Western BBQ Chicken	1 slice	230	9	35	4.5	35	710	24	1	12	1 1/2 starch, 1 lean meat, 1 fat
PAN CRUST PERSONAL PIZZA											
Chicken Rostadoro	1 pizza	910	31	31	16	85	2510	112	5	41	7 1/2 starch, 3 lean meat, 4 fat
Cheese	1 pizza	810	26	29	15	70	1880	106	4	33	7 starch, 2 high-fat meat, 2 fat
Chicken & Garlic Gourmet	1 pizza	850	27	29	13	85	2120	110	5	36	7 starch, 2 medium-fat meat, 3 fat
Gourmet Veggie	1 pizza	820	25	27	12	60	1790	114	7	32	7 1/2 starch, 2 high-fat meat, 1/2 fat

✓ = Healthiest Bets

(Continued)

PAN CRUST PERSONAL PIZZA (*Continued*)	Amount	Cal.	Fat (g)	% Cal. Fat	Sat. Fat (g)	Chol. (mg)	Sod. (mg)	Carb. (g)	Fiber (g)	Pro. (g)	Servings/Exchanges
Guinevere's Garden Delight	1 pizza	760	21	25	11	50	1850	110	6	29	7 starch, 1 high-fat meat, 2 fat
Hearty Bacon Supreme	1 pizza	940	37	35	16	85	2310	105	4	38	7 starch, 2 high-fat meat, 4 fat
Italian Garlic Supreme	1 pizza	990	43	39	19	95	2310	109	5	37	7 starch, 2 high-fat meat, 5 fat
King Arthur Supreme	1 pizza	900	34	34	15	90	2340	109	5	36	7 starch, 2 high-fat meat, 3 fat
Maui Zaui	1 pizza	820	24	26	12	70	2160	111	5	35	7 1/2 starch, 2 medium-fat meat, 2 1/2 fat
Montague's All Meat Marvel	1 pizza	1010	46	41	18	110	2630	107	4	33	7 starch, 2 high-fat meat, 6 fat
Pepperoni	1 pizza	840	29	31	15	70	2120	106	4	32	7 starch, 2 high-fat meat, 3 fat

Pepperoni Rostadoro	1 pizza	970	37	34	18	85	2610	116	5	39	7 1/2 starch, 3 high-fat meat, 2 fat
Roastin' Toastin' Chicken Club	1 pizza	940	35	34	16	90	2320	112	4	40	7 1/2 starch, 3 medium-fat meat, 3 1/2 fat
Western BBQ Chicken	1 pizza	840	25	27	19	85	2310	107	5	34	7 starch, 2 medium-fat meat, 3 fat
PAN CRUST, LARGE											
Cheese	1 slice	290	10	31	6	25	680	38	1	13	2 1/2 starch, 1 high-fat meat
Chicken & Garlic Gourmet	1 slice	320	11	31	6	35	780	39	2	15	2 1/2 starch, 1 high-fat meat, 1/2 fat
Chicken Rostadoro	1 slice	330	12	33	6	35	920	40	2	17	3 starch, 1 medium-fat meat, 1/2 fat
Gourmet Veggie	1 slice	310	11	32	5	25	670	40	2	13	3 starch, 1 medium-fat meat, 1 fat

✔ = Healthiest Bets

(*Continued*)

PAN CRUST, LARGE (*Continued*)	Amount	Cal.	Fat (g)	% Cal. Fat	Sat. Fat (g)	Chol. (mg)	Sod. (mg)	Carb. (g)	Fiber (g)	Pro. (g)	Servings/Exchanges
Guinevere's Garden Delite	1 slice	290	9	28	5	25	690	39	2	13	2 1/2 starch, 1 high-fat meat
Hawaiian	1 slice	290	9	28	5	30	770	39	2	14	2 1/2 starch, 1 high-fat meat
Hearty Bacon Supreme	1 slice	360	17	43	7	35	920	38	1	16	2 1/2 starch, 1 high-fat meat, 2 fat
Italian Garlic Supreme	1 slice	360	16	40	7	35	820	39	2	15	2 1/2 starch, 1 high-fat meat, 1 1/2 fat
King Arthur's Supreme	1 slice	340	14	37	6	35	840	39	2	15	2 1/2 starch, 1 high-fat meat, 1 fat
Maui Zaui (Polynesian Sauce)	1 slice	330	11	30	6	30	870	42	2	15	3 starch, 1 medium-fat meat, 1 fat
Maui Zaui (Zesty Red Sauce)	1 slice	320	11	31	6	30	860	40	2	16	2 1/2 starch, 1 medium-fat meat, 1 fat

Montague's All Meat Marvel	1 slice	350	16	41	6	40	860	38	2	15	2 1/2 starch, 1 high-fat meat, 1 1/2 fat
Pepperoni	1 slice	320	12	34	6	30	810	38	2	14	2 1/2 starch, 1 high-fat meat, 1 fat
Pepperoni Rostadoro	1 slice	350	14	36	7	35	940	41	2	16	3 starch, 1 high-fat meat, 1 fat
Roastin' Toastin' Chicken Club	1 slice	350	14	36	7	35	840	40	2	16	3 starch, 1 medium-fat meat, 2 fat
Western BBQ Chicken	1 slice	320	11	31	6	25	870	38	2	15	2 1/2 starch, 1 medium-fat meat, 1 fat
SALADS											
✓Caesar Salad	large	140	7	45	2.5	10	390	11	2	6	1/2 starch, 1 veg, 1 medium-fat meat
✓Caesar Salad	small	140	7	45	2.5	10	390	11	2	6	1/2 starch, 1 veg, 1 medium-fat meat

✓ = Healthiest Bets

(Continued)

SALADS (*Continued*)	Amount	Cal.	Fat (g)	% Cal. Fat	Sat. Fat (g)	Chol. (mg)	Sod. (mg)	Carb. (g)	Fiber (g)	Pro. (g)	Servings/Exchanges
✓Garden Salad	large	100	4	36	0	0	220	14	2	2	3 veg, 1/2 fat
✓Garden Salad	small	100	4	36	0	0	220	14	2	2	3 veg, 1/2 fat
SANDWICHES											
Chicken Club	1	820	39	43	14	125	2540	75	3	38	5 carb, 3 medium-fat meat, 4 1/2 fat
Ham Club	1	810	37	41	13	90	2710	76	3	36	5 starch, 3 medium-fat meat, 4 fat
RT Pizza Sandwich	1	690	34	44	15	90	2070	65	4	30	4 starch, 2 high-fat meat, 4 fat
RT Veggie Sandwich	1	680	29	38	11	55	1650	79	5	23	5 starch, 1 high-fat meat, 4 fat
Turkey Club	1	800	37	42	14	85	2290	75	3	39	5 starch, 3 medium-fat meat, 4 fat

SKINNY CRUST, LARGE											
Cheese	1 slice	180	8	40	5	25	460	17	1	10	1 starch, 1 high-fat meat
Chicken & Garlic Gourmet	1 slice	200	9	41	4.5	35	510	19	1	12	1 starch, 1 high-fat meat
Chicken Rostadoro	1 slice	220	10	41	5	30	680	20	1	12	1 starch, 1 medium-fat meat, 1 fat
✓Gourmet Veggie	1 slice	190	8	38	4.5	20	410	20	1	9	1 starch, 1 high-fat meat
Guinevere's Garden	1 slice	170	7	37	4	20	480	20	2	9	1 starch, 1 high-fat meat
Hawaiian	1 slice	180	7	35	4	25	550	20	1	10	1 starch, 1 high-fat meat
Hearty Bacon Supreme	1 slice	260	15	52	6	35	650	17	1	12	1 starch, 1 high-fat meat, 1 1/2 fat
Italian Garlic Supreme	1 slice	240	14	53	6	30	550	18	1	11	1 starch, 1 high-fat meat, 1 fat
King Arthur's Supreme	1 slice	240	14	53	6	35	660	19	1	11	1 starch, 1 high-fat meat, 1 1/2 fat

✓ = Healthiest Bets

(*Continued*)

SKINNY CRUST, LARGE (*Continued*)	Amount	Cal.	Fat (g)	% Cal. Fat	Sat. Fat (g)	Chol. (mg)	Sod. (mg)	Carb. (g)	Fiber (g)	Pro. (g)	Servings/Exchanges
Maui Zaui (Polynesian Sauce)	1 slice	210	9	39	5	25	600	21	1	11	1 1/2 starch, 1 medium-fat meat, 1/2 fat
Maui Zaui (Zesty Red Sauce)	1 slice	210	9	39	4.5	25	620	20	1	12	1 starch, 1 medium-fat meat, 1 fat
Montague's All Meat Marvel	1 slice	260	16	55	6	40	750	18	1	12	1 starch, 1 high-fat meat, 1 fat
Pepperoni	1 slice	210	11	47	5	30	590	18	1	10	1 starch, 1 high-fat meat, 1/2 fat
Pepperoni Rostadoro	1 slice	240	12	45	6	30	700	21	1	12	1 1/2 starch, 1 high-fat meat, 1/2 fat
Roastin' Toastin' Chicken Club	1 slice	230	12	47	5	30	580	19	1	12	1 starch, 1 high-fat meat, 1 fat
Western BBQ Chicken	1 slice	200	9	41	4.5	35	640	17	1	11	1 starch, 1 high-fat meat

✔ = Healthiest Bets

Sbarro

❖ Sbarro provides nutrition information for all its menu items on its Web site at www.sbarro.com.

Light 'n Lean Choice

Spaghetti and Meatballs *(split)*
Mixed Garden Salad *(no dressing included)*
Fruit Salad *(split)*

Calories....................440
Fat (g)........................13
% calories from fat..27
Saturated fat (g).....n/a
Cholesterol (mg)..........8
Sodium (mg).............883
Carbohydrate (g).........71
Fiber (g)...................10
Protein (g)..................13

Exchanges: 3 starch, 2 veg, 1 fruit, 2 fat

Healthy 'n Hearty Choice

Spinach Tomato Broccoli Stromboli
Greek Salad *(no dressing included)*

Calories....................740
Fat (g)........................29
% calories from fat..39
Saturated fat (g).....n/a
Cholesterol (mg).........11
Sodium (mg)..........1,550
Carbohydrate (g).........87
Fiber (g)...................31
Protein (g)..................29

Exchanges: 5 starch, 2 veg, 2 medium-fat meat, 3 fat

(*Continued*)

Sbarro

	Amount	Cal.	Fat (g)	% Cal. Fat	Sat. Fat (g)	Chol. (mg)	Sod. (mg)	Carb. (g)	Fiber (g)	Pro. (g)	Servings/Exchanges
DESSERTS											
Black Forest Cake	1	480	24	45	n/a	50	340	59	1	3	4 carb, 4 fat
Deluxe Carrot Cake	1	540	29	48	n/a	65	400	64	1	5	4 carb, 5 fat
Deluxe Cheese Cake	1	560	40	64	n/a	170	450	42	1	9	3 carb, 8 fat
Deluxe Milk Chocolate Cake	1	490	35	64	n/a	30	310	59	1	4	4 carb, 6 fat
DINNER PLATES											
Baked Ziti w/ Sauce	1	700	41	53	n/a	135	1220	43	4	39	3 starch, 9 fat
Chicken Francese	1	640	38	53	n/a	175	590	8	2	63	1/2 starch, 9 lean meat, 2 1/2 fat
Chicken Parmesan	1	520	22	38	n/a	175	750	16	2	64	1 starch, 8 lean meat

Chicken Portofino	1	730	48	59	n/a	225	790	7	1	63	1/2 starch, 9 lean meat, 4 1/2 fat
Chicken Vesuvio	1	690	43	56	n/a	225	810	8	1	63	1/2 starch, 9 lean meat, 3 1/2 fat
Eggplant Rollatini w/ Cheese	1	580	38	59	n/a	50	900	40	4	21	3 starch, 2 medium-fat meat, 4 1/2 fat
✓Garlic Rolls	1	170	5	26	n/a	0	370	28	0	5	2 starch, 1/2 fat
Meat Lasagna	1	650	37	51	n/a	130	1130	36	3	41	2 1/2 starch, 5 medium-fat meat, 2 fat
Meatballs	1	140	9	58	n/a	30	880	10	1	8	1/2 starch, 1 high-fat meat
Mixed Vegetables	1	190	15	71	n/a	0	330	14	4	3	3 veg, 3 fat
Pasta Milano	1	640	32	45	n/a	175	740	41	6	45	3 starch, 4 high-fat meat
Pasta Rustica	1	600	47	71	n/a	70	2288	39	5	10	2 1/2 starch, 9 fat
Penne alla Vodka	1	640	28	39	n/a	120	1000	67	5	23	4 1/2 starch, 1 high-fat meat, 4 fat
Penne w/ Sausage & Peppers	1	710	49	62	n/a	130	1690	33	4	35	2 starch, 4 high-fat meat, 3 1/2 fat

✓ = Healthiest Bets; n/a = not available

(*Continued*)

DINNER PLATES (*Continued*)	Amount	Cal.	Fat (g)	% Cal. Fat	Sat. Fat (g)	Chol. (mg)	Sod. (mg)	Carb. (g)	Fiber (g)	Pro. (g)	Servings/Exchanges
Sausage & Peppers	1	410	30	66	n/a	55	1340	19	4	17	1 starch, 2 high-fat meat, 3 fat
Spaghetti w/ Chicken Francese	1	800	37	42	n/a	110	860	64	5	49	4 starch, 7 lean meat, 4 fat
Spaghetti w/ Chicken Parmesan	1	930	36	35	n/a	175	950	75	6	75	5 starch, 8 lean meat, 2 fat
Spaghetti w/ Chicken Vesuvio	1	850	41	43	n/a	145	1100	64	4	50	4 starch, 8 lean meat, 4 fat
Spaghetti w/ Meatballs	1	680	25	33	n/a	15	1720	96	9	19	6 1/2 starch, 5 fat
Spaghetti w/ Sauce	1	820	28	31	n/a	0	890	120	10	20	8 starch, 4 fat
OTHER ITEMS											
Cheese Calzone	1	770	28	33	n/a	90	1410	87	3	39	5 1/2 starch, 3 high-fat meat, 1 1/2 fat

Pepperoni Stromboli	1	890	44	44	n/a	80	2470	82	3	39	5 1/2 starch, 3 high-fat meat, 4 fat
Spinach, Tomato, Broccoli Stromboli	1	680	24	32	n/a	35	1420	84	5	29	5 1/2 starch, 2 high-fat meat, 1 1/2 fat
PIZZA											
Cheese	1 slice	460	13	25	n/a	30	1080	60	3	24	4 starch, 2 medium-fat meat, 1/2 fat
Chicken Vegetable	1 slice	530	17	29	n/a	45	1260	69	5	24	4 1/2 starch, 1 medium-fat meat, 2 1/2 fat
Fresh Tomato	1 slice	450	14	28	n/a	25	1040	60	3	20	4 starch, 1 high-fat meat, 1 fat
Gourmet Broccoli & Spinach	1 slice	720	28	35	n/a	30	1540	99	6	29	6 1/2 starch, 1 high-fat meat, 3 fat
Gourmet Ham, Pineapple & Bacon	1 slice	680	21	28	n/a	45	1820	88	4	33	6 starch, 2 high-fat meat, 1 fat
Gourmet Meat Delight	1 slice	780	29	33	n/a	80	2250	94	4	41	6 starch, 3 high-fat meat, 1 fat

✔ = Healthiest Bets; n/a = not available

(*Continued*)

PIZZA (*Continued*)	Amount	Cal.	Fat (g)	% Cal. Fat	Sat. Fat (g)	Chol. (mg)	Sod. (mg)	Carb. (g)	Fiber (g)	Pro. (g)	Servings/Exchanges
Gourmet Mushroom	1 slice	610	20	30	n/a	20	1600	85	5	22	5 1/2 starch, 1 high-fat meat, 1 1/2 fat
Gourmet Mushroom & Spinach	1 slice	710	27	34	n/a	30	1680	87	6	29	5 1/2 starch, 2 high-fat meat, 2 fat
Gourmet Spinach & Yellow Pepper	1 slice	670	24	32	n/a	30	1470	86	5	28	5 1/2 starch, 2 medium-fat meat, 3 1/2 fat
Gourmet Tomato & Basil	1 slice	700	25	32	n/a	40	1650	87	5	28	5 1/2 starch, 2 medium-fat meat, 3 fat
Gourmet Cheese	1 slice	660	21	29	n/a	40	1460	84	4	30	5 1/2 starch, 2 medium-fat meat, 2 fat
Low Carb Cheese	1 slice	310	14	41	n/a	25	640	18	n/a	34	1 starch, 4 lean meat
Low Carb Pepperoni	1 slice	420	14	30	n/a	60	940	18	n/a	36	1 starch, 4 lean meat, 2 fat
Low Carb Sausage/ Pepperoni	1 slice	560	35	56	n/a	95	1300	18	n/a	44	1 starch, 6 medium-fat meat, 1/2 fat

Mushroom	1 slice	460	14	27	n/a	30	1310	62	4	19	4 starch, 1 high-fat meat, 1 fat
Pepperoni	1 slice	730	37	46	n/a	75	2200	61	3	35	4 starch, 3 high-fat meat, 3 fat
Sausage	1 slice	670	31	42	n/a	80	1810	60	3	35	4 starch, 3 high-fat meat, 1 1/2 fat
Stuffed Pepperoni	1 slice	960	42	39	n/a	115	3200	89	4	52	6 starch, 5 medium-fat meat, 3 fat
Stuffed Philly Cheesesteak	1 slice	830	33	36	n/a	70	2090	94	5	38	6 starch, 3 high-fat meat, 2 fat
Stuffed Spinach & Broccoli	1 slice	790	34	39	n/a	50	1610	89	5	32	6 starch, 2 high-fat meat, 3 fat
Supreme	1 slice	630	27	39	n/a	60	1720	63	3	31	4 starch, 3 high-fat meat, 1 fat
White	1 slice	570	23	36	n/a	55	1150	59	2	30	4 starch, 3 medium-fat meat, 1 1/2 fat
SALADS											
✓Caesar	1	80	5	56	n/a	5	200	6	1	2	1 veg, 1 fat
Cucumber & Tomato	1	130	11	76	n/a	0	85	9	2	1	1 veg, 2 fat

✓ = Healthiest Bets; n/a = not available

(*Continued*)

SALADS (*Continued*)	Amount	Cal.	Fat (g)	% Cal. Fat	Sat. Fat (g)	Chol. (mg)	Sod. (mg)	Carb. (g)	Fiber (g)	Pro. (g)	Servings/Exchanges
✓Fruit	1	130	1	7	n/a	0	15	32	3	2	2 fruit
✓Greek	1	60	5	75	n/a	10	130	3	0	2	1 veg, 1 fat
✓Mixed Garden	1	35	0	0	n/a	0	15	7	3	2	1 veg
Pasta Primavera	1	190	10	47	n/a	0	1180	21	2	4	1 starch, 1 veg, 2 fat
Stringbean & Tomato	1	100	7	63	n/a	0	80	9	2	1	2 veg, 1 fat

✓ = Healthiest Bets; n/a = not available

Tacos, Burritos, and All Else Mexican

RESTAURANTS

Baja Fresh Mexican Grill

Chipotle

Del Taco

Taco Bell

Taco John's

NUTRITION PROS

- Beans used in Mexican cooking, such as pinto beans and black beans, add soluble fiber. This kind of fiber allows your blood glucose to rise slowly and not as high. Beans are a terrific source of vitamins and minerals.
- In most of the fast-food Mexican restaurants, ordering is à la carte—an enchilada, a burrito, a Mexican salad. This helps you order and eat less.
- Even in the newer, slightly upscale Baja Fresh and Chipotle, you can pick and choose what you want on or left out of your order.
- High-fat items, such as guacamole, cheese, and sour cream, are added onto and not mixed into some dishes. That's a plus because you can ask the kitchen to hold or serve them on the side.
- Do opt for guacamole over sour cream, as it contains healthier monounsaturated fat rather than saturated fat and cholesterol. Calorie for calorie, it's better for you.

- Hot and spicy sauces—red sauce, green sauce, salsa, and pico de gallo—add zest without fat and calories.
- Garlic, cilantro, chilies, and onions add flavor with few calories.
- Mexican cuisine is naturally low in protein. You don't get 8-oz hunks of meat. You find a small amount of protein mixed into dishes.
- Most fast-food Mexican restaurants now fry in 100% vegetable oil. That's better than lard because it contains no cholesterol and less saturated fat. However, it may contain a few grams of trans fat. But remember, teaspoon for teaspoon, the calories are the same.
- In the fast-food Mexican restaurants, and in the slightly upscale ones such as Baja Fresh and Chipotle, the tortilla chips don't greet you at the table.

NUTRITION CONS

- Fried items seem almost unavoidable—tortilla chips, taco shells, tortilla shells (which salad might be served in), and chimichangas.
- Your carbohydrate count can escalate quickly with tortillas, beans, rice, and those hard-to-resist tortilla chips.
- Cheese—shredded, melted, or sauced—is a mainstay ingredient.
- Vegetables are few and far between—a few shreds of lettuce or pieces of tomato.
- Fruit is unavailable.
- High-fiber beans are often served refried. Some restaurants still use lard to make them.
- The bet-you-can't-eat-just-one tortilla chips are waiting at your table in most sit-down Mexican or Tex-Mex restaurants.

Healthy Tips

- ★ If the fried tortilla chips greet you when you sit down, hands off. Send them back or at least to the opposite side of the table.
- ★ Use extra salsa and other hot sauces to add flavor with very few calories.
- ★ Use salsa or another hot sauce as a salad dressing.
- ★ Don't feel you have to order an entree. Choose from appetizers and side dishes to control your portions.
- ★ Take advantage of ordering à la carte. Mix and match a healthy meal.
- ★ As a starter, try a cup of black bean soup or chili to fill you up and not out.
- ★ Make a bowl of black bean soup or chili the main course with a salad on the side.
- ★ Look for menu items that use soft tortillas rather than crispy fried ones. For example, choose a burrito or an enchilada rather than a taco or a chimichanga.
- ★ Fajitas are great to split. There's always enough for two.
- ★ Split a side dish—Mexican rice, refried beans, or black beans—to get more carbohydrates and fiber.
- ★ Take advantage of lite or nonfat sour cream if it's served.

Get It Your Way

- ★ Hold the guacamole, cheese, and sour cream, or ask for them on the side.
- ★ If a menu item is served with melted cheese, request a light helping.
- ★ Substitute black beans for refried beans (if available).
- ★ Ask for extra tomatoes and lettuce.
- ★ Request extra salsa or other zesty, low-calorie topper.

Baja Fresh Mexican Grill

❖ Baja Fresh provides nutrition information for all its menu items at www.bajafresh.com.

Light 'n Lean Choice

Charbroiled Chicken Salad
Fat-Free Salsa Verde
Black Beans *(1/2 serving)*
Guacamole *(2 oz serving)*

Calories	575	Sodium (mg)	2,330
Fat (g)	14	Carbohydrate (g)	56
% calories from fat	23	Fiber (g)	22
Saturated fat (g)	3	Protein (g)	57
Cholesterol (mg)	113		

Exchanges: 3 starch, 3 veg, 6 very lean meat, 1 fat

Healthy 'n Hearty Choice

(Split whole meal in half.)
Steak with Corn Tortilla
Pinto Beans
Rice

Calories	810	Sodium (mg)	1,965
Fat (g)	17	Carbohydrate (g)	113
% calories from fat	19	Fiber (g)	23
Saturated fat (g)	6	Protein (g)	47
Cholesterol (mg)	83		

Exchanges: 7 starch, 1 veg, 3 medium-fat meat

(Continued)

Baja Fresh Mexican Grill

	Amount	Cal.	Fat (g)	% Cal. Fat	Sat. Fat (g)	Chol. (mg)	Sod. (mg)	Carb. (g)	Fiber (g)	Pro. (g)	Servings/Exchanges
BURRITOS											
Bare	1	650	7	10	1.5	75	2410	99	22	45	6 carb, 3 lean meat
Bean & Cheese Charbroiled Chicken	1	980	33	30	14	145	2070	99	22	69	6 1/2 starch, 6 medium-fat meat, 1/2 fat
Bean & Cheese Charbroiled Steak	1	1070	41	34	18	170	2080	99	21	74	6 1/2 starch, 7 medium-fat meat, 1 fat
Bean & Cheese No Meat	1	850	31	33	14	70	1620	99	21	41	6 1/2 starch, 2 medium-fat meat, 4 fat
Enchilada Style Add-On to Burritos	1	640	40	56	17	85	1510	44	7	24	3 starch, 2 medium-fat meat, 6 fat
Enchilada Style Add-On to Dos Manos	1	640	40	56	17	85	1510	44	7	24	3 starch, 2 medium-fat meat, 6 fat

Grilled Veggie	1	810	32	36	15	75	1710	96	17	33	3 starch, 1 veg, 2 medium-fat meat, 6 fat
Veggie Bare	1	590	10	15	4	20	2050	102	21	20	6 starch, 1 veg, 2 1/2 fat
BURRITOS - CHARBROILED											
Chicken Baja Burrito	1	800	34	38	13	120	1980	70	11	54	4 1/2 starch, 6 medium-fat meat, 1 fat
Chicken Burrito Dos Manos	1	780	25	29	10	80	1880	97	15	40	6 1/2 starch, 3 lean meat, 3 fat
Chicken Burrito Mexicano	1	810	13	14	2	75	2090	119	20	51	8 starch, 4 lean meat
Chicken Burrito Ultimo	1	890	35	35	15	145	2030	87	10	56	5 1/2 starch, 6 medium-fat meat, 3 fat
Steak Baja Burrito	1	890	42	42	16	155	1990	70	10	59	4 1/2 starch, 6 medium-fat meat, 2 fat
Steak Burrito Dos Manos	1	820	29	32	12	95	1880	95	14	42	6 1/2 starch, 3 medium-fat meat, 3 fat

✓ = Healthiest Bets

(Continued)

BURRITOS - CHARBROILED (*Continued*)	Amount	Cal.	Fat (g)	% Cal. Fat	Sat. Fat (g)	Chol. (mg)	Sod. (mg)	Carb. (g)	Fiber (g)	Pro. (g)	Servings/Exchanges
Steak Burrito Dos Manos	1	820	29	32	12	95	1880	95	14	42	6 starch, 4 medium-fat meat, 2 fat
Steak Burrito Mexicano	1	900	20	20	6	100	2110	119	19	56	8 starch, 4 lean meat, 1 fat
Steak Burrito Ultimo	1	990	42	38	19	170	2040	87	9	60	5 1/2 starch, 6 medium-fat meat, 1 1/2 fat
FAJITAS											
Chicken w/ Corn Tortillas	1	870	19	20	6	125	2050	116	25	62	7 1/2 starch, 6 lean meat
Chicken w/ Flour Tortillas	1	1050	29	25	8	125	2640	133	24	75	9 starch, 9 lean meat
Steak w/ Corn Tortillas	1	1020	30	26	11	165	2090	116	23	70	7 1/2 starch, 7 lean meat, 2 fat
Steak w/ Flour Tortillas	1	1190	38	29	13	165	2680	133	24	76	9 starch, 7 lean meat, 3 1/2 fat

KIDS' FAVORITES											
Kids' Bean & Cheese Burrito	1	610	17	25	6	60	1020	92	13	20	6 starch, 1 lean meat, 2 1/2 fat
Kids' Chicken Taquitos	1	700	37	48	7	70	1000	69	5	19	4 1/2 starch, 1 lean meat, 7 fat
Kids' Nachos	1	700	33	42	12	55	720	89	6	19	6 starch, 5 fat
Kids' Quesadilla	1	610	25	37	11	55	870	72	5	20	4 1/2 starch, 1 lean meat, 4 fat
NACHOS											
Charbroiled Chicken	1	2010	105	47	38	245	6060	166	34	93	11 starch, 9 lean meat, 14 fat
Charbroiled Steak	1	2100	133	57	41	275	3050	166	33	98	11 starch, 9 medium-fat meat, 12 fat
Cheese	1	1880	103	49	37	175	2590	166	33	65	11 starch, 4 high-fat meat, 13 1/2 fat

✔ = Healthiest Bets

(*Continued*)

	Amount	Cal.	Fat (g)	% Cal. Fat	Sat. Fat (g)	Chol. (mg)	Sod. (mg)	Carb. (g)	Fiber (g)	Pro. (g)	Servings/Exchanges
QUESADILLAS											
Charbroiled Chicken	1	1240	71	52	35	145	2610	75	11	77	5 starch, 9 lean meat, 9 fat
Charbroiled Steak	1	1330	79	53	38	180	2620	75	10	81	5 starch, 9 1/2 medium-fat meat, 9 1/2 fat
Cheese	1	1110	69	56	34	170	2160	75	10	48	5 starch, 5 medium-fat meat, 9 fat
Veggie	1	1160	69	54	34	175	2330	87	13	50	5 1/2 starch, 2 veg, 4 medium-fat meat, 9 fat
SALAD DRESSINGS											
✓Fat Free Salsa Verde	1	15	0	0	0	0	370	3	1	0	free
Olive Oil Vinaigrette	1	290	21	65	0.5	0	290	2	0	0	4 fat
Ranch Dressing	1	260	26	90	6	50	460	3	0	2	5 fat

SALADS

Charbroiled Chicken	1	310	7	20	2	110	1210	18	7	46	3 veg, 6 lean meat
Charbroiled Fish	1	360	14	35	3.5	70	1020	27	11	35	1 starch, 3 veg, 4 1/2 lean meat
Charbroiled Steak	1	450	18	36	7	150	1240	18	6	54	3 veg, 7 lean meat
Chile Lime Chicken w/out dressing	1	640	16	23	6	90	1390	75	22	51	4 starch, 3 veg, 5 lean meat
Chile Lime Dressing	1	170	16	85	3	10	450	5	0	0	3 fat
Chipotle Glazed Charbroiled Chicken	1	600	22	33	6	105	1120	56	11	47	2 1/2 starch, 3 veg, 5 lean meat, 2 1/2 fat
✓Side w/out dressing	1	70	3	39	1	5	240	10	3	4	2 veg

SIDE-BY-SIDE

Side-by-Side	1	520	25	43	9	155	1700	16	11	61	1 starch, 8 lean meat

✓ = Healthiest Bets

(Continued)

	Amount	Cal.	Fat (g)	% Cal. Fat	Sat. Fat (g)	Chol. (mg)	Sod. (mg)	Carb. (g)	Fiber (g)	Pro. (g)	Servings/Exchanges
SIDE ORDERS											
✓12″ Flour Tortillas	1	350	8	21	1	0	540	58	5	10	4 starch, 1 1/2 fat
8″ Flour Tortillas	4 each	520	12	21	1.5	0	810	87	7	15	5 1/2 starch, 2 1/2 fat
Black Beans	1	360	3	8	1	5	1120	61	26	23	3 1/2 starch, 2 lean meat
Breaded Fish	1	390	16	37	2.5	30	410	25	0	30	1 1/2 starch, 4 lean meat, 1 fat
Charbroiled Chicken	1	230	4	16	0.5	125	760	0	2	48	5 lean meat
✓Charbroiled Fish	1	210	3	13	1	110	240	1	0	44	5 lean meat
Charbroiled Steak	1	330	14	38	6	145	670	0	0	48	6 lean meat, 2 fat
Chips & Guacamole	1	1320	72	49	10	0	990	145	29	20	9 1/2 starch, 12 fat
Chips & Salsa Baja	1	70	3	39	0	0	970	7	4	2	1/2 starch, 1/2 fat
Chips & Salsa Pico del Gallo	1	50	1	18	0	0	890	12	3	2	1 starch

Chips & Salsa Roja	1	70	1	13	0	0	1070	13	4	3	1 starch
Chips & Salsa Verde	1	50	0	0	0	0	1170	11	3	2	1/2 starch
✓Fresh Corn Tortillas	5 each	360	1	3	0	0	25	80	7	9	4 1/2 starch, 2 carb
Fresh Corn Tortillas Chips	1	150	7	42	0.5	0	35	18	2	2	1 starch, 1 1/2 fat
Guacamole - 2 oz	1	70	6	77	1	0	190	5	1	1	1 fat
Guacamole - 3 oz	1	110	9	74	2	0	280	7	6	2	1/2 starch, 1 fat
✓Onions, Peppers, & Chiles	1	110	0	0	0	0	330	24	6	3	1 1/2 starch, 1 veg
Pinto Beans	1	320	1	3	0	5	840	56	21	19	3 1/2 starch, 1 lean meat
Pronto Guacamole	1	550	30	49	4	0	290	61	11	8	4 starch, 1 carb, 5 1/2 fat
Rice	1	280	4	13	0.5	0	980	55	4	5	3 1/2 starch, 1 1/2 carb, 1/2 fat
Tostada Shell	1	500	28	50	3.5	0	600	44	4	7	3 starch, 1 carb, 5 1/2 fat
Wild Gulf Shrimp	1	150	2	12	0.5	335	740	1	0	31	4 1/2 lean meat

✓ = Healthiest Bets

(Continued)

	Amount	Cal.	Fat (g)	% Cal. Fat	Sat. Fat (g)	Chol. (mg)	Sod. (mg)	Carb. (g)	Fiber (g)	Pro. (g)	Servings/Exchanges
TACOS											
✓Breaded Fish Taco	1 serving	260	12	42	2	15	410	60	3	8	4 starch, 1/2 carb, 1 lean meat, 1 fat
✓Charbroiled Chicken Taco	1 serving	180	4	20	0.5	25	230	25	3	12	2 starch, 1 lean meat
✓Charbroiled Fish Taco	1 serving	250	9	32	1.5	20	390	31	6	13	2 starch, 1 lean meat, 1 fat
✓Charbroiled Steak Taco	1 serving	210	6	26	1.5	30	230	25	3	14	1 1/2 starch, 1 1/2 lean meat
✓Wild Gulf Shrimp Taco	1 serving	190	5	24	0.5	90	350	26	3	12	1 1/2 starch, 1 lean meat, 1/2 fat
TAQUITOS											
Charbroiled Chicken w/ Beans	1 order	750	36	43	13	85	1520	66	19	38	4 1/2 starch, 3 lean meat, 5 1/2 fat

Charbroiled Chicken w/ Rice	1 order	710	36	46	11	80	1480	64	9	30	4 starch, 2 1/2 lean meat, 5 1/2 fat
Charbroiled Steak w/ Beans	1 order	820	42	46	16	105	1660	39	20	40	2 1/2 starch, 4 medium-fat meat, 4 fat
Charbroiled Steak w/ Rice	1 order	790	42	48	15	105	1630	67	10	32	4 1/2 starch, 2 1/2 medium- fat meat, 6 fat
TOSTADAS											
Charbroiled Chicken	1 order	1130	52	41	14	120	2390	100	29	61	6 1/2 starch, 6 lean meat, 7 fat
Charbroiled Steak	1 order	1230	60	44	17	145	2400	100	28	65	6 1/2 starch, 6 1/2 lean meat, 5 1/2 fat
No Meat	1 order	1000	50	45	14	45	1950	100	28	32	6 starch, 1 veg, 2 medium-fat meat, 8 fat

✓ = Healthiest Bets

Chipotle

❖ Chipotle provided some nutrition information for this book. It does not provide nutrition information on its Web site, www.chipotle.com. Nutrition information in this book is provided as ingredients because Chipotle makes up your meal as you request it. The meals below show two examples of how to use Chipotle's menu items to design healthy meals.

Light 'n Lean Choice

6″ Flour Tortillas *(3)*
Chicken *(1 order, 4 oz)*
Black Beans *(1 order, 4 oz)*
Red Tomatillo Sauce *(4 T)*

Calories	677	Sodium (mg)	1,962
Fat (g)	21	Carbohydrate (g)	71
% calories from fat	28	Fiber (g)	n/a
Saturated fat (g)	2	Protein (g)	48
Cholesterol (mg)	96		

Exchanges: 4 1/2 starch, 1 veg, 4 lean meat, 1 fat

Healthy 'n Hearty Choice

6″ Flour Tortillas *(3)*
Fajita Vegetables *(1 order, 3 oz)*
Pinto Beans *(1 order, 4 oz)*
Corn Salsa *(4 T)*
Guacamole *(1/2 order, 2 oz)*

Calories 723	Sodium (mg) 2,454
Fat (g) 26	Carbohydrate (g) 100
% calories from fat 32	Fiber (g) n/a
Saturated fat (g) 2.5	Protein (g) 23
Cholesterol (mg) 0	

Exchanges: 6 starch, 3 veg, 4 fat

(*Continued*)

Chipotle

	Amount	Cal.	Fat (g)	% Cal. Fat	Sat. Fat (g)	Chol. (mg)	Sod. (mg)	Carb. (g)	Fiber (g)	Pro. (g)	Servings/Exchanges
MEATS											
Barbacoa	1 serving	285	16	51	4	74	580	1	n/a	34	5 lean meat
Carnitas	1 serving	227	12	48	3	66	873	0	n/a	29	4 lean meat
✓Chicken	1 serving	219	11	45	2	96	431	0	n/a	29	4 lean meat
✓Steak	1 serving	230	12	47	4	51	206	2	n/a	29	4 lean meat
OTHER TOPPINGS											
Cheese	1 serving	110	9	74	6	30	180	0	0	7	1 high-fat meat
Guacamole	1 serving	170	15	79	2.5	0	370	8	5	2	1/2 starch, 3 fat
Sour Cream	1 serving	120	10	75	7	10	30	2	0	2	2 fat
RICE & BEANS											
✓Black Beans	1 serving	130	1	7	0	0	318	22	n/a	9	1 1/2 starch

✓Pinto Beans	1 serving	138	1	7	0	0	374	23	n/a	9	1 1/2 carb, 1 lean meat
Rice	1 serving	240	7	26	1	0	610	42	0	4	2 1/2 starch, 1 fat
SALSA & TOMATILLO											
Corn Salsa	1 serving	100	1	9	0	0	540	22	3	3	1 1/2 starch
✓Green Tomatillo	1 serving	15	0	0	0	0	227	3	n/a	1	free
Red Tomatillo	1 serving	28	1	32	0	0	493	4	n/a	1	insufficient info. to calculate
Tomato Salsa	1 serving	25	0	0	0	0	560	6	1	1	1/2 starch
TORTILLAS & TACO SHELLS											
✓13″ Flour Tortilla	1	340	9	24	2	0	860	54	2	9	3 1/2 starch, 2 fat
✓6″ Flour Tortilla	3	300	8	24	1.5	0	720	45	2	9	3 starch, 1 1/2 fat
Chips	4 oz	490	19	35	4	0	130	71	5	7	4 1/2 starch, 4 fat
Crispy Taco Shells	4	240	9	34	2	0	40	34	2	4	2 starch, 2 fat
VEGETABLES											
✓Fajita Vegetables	1 serving	100	8	72	1	0	640	6	1	1	1 veg, 2 fat

✓ = Healthiest Bets; n/a = not available

Del Taco

❖ Del Taco provides nutrition information for all its menu items on its Web site at www.deltaco.com.

Light 'n Lean Choice

Chicken Soft Taco
1/2 Beans 'n Cheese Cup

Calories	470	Sodium (mg)	630
Fat (g)	15	Carbohydrate (g)	60
% calories from fat	29	Fiber (g)	17
Saturated fat (g)	6	Protein (g)	27
Cholesterol (mg)	35		

Exchanges: 4 starch, 2 lean meat, 1 fat

Healthy 'n Hearty Choice

Carnitas Burrito *(1)*
Rice Cup

Calories	580	Sodium (mg)	1,960
Fat (g)	23	Carbohydrate (g)	68
% calories from fat	36	Fiber (g)	4
Saturated fat (g)	13	Protein (g)	28
Cholesterol (mg)	72		

Exchanges: 4 starch, 1 veg, 2 medium-fat meat, 2 fat

Del Taco

	Amount	Cal.	Fat (g)	% Cal. Fat	Sat. Fat (g)	Chol. (mg)	Sod. (mg)	Carb. (g)	Fiber (g)	Pro. (g)	Servings/Exchanges
BREAKFAST											
Bacon & Egg Quesadilla	1	450	23	46	12	260	920	40	2	21	2 1/2 starch, 2 high-fat meat, 1 fat
Hash Brown Sticks	1	250	19	68	1	0	200	20	0	0	1 starch, 4 fat
✓Side of Bacon	2 slices	50	4	72	1.5	10	170	0	0	3	1 fat
BREAKFAST BURRITO											
✓Breakfast	1	250	11	40	6	160	520	24	1	10	1 1/2 starch, 1 high-fat meat, 1 fat
Egg & Cheese	1	450	24	48	13	530	740	29	3	23	2 starch, 2 high-fat meat, 2 fat

✓ = Healthiest Bets

(*Continued*)

BREAKFAST BURRITO (*Continued*)	Amount	Cal.	Fat (g)	% Cal. Fat	Sat. Fat (g)	Chol. (mg)	Sod. (mg)	Carb. (g)	Fiber (g)	Pro. (g)	Servings/Exchanges
Macho Bacon & Egg	1	1030	60	52	20	790	1760	82	6	40	5 1/2 starch, 4 high-fat meat, 5 fat
Steak & Egg	1	580	34	53	16	560	1270	41	3	33	3 starch, 3 high-fat meat, 1 1/2 fat
BURGERS											
Bacon Double Del Cheeseburger	1	610	39	58	14	95	1130	35	4	29	2 starch, 3 high-fat meat, 2 fat
Bun Taco	1	440	21	43	12	65	830	37	4	24	2 1/2 starch, 2 high-fat meat, 1 fat
Cheeseburger	1	330	13	35	6	35	870	37	3	16	2 1/2 starch, 1 high-fat meat, 1 fat
Del Cheeseburger	1	430	25	52	7	45	710	35	4	16	2 1/2 starch, 2 high-fat meat, 1 fat

Double Del Cheeseburger	1	560	35	56	12	85	960	35	4	26	2 1/2 starch, 3 high-fat meat, 1 1/2 fat
✓Hamburger	1	280	9	29	3	25	640	37	3	13	2 1/2 starch, 1 high-fat meat
BURRITOS											
Bean & Cheese Green	1	280	8	26	5	15	1030	38	6	11	2 1/2 carb, 1 high-fat meat
Bean & Cheese Red	1	270	8	27	5	15	1020	38	6	11	2 1/2 starch, 1 medium-fat meat
Carnitas	1	440	21	43	12	70	1050	41	3	25	3 carb, 2 high-fat meat
Chicken Works	1	520	23	40	12	65	1620	57	4	26	3 1/2 starch, 2 medium-fat meat, 2 fat
Del Beef	1	550	30	49	17	90	1090	42	3	31	3 starch, 3 medium-fat meat, 3 fat
Del Classic Chicken	1	560	36	58	13	70	1100	41	3	24	3 starch, 3 medium-fat meat, 1 1/2 fat

✓ = Healthiest Bets

(*Continued*)

BURRITOS (*Continued*)	Amount	Cal.	Fat (g)	% Cal. Fat	Sat. Fat (g)	Chol. (mg)	Sod. (mg)	Carb. (g)	Fiber (g)	Pro. (g)	Servings/Exchanges
Del Combo	1	530	22	37	13	55	1680	31	11	28	2 starch, 3 high-fat meat, 2 fat
Deluxe Del Beef	1	590	33	50	19	95	1110	45	4	32	3 starch, 3 high-fat meat, 1 fat
Deluxe Del Combo	1	570	25	39	15	60	1700	64	12	29	4 starch, 2 medium-fat meat, 3 fat
Half Pound Green	1	430	12	25	9	20	1690	59	13	20	4 starch, 1 medium-fat meat, 1 1/2 fat
Half Pound Red	1	430	12	25	9	20	1670	65	13	20	4 starch, 1 medium-fat meat, 1 1/2 fat
Macho Beef	1	1170	62	48	29	190	2190	89	7	60	6 starch, 6 high-fat meat
Macho Chicken	1	930	33	32	15	100	2990	111	15	47	7 starch, 4 medium-fat meat, 1 1/2 fat

Macho Combo	1	1050	44	38	21	115	2760	113	17	49	7 1/2 starch, 4 high-fat meat, 1 fat
Spicy Chicken	1	480	16	30	10	40	1850	66	8	23	4 1/2 carb, 2 lean meat, 1/2 fat
Steak Works	1	590	31	47	16	70	1820	58	4	27	3 1/2 starch, 3 high-fat meat
Veggie Works	1	490	18	33	11	25	1660	69	9	18	3 carb, 2 veg, 1 high-fat meat, 2 fat
FRIES											
Chile Cheese	1	670	46	62	15	45	880	51	5	17	3 1/2 starch, 2 high-fat meat, 2 1/2 fat
Deluxe Chili Cheese	1	710	49	62	16	50	880	53	6	17	3 1/2 starch, 2 high-fat meat, 5 fat
Large	1	490	32	59	5	0	380	47	5	5	3 starch, 6 fat
Macho	1	690	46	60	7	0	550	68	6	7	4 1/2 starch, 7 1/2 fat
Regular	1	350	23	59	4	0	270	34	3	3	2 starch, 4 1/2 fat

✓ = Healthiest Bets

(*Continued*)

FRIES (*Continued*)	Amount	Cal.	Fat (g)	% Cal. Fat	Sat. Fat (g)	Chol. (mg)	Sod. (mg)	Carb. (g)	Fiber (g)	Pro. (g)	Servings/Exchanges
Small	1	210	14	60	2	0	160	20	2	2	1 1/2 starch, 2 fat
NACHOS											
Macho Nachos	1	1100	63	52	24	55	2640	113	15	31	7 1/2 starch, 2 high-fat meat, 5 1/2 fat
Nachos	1	380	24	57	8	5	630	40	2	5	3 starch, 1 high-fat meat, 1 fat
QUESADILLAS											
Cheddar	1	500	27	49	20	75	860	39	2	23	2 1/2 starch, 2 high-fat meat, 2 fat
Chicken Cheddar	1	580	31	48	21	104	1240	41	2	33	3 starch, 3 high-fat meat, 1 fat
Spicy Jack	1	490	26	48	17	75	920	38	2	23	2 1/2 starch, 2 high-fat meat, 2 fat

Spicy Jack Chicken	1	570	30	47	16	105	1300	40	2	32	3 starch, 3 high-fat meat, 1 fat
SALADS											
Deluxe Chicken	1	740	34	41	15	70	2610	77	15	33	4 starch, 3 veg, 3 lean meat, 4 fat
Deluxe Taco	1	780	40	46	18	80	2250	76	14	33	4 starch, 3 veg, 3 lean meat, 5 fat
Taco	1	350	30	77	10	45	390	10	2	10	2 veg, 1 high-fat meat, 4 1/2 fat
SHAKES											
Large Chocolate	1	680	16	21	12	45	350	117	1	16	8 carb, 1 1/2 fat
Large Strawberry	1	540	8	13	6	10	280	100	1	14	6 1/2 carb, 1 fat
Large Vanilla	1	550	10	16	6	50	320	97	0	16	6 1/2 carb, 1 fat
Small Chocolate	1	520	12	21	9	35	270	89	1	12	6 carb, 1 1/2 fat

✓ = Healthiest Bets

(Continued)

SHAKES (*Continued*)	Amount	Cal.	Fat (g)	% Cal. Fat	Sat. Fat (g)	Chol. (mg)	Sod. (mg)	Carb. (g)	Fiber (g)	Pro. (g)	Servings/Exchanges
Small Strawberry	1	410	6	13	4	30	220	76	1	11	5 carb, 1 fat
Small Vanilla	1	420	7	15	5	35	250	75	0	12	5 carb, 1 fat
SIDES											
Beans 'n Cheese Cup	1	260	3	10	2	5	1810	44	16	16	2 1/2 starch, 1 medium-fat meat
Rice Cup	1	140	2	13	1	2	910	27	1	3	1 1/2 starch
TACOS											
Big Fat Chicken	1	340	13	34	4	45	840	38	3	18	2 1/2 starch, 2 lean meat, 1 fat
Big Fat Steak	1	390	19	44	6	45	960	38	3	18	2 1/2 starch, 2 medium-fat meat, 1 fat
Big Fat Taco	1	320	11	31	5	35	680	39	3	16	2 1/2 starch, 1 high-fat meat, 1/2 fat
✓Carnitas	1	170	6	32	2	25	370	18	2	9	1 starch, 1 medium-fat meat

✔Chicken Del Carbon	1	170	5	26	1	30	530	19	2	12	1 starch, 1 medium-fat meat
✔Chicken Soft	1	210	12	51	4	30	520	16	1	11	1 starch, 1 medium-fat meat, 1 fat
✔Regular	1	160	1	6	4	20	150	11	1	7	1/2 starch, 1 medium-fat meat
✔Soft	1	160	8	45	4	20	330	16	1	8	1 starch, 1 medium-fat meat
✔Steak Del Carbon	1	220	11	45	4	360	680	19	2	12	1 starch, 1 high-fat meat, 1/2 fat
✔Ultimate	1	260	17	59	8	50	470	13	2	14	1 starch, 2 medium-fat meat, 1/2 fat

✔ = Healthiest Bets

Taco Bell

❖ Taco Bell provides nutrition information for all its menu items on its Web site at www.tacobell.com.

Light 'n Lean Choice

Beef Soft Taco *(1)*
Tostada *(1)*
Pintos 'n Cheese *(1)*

Calories 570
Fat (g) 21
% calories from fat..33
Saturated fat (g) 7
Cholesterol (mg) 35
Sodium (mg) 2,000
Carbohydrate (g).........72
Fiber (g)...................16
Protein (g) 27

Exchanges: 4 1/2 starch, 1 veg, 2 lean meat, 2 fat

Healthy 'n Hearty Choice

Gordita Supreme Chicken *(1)*
Grilled Steak Soft Taco *(1)*
Pintos 'n Cheese *(1)*

Calories 640
Fat (g) 24
% calories from fat..34
Saturated fat (g) 22
Cholesterol (mg) 75
Sodium (mg) 1,790
Carbohydrate (g).........59
Fiber (g)...................10
Protein (g) 38

Exchanges: 4 starch, 1 veg, 3 lean meat, 3 fat

Taco Bell

	Amount	Cal.	Fat (g)	% Cal. Fat	Sat. Fat (g)	Chol. (mg)	Sod. (mg)	Carb. (g)	Fiber (g)	Pro. (g)	Servings/Exchanges
SIDES											
Mexican Rice	1	210	10	43	4	15	740	23	3	6	2 starch, 1 1/2 fat
BIG BELL VALUE MEAL											
1/2 lb Bean Burrito Especial	1	600	21	32	5	15	1760	82	12	21	5 1/2 starch, 1 lean meat, 3 fat
1/2 lb Beef & Potato Burrito	1	530	24	41	9	40	1670	65	4	15	4 starch, 5 fat
1/2 lb Beef Combo Burrito	1	470	19	36	7	45	1620	52	5	22	3 1/2 starch, 1 high-fat meat, 2 fat
Caramel Apple Empanada	1	290	15	47	4	4	290	37	1	3	2 1/2 carb, 2 1/2 fat
Cheesy Fiesta Potatoes	1	280	18	58	6	20	800	27	2	4	2 starch, 3 fat

✓ = Healthiest Bets

(Continued)

BIG BELL VALUE MEAL (*Continued*)	Amount	Cal.	Fat (g)	% Cal. Fat	Sat. Fat (g)	Chol. (mg)	Sod. (mg)	Carb. (g)	Fiber (g)	Pro. (g)	Servings/Exchanges
✓Double Decker Taco	1	340	14	37	5	25	810	39	5	14	2 1/2 starch, 1 high-fat meat, 1 fat
Grande Soft Taco	1	450	21	42	8	45	1410	44	2	19	3 starch, 1 high-fat meat, 2 1/2 fat
Spicy Chicken Burrito	1	430	19	40	4.5	30	1160	50	4	14	3 1/2 starch, 3 1/2 fat
✓Spicy Chicken Taco	1	180	7	35	2	20	580	21	2	10	1 1/2 starch, 1 lean meat, 1/2 fat
BURRITOS											
7-Layer	1	530	21	36	8	25	1350	66	10	18	4 1/2 starch, 4 fat
Bean	1	370	10	24	3.5	10	1200	55	8	14	3 1/2 starch, 2 fat
Chili Cheese	1	390	17	39	9	40	1080	40	3	16	2 1/2 starch, 1 high-fat meat, 2 fat
Fiesta - beef	1	390	15	35	5	25	1160	50	3	14	3 1/2 starch, 2 1/2 fat

Fiesta - chicken	1	370	12	29	3.5	30	1090	48	3	18	3 starch, 1 lean meat, 2 fat
Fiesta -steak	1	370	13	32	4	25	1080	48	4	16	3 starch, 1 high-fat meat, 1 fat
Grilled Stuffed - beef	1	720	33	41	11	55	2090	79	7	27	5 starch, 2 high-fat meat, 3 fat
Grilled Stuffed - chicken	1	680	26	34	7	70	1950	76	7	35	5 starch, 3 lean meat, 3 fat
Grilled Stuffed - steak	1	680	28	37	8	55	1940	76	8	31	5 starch, 2 high-fat meat, 2 fat
Supreme - beef	1	440	18	37	8	40	1330	52	5	17	3 1/2 starch, 1 high-fat meat, 1 1/2 fat
Supreme - chicken	1	410	14	31	6	45	1270	50	5	21	3 1/2 starch, 1 lean meat, 2 fat
Supreme - steak	1	420	16	34	7	35	1260	50	6	19	3 1/2 starch, 1 high-fat meat, 1 fat

✓ = Healthiest Bets

(*Continued*)

	Amount	Cal.	Fat (g)	% Cal. Fat	Sat. Fat (g)	Chol. (mg)	Sod. (mg)	Carb. (g)	Fiber (g)	Pro. (g)	Servings/Exchanges
CHALUPAS											
Baja - beef	1	430	27	57	8	30	760	32	2	13	2 starch, 1 high-fat meat, 4 fat
Baja - chicken	1	400	24	54	6	40	690	30	2	17	2 starch, 1 lean meat, 4 fat
Baja - steak	1	400	25	56	7	30	680	30	2	15	2 starch, 1 high-fat meat, 3 fat
Nacho Cheese - beef	1	400	25	56	7	30	680	30	2	15	2 starch, 1 high-fat meat, 3 fat
Nacho Cheese - chicken	1	380	22	52	7	20	670	33	1	12	2 starch, 1 lean meat, 4 fat
✓Nacho Cheese - steak	1	350	19	49	5	20	670	31	2	14	2 starch, 1 high-fat meat, 2 fat
Supreme - beef	1	390	24	55	10	35	600	31	1	14	2 starch, 1 high-fat meat, 3 fat

✓Supreme - chicken	1	370	20	49	8	45	530	30	1	17	2 starch, 1 lean meat, 3 1/2 fat
Supreme - steak	1	370	22	54	8	35	520	29	2	15	2 starch, 1 high-fat meat, 3 fat
FRESCO STYLE ITEMS											
✓Tostada	1	200	6	27	1	0	670	30	8	8	2 starch, 1 1/2 fat
FRESCO STYLE ITEMS - BURRITO											
Bean	1	350	8	21	2	0	1330	56	9	13	3 1/2 starch, 1 1/2 fat
Fiesta - chicken	1	350	9	23	2	25	1100	49	4	16	3 starch, 1 lean meat, 1 fat
Supreme - chicken	1	350	8	21	2	25	1370	50	6	19	3 1/2 starch, 1 lean meat, 1 fat
Supreme - steak	1	350	9	23	2.5	15	1260	50	6	17	3 1/2 starch, 1 high-fat meat
FRESCO STYLE ITEMS - ENCHIRITO											
Beef	1	270	9	30	3	20	1300	35	5	12	2 starch, 1 high-fat meat

✓ = Healthiest Bets

(Continued)

FRESCO STYLE ITEMS - ENCHIRITO (*Continued*)	Amount	Cal.	Fat (g)	% Cal. Fat	Sat. Fat (g)	Chol. (mg)	Sod. (mg)	Carb. (g)	Fiber (g)	Pro. (g)	Servings/Exchanges
Chicken	1	250	5	18	1.5	25	1230	34	5	16	2 starch, 1 medium-fat meat
Steak	1	250	7	25	2	15	1220	34	3	14	2 starch, 1 high-fat meat
FRESCO STYLE ITEMS - GORDITA											
✓Baja - beef	1	250	9	32	3	20	640	31	2	12	2 starch, 1 high-fat meat
✓Baja - chicken	1	230	6	23	1	25	570	29	2	15	2 starch, 1 medium-fat meat
✓Baja - steak	1	230	7	27	1.5	15	570	29	3	13	2 starch, 1 medium-fat meat
FRESCO STYLE ITEMS - TACO											
✓Crunchy	1	150	7	42	2.5	20	360	14	2	7	1 starch, 1 1/2 fat
✓Grilled Steak Soft	1	170	5	26	1.5	15	560	21	2	11	1 1/2 starch, 1 fat
✓Ranchero Chicken Soft	1	170	4	21	1	25	710	22	2	12	1 1/2 starch, 1 fat
✓Soft - beef	1	190	8	38	2.5	20	630	22	2	9	1 1/2 starch, 1 1/2 fat

GORDITAS - BAJA											
✔Beef	1	350	19	49	5	30	760	31	2	13	2 starch, 1 high-fat meat, 2 fat
✔Chicken	1	320	15	42	3.5	40	690	29	2	17	2 starch, 1 lean meat, 2 1/2 fat
GORDITAS - NACHO CHEESE											
✔Beef	1	300	13	39	4	20	740	32	2	12	2 starch, 1 high-fat meat, 1 fat
✔Chicken	1	270	10	33	2.5	25	670	30	2	16	2 starch, 1 lean meat, 1 1/2 fat
✔Steak	1	270	11	37	3	20	660	30	2	14	2 starch, 1 high-fat meat, 1/2 fat
GORDITAS - SUPREME											
✔Beef	1	310	16	46	7	35	600	30	2	14	2 starch, 1 high-fat meat, 1 1/2 fat

✔ = Healthiest Bets

(*Continued*)

GORDITAS - SUPREME (*Continued*)	Amount	Cal.	Fat (g)	% Cal. Fat	Sat. Fat (g)	Chol. (mg)	Sod. (mg)	Carb. (g)	Fiber (g)	Pro. (g)	Servings/Exchanges
✓Chicken	1	290	12	37	5	45	530	28	2	17	2 starch, 1 lean meat, 2 fat
✓Steak	1	320	16	45	4	30	680	29	2	15	2 starch, 1 high-fat meat, 1 1/2 fat
✓Steak	1	290	13	40	6	35	520	28	2	16	2 starch, 1 high-fat meat, 1 fat
NACHOS											
Nachos	1	320	19	53	4.5	4	530	33	2	5	2 starch, 4 fat
Nachos Bell Grande	1	780	43	50	13	35	1300	80	11	20	5 starch, 8 1/2 fat
Nachos Supreme	1	450	26	52	9	35	710	42	5	13	3 starch, 5 fat
SIDES											
✓Cinnamon Twists	1	160	5	28	1	0	150	28	0	0	2 starch
Pintos 'n Cheese	1	180	7	35	3.5	15	700	20	6	10	1 1/2 starch, 1 medium-fat meat

SPECIALTIES											
Cheese Quesadilla	1	490	28	51	13	55	1150	39	3	19	2 1/2 starch, 2 high-fat meat, 2 fat
Chicken Quesadilla	1	540	30	50	13	80	1380	40	3	28	2 1/2 starch, 3 lean meat, 4 fat
Enchirito - beef	1	380	18	43	9	45	1430	35	5	19	2 starch, 2 high-fat meat
Enchirito - chicken	1	350	14	36	7	55	1360	33	5	23	2 starch, 2 lean meat, 2 fat
Enchirito - steak	1	360	16	40	8	45	1350	33	5	21	2 starch, 2 high-fat meat
Fiesta Taco Salad	1	870	47	49	16	65	1780	80	12	31	4 1/2 starch, 2 veg, 2 high-fat meat, 6 fat
Fiesta Taco Salad w/ chips	1	630	33	47	13	65	1390	58	10	26	3 starch, 2 veg, 2 high-fat meat, 3 1/2 fat
Fiesta Taco Salad w/out shell	1	500	27	49	12	65	1520	42	10	24	2 starch, 2 veg, 2 high-fat meat, 2 fat

✔ = Healthiest Bets

(*Continued*)

SPECIALTIES (*Continued*)	Amount	Cal.	Fat (g)	% Cal. Fat	Sat. Fat (g)	Chol. (mg)	Sod. (mg)	Carb. (g)	Fiber (g)	Pro. (g)	Servings/Exchanges
Mexican Pizza	1	550	31	51	11	45	1040	47	5	21	3 starch, 2 high-fat meat, 2 1/2 fat
Meximelt	1	290	16	50	8	40	880	23	2	15	1 1/2 starch, 1 high-fat meat, 1 1/2 fat
Southwest Steak Bowl	1	700	32	41	8	55	2050	73	13	30	5 starch, 2 high-fat meat, 3 fat
Steak Quesadilla	1	540	31	52	14	70	1370	40	3	26	2 1/2 starch, 3 high-fat meat, 1 fat
✓Tostada	1	250	10	36	4	15	710	29	7	11	2 starch, 1 high-fat meat
Zesty Chicken Border Bowl	1	730	42	52	9	45	1640	65	12	23	3 1/2 starch, 3 veg, 2 lean meat, 6 1/2 fat
Zesty Chicken Border Bowl w/out dressing	1	500	19	34	4.5	30	1400	60	12	22	3 starch, 3 veg, 2 lean meat, 2 fat

TACOS

✓Crunchy	1	170	10	53	4	25	350	13	0	8	1 starch, 1 high-fat meat
✓Double Decker Supreme	1	380	18	43	5	10	820	41	5	15	3 starch, 1 high-fat meat, 1 1/2 fat
✓Grilled Steak Soft	1	280	17	55	4.5	30	650	21	1	12	1 1/2 starch, 1 high-fat meat, 1 1/2 fat
✓Ranchero Chicken Soft Taco	1	270	14	47	4	35	710	21	1	14	1 1/2 starch, 1 lean meat, 2 fat
✓Soft - beef	1	210	10	43	4	25	620	21	0	10	1 1/2 starch, 1 high-fat meat
✓Soft Supreme - beef	1	260	14	48	7	35	640	23	1	11	1 1/2 starch, 1 high-fat meat, 1 fat
✓Supreme	1	220	14	57	7	35	360	14	1	9	1 starch, 1 high-fat meat, 1 fat

✓ = Healthiest Bets

Taco John's

❖ Taco John's provides nutrition information for all its menu items on its Web site at www.tacojohns.com.

Light 'n Lean Choice

Chicken Soft Shell Taco *(1)*
Bean Burrito *(1)*

Calories	570	Sodium (mg)	1,590
Fat (g)	18	Carbohydrate (g)	62
% calories from fat	28	Fiber (g)	14
Saturated fat (g)	8	Protein (g)	29
Cholesterol (mg)	45		

Exchanges: 4 starch, 1 veg, 2 lean meat, 2 fat

Healthy 'n Hearty Choice

Chicken Fajita Burritos *(1)*
Refried Beans *(split serving, 1/2)*
Mexican Rice *(split serving, 1/2)*
Guacamole *(2 T)*

Calories	750	Sodium (mg)	2,560
Fat (g)	31	Carbohydrate (g)	88
% calories from fat	37	Fiber (g)	13
Saturated fat (g)	12	Protein (g)	33
Cholesterol (mg)	13		

Exchanges: 5 1/2 starch, 1 veg, 2 lean meat, 4 fat

Taco John's

	Amount	Cal.	Fat (g)	% Cal. Fat	Sat. Fat (g)	Chol. (mg)	Sod. (mg)	Carb. (g)	Fiber (g)	Pro. (g)	Servings/Exchanges
10 G OF FAT OR LESS											
✔Bean Burrito w/out Cheese	1	320	7	20	2	3	740	53	10	11	3 1/2 starch, 1 fat
✔Chicken Softshell Taco	1	190	6	28	3	30	760	19	4	14	1 starch, 1 lean meat, 1 fat
✔Crispy Taco	1	180	10	50	4	25	270	13	3	9	1 starch, 1 high-fat meat
Refried Beans w/out Cheese	1	340	9	24	3	0	1030	49	11	15	3 starch, 1 high-fat meat
✔Softshell Taco	1	220	10	41	5	25	470	21	4	11	1 1/2 starch, 1 high-fat meat
✔Taco Burger w/out Cheese	1	250	9	32	3	25	600	29	3	13	2 starch, 1 high-fat meat
Texas Style Chili w/out Cheese	1	210	8	34	3	20	1310	26	4	11	1 1/2 starch, 1 high-fat meat

✔ = Healthiest Bets

(*Continued*)

	Amount	Cal.	Fat (g)	% Cal. Fat	Sat. Fat (g)	Chol. (mg)	Sod. (mg)	Carb. (g)	Fiber (g)	Pro. (g)	Servings/Exchanges
BURRITOS											
Bean	1	380	12	28	5	15	830	53	10	15	3 1/2 starch, 1 high-fat meat, 1/2 fat
Beef Grilled	1	590	32	49	15	75	1240	49	9	27	3 starch, 3 high-fat meat, 1 fat
Beefy	1	430	20	42	9	55	870	41	8	22	3 starch, 2 medium-fat meat, 1 fat
Chicken & Potato	1	460	19	37	7	35	1470	54	8	18	3 1/2 starch, 1 lean meat, 3 fat
Chicken Grilled	1	590	30	46	13	95	1790	47	8	33	3 starch, 3 lean meat, 4 fat
Combination	1	400	16	36	7	35	850	47	9	18	3 starch, 1 high-fat meat, 1 1/2 fat
Crunchy Chicken & Potato	1	590	29	44	8	35	1420	62	8	20	4 starch, 1 lean meat, 5 fat

Meat & Potato	1	490	23	42	9	30	1190	55	9	15	3 1/2 starch, 4 1/2 fat
Super	1	450	20	40	9	40	920	49	10	19	3 starch, 1 high-fat meat, 2 1/2 fat
CONDIMENTS											
Bacon Ranch Dressing	4 T	170	13	69	2	15	490	14	0	1	1 starch, 2 1/2 fat
Barbecue Sauce	4 T	70	0	0	0	0	490	15	0	0	1 carb
Barbeque Dipping Sauce	4 T	50	0	0	0	0	340	14	0	0	1 carb
Chipotle Cream Sauce	4 T	300	30	90	6	20	380	4	0	n/a	6 fat
Creamy Italian Dressing	4 T	180	20	100	3	0	430	4	0	0	4 fat
Guacamole	4 T	90	9	90	3	0	360	6	n/a	0	2 fat
Honey Mustard Dipping Sauce	2 T	170	15	79	3	5	180	7	0	0	1/2 carb, 3 fat
✔Hot Sauce	2 T	5	0	0	0	0	135	1	0	0	free
House Dressing	6 T	90	10	100	2	0	360	3	0	0	2 fat

✔ = Healthiest Bets; n/a = not available

(*Continued*)

CONDIMENTS (*Continued*)	Amount	Cal.	Fat (g)	% Cal. Fat	Sat. Fat (g)	Chol. (mg)	Sod. (mg)	Carb. (g)	Fiber (g)	Pro. (g)	Servings/Exchanges
Jalapenos	4 T	15	1	60	0	0	950	3	1	1	free
✓Mild Sauce	2 T	5	0	0	0	0	140	1	0	0	free
Nacho Cheese	6 T	120	9	68	4	10	740	5	0	4	1/2 carb, 2 fat
✓Pico de Gallo	4 T	15	0	0	0	0	160	4	0	1	free
Ranch Dressing	4 T	190	21	99	3	30	470	4	0	2	4 fat
Salsa	4 T	20	0	0	0	0	390	5	0	0	free
Sour Cream	4 T	120	12	90	7	58	30	2	0	2	2 1/2 fat
✓Super Hot Sauce	2 T	10	0	0	0	0	25	2	0	1	free
Sweet and Sour Dipping Sauce	2 T	60	0	0	0	0	140	14	0	0	1 carb
DESSERTS											
Apple Grande	1	240	9	34	3	5	220	36	0	5	2 carb, 2 fat

Choco Taco	1	300	15	45	7	15	110	38	1	4	2 1/2 carb, 3 fat
Churros	1	230	11	43	2	10	120	31	1	2	2 carb, 2 fat
✓Elf Grahams (Kids Meal)	1	60	2	30	0	0	50	9	0	1	1/2 carb
✓Giant Goldfish Grahams	1	120	5	38	1	0	105	19	0	1	1 carb, 1 fat
LOCAL FAVORITES											
✓Bean Tostada	1	160	6	34	2	5	250	19	3	6	1 starch, 1 1/2 fat
Beef & Bean Chimi Platter	1	760	34	40	11	50	1930	88	9	27	6 starch, 1 high-fat meat, 4 1/2 fat
Beef Enchilada Platter	1	780	37	43	15	70	2460	80	11	32	5 starch, 2 high-fat meat, 4 fat
Beefy Cheesy Taco Bravo	1	410	22	48	9	50	850	35	6	18	2 starch, 2 high-fat meat, 1 fat
Cheese Crisp	1	210	14	60	7	35	260	11	1	10	1 starch, 1 high-fat meat, 1 fat

✓ = Healthiest Bets

(*Continued*)

LOCAL FAVORITES (*Continued*)	Amount	Cal.	Fat (g)	% Cal. Fat	Sat. Fat (g)	Chol. (mg)	Sod. (mg)	Carb. (g)	Fiber (g)	Pro. (g)	Servings/Exchanges
Chicken Enchilada Platter	1	700	32	41	13	65	2460	73	9	30	5 starch, 2 lean meat, 4 1/2 fat
Chili Enchilada	1	740	38	46	12	75	1470	71	8	31	4 starch, 3 high-fat meat, 2 1/2 fat
Chili Potato Oles	1	610	36	53	11	25	2290	59	7	13	4 starch, 6 1/2 fat
Chilito	1	430	22	46	12	60	1040	38	7	20	2 1/2 starch, 2 high-fat meat, 1 fat
Double Enchilada	1	720	40	50	18	105	2090	54	11	37	3 1/2 starch, 3 high-fat meat, 3 fat
El Grande Chicken Taco	1	380	20	47	7	60	1010	28	2	22	2 starch, 2 lean meat, 2 1/2 fat
El Grande Taco	1	510	32	56	11	75	920	32	4	24	2 starch, 3 high-fat meat, 1 1/2 fat
Mexi Rolls	1	480	30	56	10	50	1270	33	3	20	2 starch, 2 high-fat meat, 3 fat

Mexi Rolls w/out nacho cheese	1	370	21	51	6	40	530	29	3	16	2 starch, 1 high-fat meat, 2 1/2 fat
✓Tostada	1	180	10	50	4	25	270	14	3	9	1 starch, 1 high-fat meat
LOCAL FAVORITES - BURRITOS											
Chicken Fajita	1	340	11	29	5	50	1120	39	7	22	2 1/2 starch, 2 lean meat, 1 fat
Chicken Festiva	1	530	24	41	7	50	1300	58	8	21	3 1/2 starch, 1 lean meat, 4 fat
El Grande	1	720	36	45	17	90	1640	67	10	32	4 1/2 starch, 3 high-fat meat, 1 1/2 fat
El Grande Chicken	1	660	28	38	13	100	2210	64	9	39	4 starch, 4 lean meat, 3 fat
Ranch - Beef	1	420	22	47	7	45	860	41	8	17	3 starch, 1 high-fat meat, 2 1/2 fat
Ranch - Chicken	1	390	18	42	6	50	1140	40	7	20	2 1/2 starch, 2 lean meat, 2 fat

✓ = Healthiest Bets

(*Continued*)

LOCAL FAVORITES (*Continued*)	Amount	Cal.	Fat (g)	% Cal. Fat	Sat. Fat (g)	Chol. (mg)	Sod. (mg)	Carb. (g)	Fiber (g)	Pro. (g)	Servings/Exchanges
Smothered	1	500	21	38	10	50	1330	56	11	23	3 1/2 starch, 1 high-fat meat, 2 1/2 fat
Smothered Platter	1	830	33	36	13	55	2230	102	16	33	6 1/2 starch, 2 high-fat meat, 3 fat
PROMOTIONAL ITEMS - MEXICAN SHREDDED BEEF											
Grilled Burrito	1	530	25	42	11	75	1870	49	7	28	3 starch, 3 high-fat meat
Quesadilla	1	580	31	48	15	95	2100	44	6	29	3 starch, 3 high-fat meat, 1 fat
✓Softshell Taco	1	230	9	35	4	40	770	21	3	16	1 1/2 starch, 2 lean meat, 1/2 fat
SIDES											
Crunchy Chicken Side	1	450	27	54	4	60	1040	24	0	29	1 1/2 starch, 3 lean meat, 3 1/2 fat

Mexican Rice	1	240	8	30	2	0	850	35	0	4	2 starch, 2 fat
Nachos	1	380	23	54	6	10	970	38	0	6	2 1/2 starch, 4 1/2 fat
Potato Oles - kid's meal	1	300	18	54	4	0	880	33	3	3	2 starch, 3 fat
Potato Oles - large	1	790	47	54	11	0	2290	86	8	7	5 1/2 starch, 8 fat
Potato Oles - medium	1	620	36	52	8	0	1780	67	6	5	4 1/2 starch, 6 fat
Potato Oles - small	1	440	26	53	6	0	1270	48	5	4	3 starch, 5 fat
Potato Oles w/ Nacho Cheese	1	550	35	57	10	10	2000	52	5	7	3 1/2 starch, 6 fat
Refried Beans	1	400	14	32	5	15	1110	50	11	18	3 1/2 starch, 3 fat
✓Side Salad w/out dressing	1	80	5	56	2	5	50	6	1	3	1 veg, 1 fat
Texas Style Chili	1	270	12	40	6	35	1400	26	4	15	1 1/2 starch, 1 high-fat meat, 1 fat
SPECIALTIES											
Cheese Quesadilla	1	480	28	53	15	50	960	39	6	20	2 1/2 starch, 2 high-fat meat, 2 fat

✓ = Healthiest Bets

(*Continued*)

SPECIALTIES (*Continued*)	Amount	Cal.	Fat (g)	% Cal. Fat	Sat. Fat (g)	Chol. (mg)	Sod. (mg)	Carb. (g)	Fiber (g)	Pro. (g)	Servings/Exchanges
Chicken Quesadilla	1	540	29	48	15	75	1430	41	7	29	3 starch, 3 lean meat, 3 1/2 fat
Chicken Taco Salad w/out dressing	1	530	27	46	11	70	1330	45	3	27	2 starch, 3 veg, 3 lean meat, 3 fat
Potato Oles Bravo	1	580	36	56	11	20	1760	55	6	9	3 1/2 starch, 7 fat
Super Nachos	1	830	51	55	17	60	1730	73	5	22	5 starch, 10 fat
Super Potato Oles	1	980	63	58	22	60	3950	82	10	22	5 1/2 starch, 12 fat
Taco Salad w/out dressing	1	580	32	50	13	60	960	46	4	23	3 starch, 2 veg, 2 high-fat meat, 2 1/2 fat
SPECIALTIES - FESTIVA SALAD											
Chicken w/out dressing	1	580	24	37	10	65	1190	60	11	29	3 starch, 3 veg, 3 lean meat, 2 1/2 fat

✔Chicken w/out dressing & tortilla	1	380	20	47	8	65	820	25	5	24	1/2 starch, 3 veg, 3 lean meat, 2 fat
Crunchy Chicken w/out dressing	1	750	37	44	11	60	1140	71	10	33	3 1/2 starch, 3 veg, 3 lean meat, 5 fat
✔Crunchy Chicken w/out dressing & tortilla	1	550	33	54	10	60	770	36	4	27	1 1/2 starch, 3 veg, 3 lean meat, 4 1/2 fat
TACOS											
✔Beef Taco in a Bag	1	180	12	60	6	40	420	6	2	12	1/2 starch, 1 high-fat meat, 1 fat
✔Chicken Softshell Taco	1	190	6	28	3	30	760	19	4	14	1 starch, 1 lean meat, 1 fat
✔Chicken Taco in a Bag	1	140	7	45	4	50	790	4	1	17	2 lean meat, 1/2 fat
✔Crispy Taco	1	180	10	50	4	25	270	13	3	9	1 starch, 1 high-fat meat
✔Low Carb Beef Softshell Taco	1	190	10	47	4	25	520	16	11	12	1 starch, 1 high-fat meat

✔ = Healthiest Bets

(Continued)

TACOS (*Continued*)	Amount	Cal.	Fat (g)	% Cal. Fat	Sat. Fat (g)	Chol. (mg)	Sod. (mg)	Carb. (g)	Fiber (g)	Pro. (g)	Servings/Exchanges
✔Low Carb Chicken Softshell Taco	1	160	6	34	3	30	800	15	10	15	1 starch, 1 medium-fat meat
✔Softshell Taco	1	220	10	41	5	25	470	21	4	11	1 1/2 starch, 1 high-fat meat
✔Taco Bravo	1	340	14	37	5	25	650	39	8	15	2 1/2 starch, 1 high-fat meat, 1 fat
✔Taco Burger	1	280	12	39	5	35	600	28	3	14	2 starch, 1 medium-fat meat,1/2 fat

✔ = Healthiest Bets

Sweets, Desserts, and Frozen Treats

RESTAURANTS

Baskin Robbins
Cold Stone Creamery
Freshëns Premium Yogurt
Häagen-Dazs Ice Cream Café
Mrs. Fields Cookies
TCBY

The Scoop: Nutrition information is for 4-fluid-ounce servings. Yes, that's small, but it is the industry standard. In many cases the nutrition information is only for vanilla or several other flavors. Flavors that have nuts, fudge, or chocolate pieces will most likely have more calories. Several companies base their nutrition information on an average of all flavors.

No meals are provided for this chapter because these foods are usually eaten as a snack or in addition to a meal.

NUTRITION PROS

- Small portions are an option.
- Some restaurants offer a kiddie size. That's sometimes enough to satisfy your sweet tooth.
- Healthier toppings are easy to spot: fresh fruit, granola, nuts, or raisins.
- Low-fat, fat-free, and/or sugar-free frozen treats abound.

- Desserts are easy to split. Just ask for two forks or spoons.
- You can watch the server's every move. Make sure they do what you want.

NUTRITION CONS

- Overindulgence is easy.
- Unhealthy toppers are plentiful: candy bar pieces, cookies, hot fudge, or butterscotch.
- Sometimes the low-fat, fat-free, and/or sugar-free desserts are not that much lower in calories than the regular varieties. Check it out.
- Often the low-fat or fat-free products are higher in carbohydrate. The fat gets swapped for the carbohydrate.
- Fruit smoothies or shakes are often light on the "real fruit" and heavy on the sugar.

Healthy Tips

★ Don't think kiddie size is just for kids. It's a great small size for calorie and carbohydrate counters too.

★ Order one dessert and two spoons. Just a few bites often quiets your sweet tooth.

Get It Your Way

★ Low-fat or fat-free; frozen yogurt, light ice cream, or sorbet; and kiddie and small—options are aplenty for healthful eating.

Baskin Robbins

❖ Baskin Robbins provides nutrition information for all its menu items on its Web site at www.baskinrobbins.com.

Baskin Robbins

	Amount	Cal.	Fat (g)	% Cal. Fat	Sat. Fat (g)	Chol. (mg)	Sod. (mg)	Carb. (g)	Fiber (g)	Pro. (g)	Servings/Exchanges
BLASTS											
Cappuccino Blast Regular w/ whipped cream	16 oz	320	14	39	9	55	110	44	0	6	2 starch, 1 carb, 3 fat
✓Cappuccino Nonfat Blast	16 oz	210	0	0	0	5	120	45	0	7	2 starch, 1 carb
Chocolate Blast Regular	16 oz	450	12	24	8	45	140	81	0	6	2 starch, 2 carb, 2 1/2 fat
Chocolate Blast Regular	24 oz	680	19	25	12	65	210	123	0	10	3 starch, 3 carb, 4 fat
Mintopia Blast Regular	16 oz	430	17	36	10	50	125	63	1	7	2 starch, 2 carb, 3 1/2 fat
Mocha Blast	16 oz	350	12	31	7	45	90	47	0	5	2 starch, 1 carb, 2 1/2 fat
Turtle Blast Regular	16 oz	540	17	28	10	50	330	92	0	7	2 starch, 4 carb, 2 1/2 fat

✓ = Healthiest Bets

(*Continued*)

	Amount	Cal.	Fat (g)	% Cal. Fat	Sat. Fat (g)	Chol. (mg)	Sod. (mg)	Carb. (g)	Fiber (g)	Pro. (g)	Servings/Exchanges
FROZEN YOGURT											
✓Butter Pecan No Sugar Added Nonfat Soft Serve	1/2 cup	90	0	0	0	5	90	17	1	4	1 starch
✓Café Mocha Nonfat Soft Serve	1/2 cup	90	0	0	0	5	85	18	1	4	1 carb
✓Chocolate No Sugar Added Nonfat Soft Serve	1/2 cup	80	0	0	0	0	80	15	0	4	1 carb
✓Chocolate Nonfat Soft Serve	1/2 cup	120	0	0	0	0	85	25	1	4	1 1/2 carb
Maui Brownie Low Fat	1/2 cup	210	4	17	1.5	10	140	39	1	6	2 1/2 carb, 1 fat
✓Peppermint Nonfat Soft Serve	1/2 cup	110	0	0	0	0	75	24	0	4	1 1/2 starch

Perils of Praline Low Fat	1/2 cup	190	4	19	1.5	5	170	37	1	5	2 1/2 carb, 1/2 fat
Raspberry Cheese Louise Low Fat	1/2 cup	190	4	19	2.5	10	150	36	1	5	2 carb, 1 fat
✓Red Raspberry Nonfat Soft Serve	1/2 cup	110	0	0	0	0	75	25	0	4	1 1/2 carb
✓Strawberry Patch No Sugar Added Nonfat Soft Serve	1/2 cup	90	0	0	0	5	90	17	1	4	1 carb
✓Vanilla No Sugar Added Nonfat Soft Serve	1/2 cup	90	0	0	0	5	90	17	1	4	1 carb
Vanilla Nonfat	1/2 cup	150	0	0	0	5	105	32	0	6	2 carb
✓Vanilla Nonfat Soft Serve	1/2 cup	110	0	0	0	0	80	23	0	4	1 1/2 carb
LOW FAT ICE CREAM											
Espresso 'n Cream	1/2 cup	180	4	20	1.5	10	120	32	1	5	2 carb, 1 fat

✓ = Healthiest Bets

(*Continued*)

	Amount	Cal.	Fat (g)	% Cal. Fat	Sat. Fat (g)	Chol. (mg)	Sod. (mg)	Carb. (g)	Fiber (g)	Pro. (g)	Servings/Exchanges
NO SUGAR ADDED ICE CREAM											
✔Berries 'n Banana Low Fat	1/2 cup	110	2	16	1	10	125	25	1	5	1 1/2 carb, 1/2 fat
✔Chocolate Chip Low Fat	1/2 cup	170	5	26	3.5	10	11	30	1	4	2 carb, 1 fat
Mad About Chocolate Low Fat	1/2 cup	160	4	23	3	10	125	35	1	5	2 carb, 1 fat
✔Pineapple Coconut Low Fat	1/2 cup	150	2	12	1.5	10	105	27	0	4	1 1/2 carb, 1/2 fat
Tin Roof Low Fat	1/2 cup	190	3	14	1.5	10	105	34	1	4	2 carb, 1/2 fat
NO SUGAR ADDED ICE CREAMS											
✔Chocolate Chocolate Chip	1/2 cup	150	5	30	3.5	10	140	30	1	6	2 carb, 1 fat
REGULAR DELUXE ICE CREAMS											
✔Banana Nut	1/2 cup	260	16	55	7	45	75	27	1	5	1 1/2 carb, 3 fat

Bananas 'n Strawberry	1/2 cup	220	9	37	6	35	70	35	0	3	2 carb, 2 fat
Baseball Nut	1/2 cup	270	14	47	8	45	100	32	0	5	2 carb, 2 fat
Black Walnut	1/2 cup	280	19	61	9	50	90	25	1	6	1 1/2 carb, 3 1/2 fat
Blueberry Cheesecake	1/2 cup	270	14	47	8	55	125	32	0	5	2 carb, 3 fat
Bobsled Brownie	1/2 cup	320	17	48	8	45	130	37	2	5	2 1/2 carb, 3 fat
Candy Cookie Commotion	1/2 cup	300	16	48	9	45	150	36	1	5	2 carb, 3 fat
Chocoholic's Resolution	1/2 cup	300	16	48	9	45	130	38	0	5	2 1/2 carb, 3 fat
Chocolate	1/2 cup	260	14	48	9	50	130	33	0	5	2 carb, 3 fat
Chocolate Almond	1/2 cup	310	18	52	9	45	120	32	1	7	2 carb, 3 1/2 fat
Chocolate Chip	1/2 cup	270	16	53	10	55	95	28	1	5	2 carb, 3 fat
Chocolate Chip Cookie Dough	1/2 cup	290	15	47	9	55	130	36	1	5	2 carb, 3 fat
Chocolate Fudge	1/2 cup	270	15	50	10	50	140	35	0	4	2 carb, 3 fat

✓ = Healthiest Bets

(Continued)

REGULAR DELUXE ICE CREAMS (*Continued*)	Amount	Cal.	Fat (g)	% Cal. Fat	Sat. Fat (g)	Chol. (mg)	Sod. (mg)	Carb. (g)	Fiber (g)	Pro. (g)	Servings/Exchanges
Chocolate Mousse Royale	1/2 cup	300	17	51	8	40	120	37	1	5	2 1/2 carb, 3 1/2 fat
Chocolate Ribbon	1/2 cup	240	12	45	8	45	85	31	0	4	2 carb, 2 1/2 fat
Cinnamon Bun Swirl	1/2 cup	280	12	39	8	50	115	39	0	4	2 1/2 carb, 2 1/2 fat
Egg Nog	1/2 cup	250	13	47	8	70	90	31	0	5	2 carb, 2 1/2 fat
French Vanilla	1/2 cup	280	18	58	11	120	85	26	0	4	1 1/2 carb, 3 1/2 fat
Fudge Brownie	1/2 cup	300	19	57	11	45	140	35	1	5	2 carb, 4 fat
German Chocolate Cake	1/2 cup	300	16	48	9	45	150	36	1	5	2 carb, 3 fat
Gold Metal Ribbon	1/2 cup	260	13	45	8	45	150	34	0	5	2 carb, 2 1/2 fat
Honest to Goodnuts	1/2 cup	300	14	42	8	40	135	38	0	5	2 1/2 carb, 3 fat
Jamoca Almond	1/2 cup	270	15	50	7	40	80	31	1	6	2 carb, 3 fat
Jamoca Roca	1/2 cup	280	14	45	9	45	130	33	0	4	2 carb, 3 fat

Key Lime Pie	1/2 cup	270	14	47	8	45	135	33	0	5	2 carb, 3 fat
Lemon Custard	1/2 cup	260	13	45	8	75	105	30	0	5	2 carb, 2 1/2 fat
Love Gone Sour	1/2 cup	270	14	47	8	55	115	32	0	5	2 carb, 3 fat
Love Potion #31	1/2 cup	270	14	47	9	45	90	34	1	4	2 carb, 3 fat
Macadamia Nuts 'n Cream	1/2 cup	270	18	60	9	55	90	25	1	5	1 1/2 carb, 3 1/2 fat
Mint Chocolate Chip	1/2 cup	270	16	53	10	55	95	28	1	5	2 carb, 3 fat
New York Cheesecake	1/2 cup	280	16	51	10	50	135	31	0	5	2 carb, 3 fat
Nutcracker Sweet	1/2 cup	300	18	54	8	45	135	31	1	5	2 carb, 3 1/2 fat
Nutty Coconut	1/2 cup	300	20	60	9	45	90	28	1	6	2 carb, 4 fat
Oatmeal Cookie	1/2 cup	270	12	40	7	45	115	37	0	4	2 1/2 carb, 2 1/2 fat
Old Fashion Butter Pecan	1/2 cup	280	18	58	9	50	95	24	1	5	1 1/2 carb, 3 1/2 fat
Oregon Blackberry	1/2 cup	240	12	45	8	50	85	28	0	4	2 carb, 2 1/2 fat

✔ = Healthiest Bets

(Continued)

REGULAR DELUXE ICE CREAMS (*Continued*)	Amount	Cal.	Fat (g)	% Cal. Fat	Sat. Fat (g)	Chol. (mg)	Sod. (mg)	Carb. (g)	Fiber (g)	Pro. (g)	Servings/Exchanges
Oreo Cookies 'n Cream	1/2 cup	280	15	48	8	50	150	32	1	5	2 carb, 3 fat
Original Cinn	1/2 cup	290	13	40	8	45	130	39	0	4	2 1/2 carb, 2 1/2 fat
Peanut Butter 'n Chocolate	1/2 cup	320	20	56	9	45	180	31	1	7	2 carb, 4 fat
Peppermint	1/2 cup	270	14	47	9	50	85	32	0	4	2 carb, 3 fat
Pink Bubblegum	1/2 cup	260	12	42	8	50	80	36	0	4	2 carb, 2 1/2 fat
Pistachio Almond	1/2 cup	290	19	59	9	50	85	25	1	7	1 1/2 carb, 4 fat
Pralines 'n Cream	1/2 cup	270	14	47	8	45	170	34	0	4	2 carb, 3 fat
✓Pumpkin Pie	1/2 cup	230	12	47	7	45	90	29	0	4	2 carb, 2 1/2 fat
Quarterback Crunch	1/2 cup	290	16	50	11	45	140	33	0	4	2 carb, 3 fat
Reese's Peanut Butter Cup	1/2 cup	300	18	54	10	50	130	31	0	6	2 carb, 3 fat
Rocky Road	1/2 cup	290	15	47	8	45	120	36	1	5	2 carb, 3 fat

Strawberry Cheesecake	1/2 cup	270	12	40	9	55	115	32	0	5	2 carb, 2 1/2 fat
Tax Crunch	1/2 cup	300	18	54	8	45	135	32	1	5	2 carb, 3 fat
Trici Oreo Treat	1/2 cup	300	16	48	9	45	150	36	1	5	2 carb, 3 fat
True Blue Ginger	1/2 cup	270	13	43	8	50	140	33	0	4	2 carb, 2 1/2 fat
Truffle in Paradise	1/2 cup	330	21	57	12	50	75	32	1	5	2 carb, 4 fat
Vanilla	1/2 cup	260	16	55	10	65	70	26	0	4	1 1/2 carb, 3 fat
Very Berry Strawberry	1/2 cup	220	11	45	7	10	70	28	0	4	2 carb, 2 fat
Winter White Chocolate	1/2 cup	270	14	47	10	40	95	32	1	4	2 carb, 3 fat
World Class Chocolate	1/2 cup	270	15	50	8	45	115	33	0	5	2 carb, 3 fat
SHAKES											
Chocolate Shake w/ Chocolate Ice Cream	24 oz	990	39	35	24	125	440	159	1	20	1 1/2 carb, 9 fat
Chocolate Shake w/ Vanilla Ice Cream	16 oz	690	33	43	21	130	210	85	0	13	5 carb, 6 1/2 fat

✔ = Healthiest Bets

(Continued)

SHAKES (*Continued*)	Amount	Cal.	Fat (g)	% Cal. Fat	Sat. Fat (g)	Chol. (mg)	Sod. (mg)	Carb. (g)	Fiber (g)	Pro. (g)	Servings/Exchanges
Chocolate w/ Chocolate Ice Cream	16 oz	620	30	44	18	105	300	81	1	15	5 carb, 6 fat
Chocolate w/ Vanilla Ice Cream	24 oz	1000	45	41	28	175	290	133	0	19	9 carb, 9 fat
Espresso Shake	24 oz	790	45	51	28	175	300	80	0	19	5 carb, 9 fat
Vanilla Regular	16 oz	680	33	44	21	130	380	81	0	13	5 carb, 6 1/2 fat
Vanilla Shake	24 oz	980	45	41	28	175	640	125	0	19	8 carb, 9 fat
SHERBETS & ICES											
Blue Raspberry Sherbet	1/2 cup	160	2	11	1.5	10	40	34	0	1	2 carb
Daiquiri Ice	1/2 cup	130	0	0	0	0	15	34	0	0	2 carb
Margarita Ice	1/2 cup	130	0	0	0	0	15	34	0	0	2 carb
Orange Sherbet	1/2 cup	160	2	11	1.5	10	40	34	0	1	2 carb

Rainbow Sherbet	1/2 cup	160	2	11	1.5	10	40	34	0	1	2 carb
Red Raspberry Sherbet	1/2 cup	160	2	11	1.5	10	40	36	0	1	2 carb
Watermelon Ice	1/2 cup	130	0	0	0	0	15	34	0	0	2 carb
SMOOTHIES											
Peach Smoothie w/ soft serve yogurt	16 oz	350	1	3	0.5	5	140	80	3	7	5 carb
Peach Smoothie w/ yogurt	16 oz	360	1	3	0	5	150	83	3	8	5 1/2 carb
Strawberry Banana Smoothie w/ soft serve yogurt	16 oz	360	1	3	0.5	5	150	84	3	7	5 1/2 carb
Strawberry Banana Smoothie w/ yogurt	16 oz	370	1	2	0.5	5	160	87	3	8	5 1/2 carb
Strawberry Smoothie w/ soft serve yogurt	16 oz	330	1	3	0.5	5	150	77	3	7	5 carb

✔ = Healthiest Bets

(Continued)

SMOOTHIES (*Continued*)	Amount	Cal.	Fat (g)	% Cal. Fat	Sat. Fat (g)	Chol. (mg)	Sod. (mg)	Carb. (g)	Fiber (g)	Pro. (g)	Servings/Exchanges
Strawberry Smoothie w/ yogurt	16 oz	340	1	3	0	5	160	79	3	8	5 carb
Wildberry Banana Smoothie w/ soft serve yogurt	16 oz	390	2	5	1	5	105	92	3	5	6 carb
Wildberry Banana Smoothie w/ yogurt	16 oz	380	1	2	0	0	100	93	3	5	6 carb
SUNDAES											
2 Scoop Hot Fudge Sundae	1	530	29	49	19	85	200	62	0	8	4 carb, 6 fat
3 Scoop Hot Fudge Sundae	1	750	41	49	27	125	280	86	0	11	5 1/2 carb, 8 fat
Banana Royale	1	630	27	39	16	85	250	91	5	9	6 carb, 5 1/2 fat
Banana Split	1	1030	39	34	23	135	190	168	7	12	11 carb, 4 fat

✔ = Healthiest Bets

Cold Stone Creamery

Cold Stone Creamery provides nutrition information for all its menu items on its Web site at www.coldstonecreamery.com.

(Continued)

Cold Stone Creamery

	Amount	Cal.	Fat (g)	% Cal. Fat	Sat. Fat (g)	Chol. (mg)	Sod. (mg)	Carb. (g)	Fiber (g)	Pro. (g)	Servings/Exchanges
ADULT CAKES - 8″ ROUND											
Celebration Sensation	1.5″ slice	350	17	44	10	50	240	46	0	4	3 carb, 3 fat
Chocolate Chipper	1.5″ slice	430	24	50	11	50	210	49	3	6	3 carb, 5 fat
Coffeehouse Crunch	1.5″ slice	500	29	52	10	50	270	57	2	6	4 carb, 6 fat
Cookie Dough Delirium	1.5″ slice	400	20	45	11	60	230	51	0	5	3 1/2 carb, 4 fat
Cookies & Creamery	1.5″ slice	380	19	45	11	50	280	47	1	6	3 carb, 4 fat
Midnight Delight	1.5″ slice	500	27	49	11	55	240	59	4	7	4 carb, 5 1/2 fat
MMMMMM Chip	1.5″ slice	370	19	46	11	50	230	45	2	5	3 carb, 4 fat
Peanut Butter Playground	1.5″ slice	470	27	52	11	50	240	52	3	7	3 1/2 carb, 5 1/2 fat
Snicker's Supreme	1.5″ slice	480	27	51	11	50	240	57	3	7	3 carb, 5 1/2 fat

Strawberry Passion	1.5″ slice	380	19	45	10	50	260	49	1	5	3 carb, 4 fat
Zebra Stripes	1.5″ slice	390	21	48	13	55	220	46	1	6	3 carb, 4 fat
Zebra Stripes Dark	1.5″ slice	470	27	52	12	60	200	53	2	6	3 1/2 carb, 5 fat
ICE CREAM											
Amaretto	6 oz	390	24	55	15	95	95	40	0	6	2 1/2 carb, 5 fat
Banana	6 oz	370	22	54	14	85	85	40	0	6	2 1/2 carb, 4 fat
Black Cherry	6 oz	390	22	51	14	90	95	43	0	6	3 carb, 4 fat
Butter Pecan	6 oz	400	23	52	14	110	95	42	0	6	2 1/2 carb, 4 1/2 fat
Cake Batter	6 oz	420	23	49	14	85	180	48	0	6	3 carb, 4 1/2 fat
Candy Cane	6 oz	420	22	47	14	85	90	50	0	6	3 carb, 4 fat
Cheesecake	6 oz	390	22	51	14	85	95	44	0	6	3 carb, 4 fat
Chocolate	6 oz	390	24	55	15	90	115	39	1	7	2 carb, 5 fat
Cinnamon	6 oz	400	24	54	15	95	95	41	0	6	3 carb, 5 fat

✔ = Healthiest Bets

(*Continued*)

ICE CREAM (*Continued*)	Amount	Cal.	Fat (g)	% Cal. Fat	Sat. Fat (g)	Chol. (mg)	Sod. (mg)	Carb. (g)	Fiber (g)	Pro. (g)	Servings/Exchanges
Coconut	6 oz	390	23	53	15	90	90	39	0	6	2 1/2 carb, 4 1/2 fat
Coffee	6 oz	400	24	54	15	95	95	40	0	6	3 carb, 4 1/2 fat
Egg Nog	6 oz	400	22	50	14	90	95	46	0	6	3 carb, 4 fat
French Vanilla	6 oz	400	23	52	14	115	95	44	0	6	3 carb, 4 1/2 fat
Irish Cream	6 oz	390	24	55	15	95	95	40	0	6	3 carb, 5 fat
Macadamia Nut	6 oz	390	24	55	15	95	95	40	0	6	3 carb, 5 fat
Mango	6 oz	370	22	54	14	85	85	39	0	6	2 1/2 carb, 4 fat
Mint	6 oz	400	23	52	14	90	90	43	0	6	3 carb, 4 1/2 fat
Mocha	6 oz	390	24	55	15	90	115	40	1	7	3 carb, 4 1/2 fat
Orange Dreams	6 oz	370	22	54	14	90	90	38	0	6	2 1/2 carb, 4 fat
Oreo Cookie	6 oz	430	25	52	15	90	170	46	0	6	3 carb, 5 fat
Peanut Butter	6 oz	430	28	59	15	90	140	40	0	8	3 carb, 5 fat

Pecan Praline	6 oz	390	22	51	14	85	105	43	0	6	3 carb, 5 1/2 fat
Pistachio	6 oz	390	24	55	15	95	90	40	0	6	3 carb, 4 1/2 fat
Pumpkin	6 oz	390	22	51	14	90	95	41	0	6	3 carb, 4 fat
Raspberry	6 oz	390	22	51	14	90	90	43	0	6	3 carb, 4 fat
Sinless Sweet Cream	6 oz	160	0	0	0	4	135	41	0	7	3 carb
Strawberry	6 oz	380	22	52	14	90	90	41	0	6	3 carb, 4 fat
Sweet Cream	6 oz	390	24	55	15	95	95	40	0	6	3 carb, 4 fat
Vanilla Bean	6 oz	400	23	52	15	90	90	39	0	6	3 carb, 5 fat
White Chocolate	6 oz	390	24	55	15	95	90	40	0	6	2 1/2 carb, 4 fat
KIDS' CAKES - 8″ ROUND											
Barbie	1.5″ slice	360	19	48	12	55	190	44	0	4	3 carb, 4 fat
Blue's Clues	1.5″ slice	350	18	46	11	50	190	45	0	4	3 carb, 3 1/2 fat
Harry Potter	1.5″ slice	350	19	49	12	50	230	43	1	5	3 carb, 4 fat

✔ = Healthiest Bets

(*Continued*)

KIDS' CAKES - 8″ ROUND (*Continued*)	Amount	Cal.	Fat (g)	% Cal. Fat	Sat. Fat (g)	Chol. (mg)	Sod. (mg)	Carb. (g)	Fiber (g)	Pro. (g)	Servings/Exchanges
Hot Wheels	1.5″ slice	350	18	46	11	50	190	45	0	4	3 carb, 3 1/2 fat
Lizzie McGuire	1.5″ slice	360	19	48	12	50	220	43	0	5	3 carb, 4 fat
Nemo	1.5″ slice	350	18	46	11	50	190	45	0	4	3 carb, 3 1/2 fat
Spider Man	1.5″ slice	360	19	48	12	55	190	44	0	4	3 carb, 4 fat
Sponge Bob	1.5″ slice	360	19	48	12	50	200	45	0	4	3 carb, 4 fat
Winnie the Pooh	1.5″ slice	350	18	46	11	50	190	45	1	4	3 carb, 3 1/2 fat
MIX-INS/CANDY											
Almond Joy Candy	1 piece	160	9	51	6	0	50	20	2	1	1 carb, 2 fat
Butterfinger Candy	1/2 bar	140	6	39	3	0	60	20	1	4	1 carb, 1 fat
Chocolate Chips	2 T	130	7	48	4.5	0	55	15	0	2	1 carb, 1 1/2 fat
Gumballs	2 T	120	0	0	0	0	0	34	0	0	2 carb
Gummi Bears	2 T	120	0	0	0	0	15	30	0	0	2 carb

Heath Candy Bar	1 bar	110	7	57	0	0	75	12	0	1	1 carb, 1 fat
Kit Kat Candy Bar	1/2 bar	100	5	45	3.5	0	15	13	0	1	1 carb, 1 fat
Krackel Candy Bar	1/2 bar	130	7	48	4.5	4	35	15	1	2	1 carb, 1 fat
M&M Candy	2 T	170	7	37	4.5	4	20	25	1	2	1 1/2 carb, 1 fat
Nestle Crunch Bar	1/2 bar	130	7	48	1	4	35	16	1	2	1 carb, 1 fat
Peanut M&M's	2 T	150	8	48	3.5	4	30	18	1	3	1 carb, 1 1/2 fat
Reese's Peanut Butter Cup	1 piece	190	11	52	4	0	110	19	1	4	1 carb, 2 fat
Reese's Pieces	2 T	170	7	37	6	0	50	21	1	5	1 1/2 carb, 1 fat
Snickers Candy	1/2 bar	170	9	48	3	4	95	21	1	3	1 1/2 carb, 2 fat
Twix Candy	1 piece	150	7	42	2.5	0	60	20	0	1	1 1/2 carb, 1 fat
White Chocolate Chips	2 T	160	9	51	8	4	45	18	0	2	1 carb
York Peppermint Patties	2 pieces	120	2	15	1.5	0	5	24	1	1	1 1/2 carb

✔ = Healthiest Bets

(Continued)

	Amount	Cal.	Fat (g)	% Cal. Fat	Sat. Fat (g)	Chol. (mg)	Sod. (mg)	Carb. (g)	Fiber (g)	Pro. (g)	Servings/Exchanges
MIX-INS/FRUIT											
✓Apple Pie Filling	1 spoon mix-in	60	0	0	0	0	25	16	1	0	1 carb
✓Bananas	1/2	60	0	0	0	0	0	14	1	1	1 carb
✓Black Cherries	1 1/2 T	80	0	0	0	0	30	19	0	0	1 carb
✓Blackberries	1 1/2 T	10	0	0	0	0	0	2	1	0	free
✓Blueberries	1 1/2 T	10	0	0	0	0	0	2	0	0	free
✓Cherry Pie Filling	1 1/2 T	50	0	0	0	0	0	13	0	0	1 carb
✓Maraschino Cherries	1	5	0	0	0	0	0	1	0	0	free
✓Peach Pie Filling	2 T	60	0	0	0	0	25	16	1	0	1 carb
✓Pineapple Chunks	1 1/2 T	15	0	0	0	0	0	4	0	0	free
✓Raisins	2 T	80	0	0	0	0	0	20	1	1	1 fruit

✓Raspberries	1 1/2 T	15	0	0	0	0	0	4	1	1	free
✓Strawberries	1 1/2 T	0	0	0	0	0	7	1	0	free	
MIX-INS/NUTS											
Cashews	2 T	170	14	74	3	0	190	9	1	5	1/2 carb, 3 fat
Macadamia Nuts	2 T	180	19	95	3	0	65	3	2	2	4 fat
Peanuts	2 T	200	17	77	2.5	0	150	7	3	9	1/2 carb, 3 1/2 fat
Pecan Pralines	2 T	210	21	90	1.5	0	230	5	2	2	4 fat
Pecans	2 T	140	14	90	1	0	150	3	1	1	3 fat
Pistachio Nuts	2 T	210	18	77	2.5	0	0	10	4	5	1 carb, 3 fat
Roasted Almonds	2 T	190	17	81	1.5	0	230	5	3	6	1/2 carb, 3 1/2 fat
Sliced Almonds	2 T	210	20	86	2	0	0	6	4	7	1/2 carb, 4 fat
Walnuts	2 T	130	12	83	1	0	0	4	1	3	1/2 carb, 2 1/2 fat

✓ = Healthiest Bets

(Continued)

	Amount	Cal.	Fat (g)	% Cal. Fat	Sat. Fat (g)	Chol. (mg)	Sod. (mg)	Carb. (g)	Fiber (g)	Pro. (g)	Servings/Exchanges
MIX-INS/OTHER											
Brownies	1 piece	180	6	30	2	5	190	29	1	2	2 carb, 1 fat
Coconut	2 T	80	5	56	4.5	0	10	7	1	0	1/2 carb, 1 fat
Cookie Dough	1 piece	180	8	40	2.5	10	85	25	1	2	1 1/2 carb, 1 1/2 fat
✓Graham Cracker Pie Crust	2 T	110	3	25	0	0	160	19	1	2	1 carb, 1/2 fat
✓Granola	2 T	120	2	15	0	0	30	23	2	2	1 1/2 carb
Marshmallows	2 T	100	0	0	0	0	10	24	0	1	1 1/2 carb
✓Nilla Wafers	3	70	3	39	0	5	50	11	0	1	1 carb
Oreo Cookies	2	120	5	38	1	0	170	17	1	2	1 carb, 1 fat
Oreo Pie Crust	2 T	180	8	40	1.5	0	190	19	0	0	1 carb, 2 fat
Peanut Butter	1 1/2 T	150	13	78	2.5	0	115	5	1	6	1 high-fat meat, 1 fat
Toasted Coconut	2 T	180	14	70	13	0	1	13	1	2	1 carb, 3 fat

Yellow Sponge Cake	1 piece	70	1	13	0	25	60	15	0	1	1 carb
NON-FAT/LOWFAT FROZEN YOGURT											
Cheesecake	6 oz	230	0	0	0	0	150	48	0	9	3 carb
Chocolate	6 oz	230	2	8	1	0	140	48	3	11	3 carb
Coffee	6 oz	220	0	0	0	0	150	45	0	10	3 carb
Sweet Cream	6 oz	220	0	0	0	0	150	45	0	9	3 carb
SORBET											
Lemon	6 oz	180	0	0	0	0	20	48	0	0	2 1/2 carb
Raspberry	6 oz	200	0	0	0	0	20	50	0	0	2 1/2 carb
TOPPINGS											
✓Chocolate Sprinkles	2 T	25	0	0	0	0	0	6	0	0	1/2 carb
✓Cinnamon	1/8 teasp	15	0	0	0	0	0	4	3	0	free
Fat Free Butterscotch	2 T	80	0	0	0	0	85	19	0	1	1 carb

✓ = Healthiest Bets

(*Continued*)

TOPPINGS (*Continued*)	Amount	Cal.	Fat (g)	% Cal. Fat	Sat. Fat (g)	Chol. (mg)	Sod. (mg)	Carb. (g)	Fiber (g)	Pro. (g)	Servings/Exchanges
✓Fat Free Caramel	2 T	80	0	0	0	0	85	19	0	1	1 carb
✓Fat Free Fudge	2 T	80	0	0	0	0	15	20	0	1	1 carb
Honey	2 T	90	0	0	0	0	0	25	0	0	1 carb
Marshmallow Crème	2 T	100	0	0	0	0	20	24	0	0	1 1/2 carb
✓Rainbow Sprinkles	2 T	25	0	0	0	0	0	6	0	0	1/2 carb
Rich's Whipped Topping	1 dollop	50	4	72	3.5	0	0	4	0	0	1 fat
Smucker's Caramel	2 T	100	0	0	0	0	85	24	0	0	1 1/2 carb
Smucker's Fudge	2 T	110	3	25	0	0	45	18	0	2	1 carb, 1/2 fat
WAFFLE PRODUCTS											
Dipped Waffle	1 each	310	15	44	7	5	70	46	2	4	3 carb, 3 fat
Dipped Waffle w/ Candy	1 each	390	20	46	7	5	130	55	2	5	3 1/2 carb, 2 1/2 fat
Waffle Cone or Bowl	1 each	160	4	23	1	5	70	29	0	3	2 carb

✓ = Healthiest Bets

Freshëns Premium Yogurt

❖ Freshëns Premium Yogurt provides nutrition information for some of its menu items on its Web site at www.freshens.com.

(Continued)

Freshëns Premium Yogurt

	Amount	Cal.	Fat (g)	% Cal. Fat	Sat. Fat (g)	Chol. (mg)	Sod. (mg)	Carb. (g)	Fiber (g)	Pro. (g)	Servings/Exchanges
GOURMET PRETZELS											
Pretzel	1	510	6	11	0.5	0	780	98	4	14	6 1/2 starch
HAND-DIPPED ICE CREAM											
✓All Flavors (average)	1/2 cup	150	9	54	n/a	n/a	68	22	n/a	5	1 1/2 carb, 1 fat
SMOOTHIES											
Berry Berry	21 oz	260	0	0	n/a	0	14	66	3	1	4 carb
Caribbean Craze	21 oz	315	0	0	n/a	0	17	79	3	1	5 carb
Cayman Cooler	21 oz	320	0	0	n/a	0	28	82	2	1	5 carb
Club Trim	21 oz	291	0	0	n/a	0	26	72	2	1	4 carb
Fitness Fuel	21 oz	521	5	9	n/a	24	230	81	3	27	5 carb, 2 lean meat

Immune Support	21 oz	377	3	7	n/a	10	63	84	2	3	5 carb
Jamaican Jammer	21 oz	378	0	0	n/a	14	160	69	3	11	4 carb, 1 lean meat
Maui Mango	21 oz	354	0	0	n/a	0	29	90	2	1	6 carb
Mocha Coffee	21 oz	385	3	7	n/a	15	437	74	0	7	5 carb
Mystic Mango	21 oz	407	3	7	n/a	10	75	93	2	2	6 carb
Orange Shooter	21 oz	338	3	8	n/a	10	63	76	1	2	5 carb
Orange Sunrise	21 oz	367	3	7	n/a	10	63	82	2	3	5 carb
Peach Sunset	21 oz	388	0	0	n/a	0	33	96	3	1	6 carb
Peachy Pineapple	21 oz	415	1	2	n/a	14	173	78	2	10	5 carb
Peanut Butter Chocolate	21 oz	312	20	58	n/a	45	454	14	2	21	1 carb, 2 high-fat meat, 1 fat
Pina Collider	21 oz	451	4	8	n/a	14	170	79	3	11	5 carb, 1 lean meat
Pineapple Passion	21 oz	389	4	9	n/a	0	27	90	2	1	6 carb

✓ = Healthiest Bets; n/a = not available

(Continued)

SMOOTHIES (*Continued*)	Amount	Cal.	Fat (g)	% Cal. Fat	Sat. Fat (g)	Chol. (mg)	Sod. (mg)	Carb. (g)	Fiber (g)	Pro. (g)	Servings/Exchanges
Raspberry Royale	21 oz	346	0	0	n/a	0	26	86	4	2	5 carb
Rockin' Raspberry	21 oz	332	1	3	n/a	14	157	58	4	11	4 carb
Strawberry Shooter	21 oz	251	0	0	n/a	0	15	65	1	1	4 carb
Strawberry Squeeze	21 oz	313	1	3	n/a	14	158	55	1	10	3 carb
Vanilla Coffee	21 oz	438	3	6	n/a	15	432	90	0	7	6 carb
Vanilla Fudge	21 oz	275	17	56	n/a	45	427	13	1	19	1 carb, 2 high-fat meat
SOFT-SERVE YOGURT											
✔All Flavors (average)	1/2 cup	100	0	0	n/a	10	76	19	n/a	4	1 1/2 carb

✔ = Healthiest Bets; n/a = not available

Häagen-Dazs Ice Cream Café

❖ Häagen-Dazs Ice Cream Café provides nutrition information for most of its menu items on its Web site at www.haagendazs.com.

(*Continued*)

Häagen-Dazs Ice Cream Café

	Amount	Cal.	Fat (g)	% Cal. Fat	Sat. Fat (g)	Chol. (mg)	Sod. (mg)	Carb. (g)	Fiber (g)	Pro. (g)	Servings/Exchanges
FROZEN YOGURT											
Chocolate Fudge Brownie	1/2 cup	200	3	14	1.5	35	140	35	2	9	2 carb, 1 fat
Coffee	1/2 cup	200	5	23	2.5	65	50	31	0	8	2 carb, 1 fat
Dulce de Leche	1/2 cup	190	3	14	2	5	75	35	0	6	2 carb, 1 fat
Strawberry	1/2 cup	140	0	0	0	4	40	31	0	5	2 carb
Strawberry Banana	1/2 cup	160	2	11	1	30	25	31	0	3	2 carb
Vanilla	1/2 cup	200	5	23	2.5	65	55	31	0	9	2 carb, 1 fat
Vanilla Raspberry Swirl	1/2 cup	170	3	16	1.5	30	30	31	0	5	2 carb
ICE CREAM											
Bailey's Irish Cream	1/2 cup	270	17	57	10	115	70	23	0	5	1 1/2 carb, 3 1/2 fat

Bananas Foster	1/2 cup	260	15	52	9	100	90	28	0	4	2 carb, 2 fat
Black Walnut	1/2 cup	300	22	66	11	105	85	21	0	5	1 1/2 carb, 4 fat
Butter Pecan	1/2 cup	310	23	67	11	110	110	21	0	5	1 1/2 carb, 4 1/2 fat
Café Mocha Frappe	1/2 cup	310	19	55	12	125	75	30	0	5	2 carb, 3 1/2 fat
Cherry Vanilla	1/2 cup	240	15	56	9	100	60	23	0	4	1 1/2 carb, 2 1/2 fat
Chocolate	1/2 cup	270	18	60	11	115	60	22	1	5	1 1/2 carb, 3 1/2 fat
Chocolate Chocolate Chip	1/2 cup	300	20	60	12	105	55	26	2	5	1 1/2 carb, 4 fat
Chocolate Mousse	1/2 cup	310	19	55	12	125	75	30	0	5	2 carb, 3 1/2 fat
Chocolate Peanut Butter	1/2 cup	360	24	60	11	100	100	27	2	8	2 carb, 4 1/2 fat
Chocolate Raspberry Torte	1/2 cup	270	15	50	9	95	65	29	1	4	2 carb, 2 1/2 fat
Coffee	1/2 cup	270	18	60	11	120	70	21	0	5	1 1/2 carb, 3 1/2 fat

✓ = Healthiest Bets

(Continued)

ICE CREAM (*Continued*)	Amount	Cal.	Fat (g)	% Cal. Fat	Sat. Fat (g)	Chol. (mg)	Sod. (mg)	Carb. (g)	Fiber (g)	Pro. (g)	Servings/Exchanges
Cookie & Cream	1/2 cup	270	17	57	10	105	95	23	0	5	1 1/2 carb, 3 1/2 fat
Cookie Dough Chip	1/2 cup	310	20	58	12	95	125	29	0	4	2 carb, 3 1/2 fat
Crème Brulee	1/2 cup	280	19	61	12	120	75	23	0	4	1 1/2 carb, 2 1/2 fat
Dulce De Leche	1/2 cup	290	17	53	10	100	95	28	0	5	2 carb, 3 fat
French Vanilla Mousse	1/2 cup	310	20	58	12	130	75	29	0	4	2 carb, 3 1/2 fat
Macadamia Brittle	1/2 cup	300	20	60	12	110	110	25	0	4	1 1/2 carb, 3 fat
Mango	1/2 cup	250	14	50	8	85	50	28	0	4	2 carb, 2 fat
Mint Chip	1/2 cup	300	19	57	12	105	85	26	0	5	1 1/2 carb, 4 fat
Mocha Almond Fudge	1/2 cup	340	23	61	12	100	85	28	0	5	2 carb, 4 fat
Peaches & Cream	1/2 cup	240	12	45	7	75	55	29	0	3	2 carb, 2 fat
Peanut Butter Fudge	1/2 cup	340	23	61	11	95	95	25	1	7	1 1/2 carb, 5 fat
Pineapple Coconut	1/2 cup	230	13	51	8	90	55	25	0	4	1 1/2 carb, 2 1/2 fat

Pistachio	1/2 cup	290	20	62	11	110	80	22	0	5	1 1/2 carb, 4 fat
Rum Raisin	1/2 cup	270	17	57	10	110	60	22	0	4	1 1/2 carb, 3 1/2 fat
Strawberry	1/2 cup	250	16	58	10	95	65	23	0	4	1 1/2 carb, 3 fat
Strawberry Cheese Cake	1/2 cup	270	16	53	10	100	130	28	0	4	2 carb, 2 1/2 fat
Tres Leches	1/2 cup	290	19	59	12	105	55	26	0	4	1 1/2 carb, 4 fat
Vanilla	1/2 cup	270	18	60	11	120	70	21	0	5	1 1/2 carb, 3 1/2 fat
Vanilla Caramel Brownie	1/2 cup	300	18	54	11	105	100	30	0	5	2 carb, 3 fat
Vanilla Chocolate Chip	1/2 cup	310	20	58	12	105	75	26	1	5	1 1/2 carb, 4 fat
Vanilla Fudge	1/2 cup	290	18	56	12	100	95	26	0	5	1 1/2 carb, 4 fat
Vanilla Swiss Almond	1/2 cup	300	20	60	11	105	75	24	0	5	1 1/2 carb, 4 fat
White Chocolate Raspberry Truffle	1/2 cup	310	18	52	10	105	65	32	1	5	2 carb, 3 1/2 fat

✔ = Healthiest Bets

(Continued)

	Amount	Cal.	Fat (g)	% Cal. Fat	Sat. Fat (g)	Chol. (mg)	Sod. (mg)	Carb. (g)	Fiber (g)	Pro. (g)	Servings/Exchanges
ICE CREAM/SORBET BARS											
Chocolate & Dark Chocolate	1	290	20	62	12	70	35	23	2	4	1 1/2 carb, 4 fat
✓Chocolate Sorbet	1	80	0	0	0	0	50	20	1	1	1 carb
Coffee & Almond Crunch	1	310	22	64	12	75	65	23	0	4	1 1/2 carb, 4 fat
Dulce de Leche	1	300	19	57	12	60	70	28	0	4	2 carb, 3 fat
✓Raspberry Sorbet & Vanilla Frozen Yogurt	1	90	0	0	0	0	12	21	0	2	1 carb
Strawberry Cheese Cake	1	370	25	61	14	95	100	30	1	4	2 carb, 2 fat
Vanilla & Almonds	1	320	12	34	12	75	55	22	0	5	1 1/2 carb, 4 fat
Vanilla & Dark Chocolate	1	280	20	64	12	70	40	22	0	4	1 1/2 carb, 3 1/2 fat
Vanilla & Milk Chocolate	1	280	20	64	12	75	50	20	0	4	1 1/2 carb, 3 1/2 fat
Vanilla Caramel & Pecans	1	360	26	65	14	65	105	27	0	4	2 carb, 4 1/2 fat

SORBET

✓Chocolate	1/2 cup	130	0.5	3	0	0	70	28	2	2	2 carb
Mango	1/2 cup	120	0	0	0	0	0	31	0	0	2 carb
✓Orange	1/2 cup	120	0	0	0	0	0	30	0	0	2 carb
Orchard Peach	1/2 cup	130	0	0	0	0	0	33	0	0	2 carb
✓Raspberry	1/2 cup	120	0	0	0	0	0	30	2	0	2 carb
✓Strawberry	1/2 cup	120	0	0	0	0	0	30	1	0	2 carb
Zesty Lemon	1/2 cup	120	0	0	0	0	0	31	0	0	2 carb

✓ = Healthiest Bets

Mrs. Fields Cookies

❖ Mrs. Fields Cookies provides nutrition information for most of its products on its Web site at www.mrsfields.com.

Mrs. Fields Cookies

	Amount	Cal.	Fat (g)	% Cal. Fat	Sat. Fat (g)	Chol. (mg)	Sod. (mg)	Carb. (g)	Fiber (g)	Pro. (g)	Servings/Exchanges
BITE-SIZE NIBBLER COOKIES											
✓Butter	2	110	5	41	3	15	90	15	0	1	1 carb, 1 fat
✓Chewy Chocolate Fudge	2	110	5	41	3.5	10	130	15	0	1	1 carb, 1 fat
✓Cinnamon Sugar	2	120	5	38	3	15	90	17	0	1	1 carb, 1 fat
✓Debra's Special	2	100	5	45	2	10	80	13	0	1	1 carb, 1 fat
✓M&M	2	110	5	41	3.5	15	55	16	0	1	1 carb, 1 fat
✓Milk Chocolate	2	110	5	41	3	15	70	15	0	1	1 carb, 1 fat
✓Milk Chocolate w/ Walnuts	2	120	6	45	3	10	65	14	0	1	1 carb, 1 fat
✓Peanut Butter	2	110	6	49	2.5	15	95	13	0	2	1 carb, 1 fat

✓ = Healthiest Bets

(Continued)

BITE-SIZE NIBBLER COOKIES (*Continued*)	Amount	Cal.	Fat (g)	% Cal. Fat	Sat. Fat (g)	Chol. (mg)	Sod. (mg)	Carb. (g)	Fiber (g)	Pro. (g)	Servings/Exchanges
✓Semi - Sweet Chocolate	2	110	5	41	3	10	60	15	0	1	1 carb
✓Triple Chocolate	2	110	6	49	3	15	65	15	0	1	1 carb, 1 fat
✓White Chocolate Macadamia	2	120	7	53	3.5	10	60	13	0	1	1 carb, 1 fat
BROWNIES											
Double Fudge	1	360	19	48	11	80	240	49	2	4	3 carb, 3 fat
Frosted Fudge	1	440	21	43	12	80	265	62	2	4	4 carb, 2 1/2 fat
Pecan Fudge Brownie	1	340	21	56	9	70	220	40	2	4	2 1/2 starch, 3 fat
Pecan Pie Brownie	1	340	20	53	9	70	220	40	2	5	2 1/2 starch, 3 fat
Walnut Fudge Brownie	1	380	23	54	10	80	240	45	0	5	3 carb, 4 fat
BUNDT CAKES											
Banana Walnut w/ Chocolate Chips	1 piece	370	22	54	7	35	240	39	3	6	2 1/2 starch, 4 fat

Blueberry	1 piece	270	12	40	5	50	330	36	1	4	2 1/2 carb, 2 fat
Chocolate	1 piece	350	21	54	4.5	40	300	35	3	6	2 1/2 carb, 3 fat
Chocolate Chip	1 piece	350	17	44	8	50	330	45	0	4	3 carb, 2 1/2 fat
Raspberry Pecan Chocolate Chip	1 piece	270	12	40	5	50	330	36	0	4	2 1/2 carb, 1 1/2 fat
COOKIES											
Butter Toffee	1	290	13	40	8	55	190	40	0	3	2 1/2 carb, 2 1/2 fat
Cinnamon Sugar	1	300	12	36	8	50	250	41	0	3	3 carb, 1 1/2 fat
Coconut & Macadamia	1	280	13	42	5	20	220	39	0	3	2 1/2 carb, 2 fat
Debra's Special	1	280	12	39	6	10	180	39	2	4	2 1/2 carb, 2 fat
Milk Chocolate & Walnut	1	320	17	48	9	40	180	37	1	4	2 1/2 carb, 3 fat
Milk Chocolate Macadamia	1	320	18	51	9	40	180	36	0	4	2 1/2 carb, 3 fat
Milk Chocolate w/out Nuts	1	280	13	42	8	40	180	38	0	3	2 1/2 carb, 2 fat

✔ = Healthiest Bets

(*Continued*)

COOKIES (*Continued*)	Amount	Cal.	Fat (g)	% Cal. Fat	Sat. Fat (g)	Chol. (mg)	Sod. (mg)	Carb. (g)	Fiber (g)	Pro. (g)	Servings/Exchanges
Oatmeal Chocolate Chip	1	280	13	42	8	35	140	40	0	3	2 1/2 carb, 2 fat
Oatmeal, Raisins & Walnuts	1	280	12	39	6	40	180	39	2	4	2 1/2 carb, 2 fat
Peanut Butter	1	310	16	46	8	45	260	34	0	5	2 1/2 carb, 3 fat
Peanut Butter w/ Milk Chocolate Chips	1	300	17	51	8	40	160	35	0	5	2 1/2 carb, 3 fat
Semi-Sweet Chocolate	1	280	14	45	8	30	160	40	1	2	2 1/2 carb, 2 1/2 fat
Semi-Sweet Chocolate & Walnuts	1	310	16	46	8	35	180	38	2	3	2 1/2 carb, 3 fat
Snickerdoodle Jumbo	1	640	29	41	17	110	540	90	2	7	6 carb, 5 fat
White Chocolate Macadamia	1	310	17	49	9	35	170	37	0	4	2 1/2 carb, 3 fat

✔ = Healthiest Bets

TCBY

❖ TCBY provides nutrition information for some of its items on its Web site at www.tcby.com.

(*Continued*)

TCBY

	Amount	Cal.	Fat (g)	% Cal. Fat	Sat. Fat (g)	Chol. (mg)	Sod. (mg)	Carb. (g)	Fiber (g)	Pro. (g)	Servings/Exchanges
HAND-DIPPED PREMIUM ICE CREAM											
Butter Pecan	1/2 cup	260	20	69	8	45	130	17	0	3	1 carb, 4 fat
Chewy Chocolate Fudge	1/2 cup	200	14	63	8	50	50	18	0	3	1 carb, 3 fat
Chocolate Chocolate	1/2 cup	210	13	56	8	50	50	21	0	4	1 1/2 carb, 2 1/2 fat
Lemon Meringue Pie	1/2 cup	230	12	47	7	55	65	29	0	3	2 carb, 2 1/2 fat
Mint Chocolate	1/2 cup	230	15	59	9	50	45	23	0	3	1 1/2 carb, 3 fat
Oatmeal Raisin	1/2 cup	220	12	49	7	45	90	25	0	3	1 1/2 carb, 2 1/2 fat
Pralines & Cream	1/2 cup	210	13	56	8	45	65	22	0	3	1 1/2 carb, 2 1/2 fat
Vanilla Bean	1/2 cup	210	13	56	8	55	45	17	0	3	1 carb, 2 1/2 fat
Very Berry Strawberry	1/2 cup	180	11	55	7	40	45	19	0	3	1 carb, 2 fat

White Chunk Macadamia	1/2 cup	250	16	58	8	45	75	23	0	3	1 1/2 carb, 3 fat
SMOOTHIES W/ YOGURT											
A Lotta Coloda	20 oz	380	12	28	11	0	20	69	3	2	4 1/2 carb, 2 1/2 fat
A Lotta Coloda	32 oz	710	17	22	13	10	95	142	4	7	9 1/2 carb, 3 1/2 fat
A Lotta Coloda	20 oz	550	17	28	14	0	95	99	3	6	6 1/2 carb, 3 1/2 fat
Berry Slim	32 oz	600	4	6	2.5	10	85	143	4	6	9 1/2 carb, 1/2 fat
Berry Slim	20 oz	410	3	7	2	10	50	95	2	5	6 1/2 carb, 1/2 fat
Healthy Balance	20 oz	410	3	7	2	10	50	95	2	5	6 1/2 carb, 1/2 fat
Healthy Balance	32 oz	590	4	6	2.5	10	85	138	4	6	9 carb, 1/2 fat
Healthy Balance	20 oz	300	0	0	0	0	5	75	2	1	5 carb
Holy-Cal	20 oz	470	3	6	1.5	10	65	114	3	4	7 1/2 carb, 1/2 fat
Holy-Cal	32 oz	610	4	6	2.5	10	90	149	4	6	10 carb, 1/2 fat
Holy-Cal	20 oz	360	0	0	0	0	25	94	3	1	6 1/2 carb

✔ = Healthiest Bets

(Continued)

SMOOTHIES W/ YOGURT (*Continued*)	Amount	Cal.	Fat (g)	% Cal. Fat	Sat. Fat (g)	Chol. (mg)	Sod. (mg)	Carb. (g)	Fiber (g)	Pro. (g)	Servings/Exchanges
Peachy Lean	20 oz	470	3	6	1.5	10	70	116	0	4	7 1/2 carb, 1/2 fat
Peachy Lean	20 oz	360	0	0	0	0	30	96	0	1	6 1/2 carb
Peachy Lean	32 oz	620	4	6	5.5	10	100	151	1	6	10 carb, 1/2 fat
Raspberry DeLITE	20 oz	360	3	8	1.5	10	50	85	4	4	5 carb, 1/2 fat
Raspberry DeLITE	32 oz	510	5	9	2.5	10	80	116	7	6	7 1/2 carb, 1 fat
Raspberry Revitalizer	32 oz	530	4	7	2	10	75	124	4	6	8 carb, 1/2 fat
Raspberry Revitalizer	20 oz	370	3	7	1.5	10	50	84	3	5	5 1/2 carb, 1/2 fat
Raspberry Revitalizer	20 oz	300	0	0	0	0	0	79	6	2	5 carb
Tropical Refresher	32 oz	520	4	7	2.5	10	85	121	2	6	8 carb, 1/2 fat
Tropical Refresher	20 oz	370	3	7	1.5	10	50	87	1	4	5 1/2 carb, 1/2 fat
Tropical Refresher	20 oz	240	0	0	0	0	20	61	2	1	4 carb
Workout Whey	20 oz	340	0	0	0	0	25	92	1	1	6 carb

Workout Whey	20 oz	460	3	6	1.5	10	85	112	1	4	7 1/2 carb, 1/2 fat
Workout Whey	32 oz	600	5	8	2.5	10	95	145	2	6	9 1/2 carb, 1 fat
SMOOTHIES W/OUT YOGURT											
A Lotta-Colada	32 oz	620	15	22	13	10	75	112	3	6	7 1/2 carb, 3 fat
Berry Slim	20 oz	300	0	0	0	0	5	75	2	1	5 carb
Berry Slim	32 oz	450	1	2	0	0	25	116	4	2	7 1/2 carb
Healthy Balance	32 oz	450	1	2	0	0	30	116	4	2	7 1/2 carb
Holy-Cal	32 oz	450	0	0	0	0	35	118	3	1	8 carb
Peachy Lean	32 oz	470	0	0	0	0	45	124	1	1	8 carb
Raspberry DeLITE	20 oz	240	0	0	0	0	15	59	3	2	4 carb
Raspberry DeLITE	32 oz	300	0	0	0	0	25	74	4	2	5 carb
Raspberry Revitalizer	32 oz	470	1	2	0	0	25	118	8	2	8 carb
Tropical Refresher	32 oz	350	0	0	0	0	35	92	3	1	6 carb

✓ = Healthiest Bets

(*Continued*)

SMOOTHIES W/OUT YOGURT (*Continued*)	Amount	Cal.	Fat (g)	% Cal. Fat	Sat. Fat (g)	Chol. (mg)	Sod. (mg)	Carb. (g)	Fiber (g)	Pro. (g)	Servings/Exchanges
Workout Whey	32 oz	450	1	2	0	0	40	119	2	1	8 carb
SOFT-SERVE FROZEN YOGURT											
✔96 Fat Free Frozen Yogurt	1/2 cup	140	3	19	2	15	60	23	0	4	1 1/2 carb, 1/2 fat
✔No Sugar Added Nonfat Frozen Yogurt	1/2 cup	90	0	0	0	0	35	20	0	4	1 1/2 carb
✔Nonfat & Nondairy Sorbet	1/2 cup	100	0	0	0	0	30	24	0	0	1 1/2 carb
✔Nonfat Frozen Yogurt	1/2 cup	110	0	0	0	0	60	23	0	4	1 1/2 carb

✔ = Healthiest Bets

Other Books by Hope Warshaw from the American Diabetes Association

Diabetes Meal Planning Made Easy, 2nd edition
Hope Warshaw, MMSc, RD, CDE

The diabetes food pyramid doesn't have to be complicated. With this book, it's easy to follow and can help simplify your life. Learn how to:

- easily eat more fruits and vegetables
- skim off nasty fat grams
- eat like a champion away from home.

235 pages, softcover.
#4706-02 Nonmember: $14.95 Member: $12.95

Complete Guide to Carb Counting, 2nd edition
Hope S. Warshaw, MMSc, RD, CDE, and
Karmeen Kulkarni, MS, RD, CDE

Learn how to count carbs easily and effortlessly for improved blood sugar control, effective weight loss, and proper nutrition. End the confusion of how to count, what counts, and how much counts with the tools and techniques in this newly updated edition. Even if you purchased the earlier edition, this book is a must-have because it begins where the previous one left off. New chapters include:

- carb counting for insulin pump users
- a whole week of meal plans
- and much more.

262 pages, softcover.
#4715-02 One low price: $16.95

The Diabetes Food and Nutrition Bible
Hope S. Warshaw, MMSc, RD, CDE, and
Robyn Webb, MS

Get the nutrition advice you need and the flavor-rich recipes you crave. Learn about foods that can protect and heal, and get scrumptious recipes to work into your eating plan.

What you learn can have a dramatic effect on the way you eat, what you eat, and how long you live.

325 pages, softcover.
#4714-01 Nonmember: $18.95 Member: $16.95

Order online at http://store.diabetes.org or call toll-free at 1-800-232-6733.